Date Due

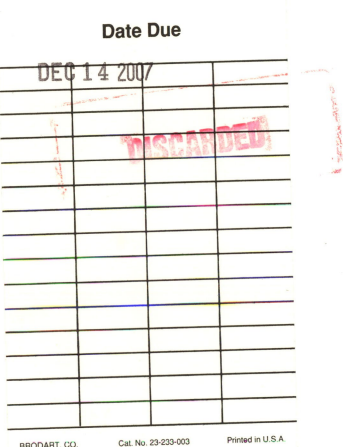

BRODART, CO.   Cat. No. 23-233-003   Printed in U.S.A.

GENERAL SONOGRAPHY
A Clinical Guide

BETH ANDERHUB, MEd, RT, CNMT, RDMS
Director, Ultrasonography Program,
St. Louis Community College–Forest Park,
St. Louis, Missouri

*with **553** illustrations*

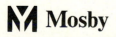 **Mosby**

St. Louis   Baltimore   Berlin   Boston   Carlsbad   Chicago   London   Madrid
Naples   New York   Philadelphia   Sydney   Tokyo   Toronto

Editor: Jeanne Rowland
Project Manager: Dana Peick
Manufacturing Supervisor: Theresa Fuchs
Design Manager: Susan Lane
Cover photograph: Doug Miner

Printed in the United States of America
Composition by Carlisle Communications, Ltd.
Printing/binding by Maple Vail

Mosby-Year Book, Inc.
11830 Westline Industrial Drive
St. Louis, Missouri 63146

Library of Congress Cataloging in Publication Data

Anderhub, Beth.
    General sonography : a clinical guide / Beth Anderhub. — 1st ed.
        p. cm.
    Includes bibliographical references and index.
    ISBN 0-8016-7421-2
    1. Diagnosis, Ultrasonic. 2. Diagnostic imaging. I. Title.
    [DNLM: 1. Ultrasonography—methods. 2. Diagnostic Imaging. WN
200 A546g 1995]
RC78.7.U4A63   1995
616.07'544—dc20
                                                        94-32304
                                                        CIP

95 96 97 98 99   /   9 8 7 6 5 4 3 2 1

preface

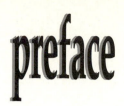

The field of diagnostic medical sonography has matured and experienced rapid development since I first entered the field in 1975. High resolution, real-time equipment has replaced B-scan units. Pulsed and color-flow Doppler have improved and enhanced the diagnostic utility of the modality. These advances have remarkably broadened the responsibilities and the knowledge base of today's sonographer. The diversity of this required knowledge ranges from ultrasound physics and instrumentation to sectional anatomy, physiology, pathology, pathophysiology, clinical signs and symptoms, normal and abnormal sonographic patterns, and terminates with the differential diagnosis.

During the past 11 years, I have taught over 140 students in the ultrasound program at St. Louis Community College. In addition, I have instructed hundreds of sonographers through shorter courses held throughout the country. Time and again, students have expressed frustration at mastering the overwhelming amount of material required to perform the routine duties of a sonographer. The greatest challenge lies in quickly recalling the information, reordering it according to the patient's clinical history, and applying it during the sonographic examination. I explain to my students that mastering this material boils down to learning how to "think like a sonographer." Teaching the reader to think like a sonographer is the primary goal of this book.

Each student must initially master each subject area—normal anatomy and physiology, pathology, clinical signs and symptoms, normal sonographic patterns, and abnormal pattern classification. At this level the student must understand the logic behind the theories and facts. This understanding, in turn, facilitates comprehension and the ordering and linking of the material, so that the student can move up to the next levels of learning, called application and synthesis. At these levels the student must recall, recombine, and apply the information while performing the sonographic examination. The final skill involves forming a preliminary differential diagnosis and obtaining additional images that will allow the interpreting physician to make a more refined formal diagnosis. I explain to my students that this final task resembles the role of a detective—searching for clues in the clinical history and the displayed sonographic patterns and using these clues to decide where else to look. This book is intended to emulate this learning process. The basic knowledge areas are presented in the earliest sections of each chapter. The sections on specific pathologic processes encompass the application and synthesis levels.

Instructors in formal educational programs will find this book appropriate for introductory courses on the imaging applications for abdominal, obstetric, gynecologic, and superficial-parts sonography. I have attempted to provide an easy-to-read writing style and a logical organization with extensive use of subheadings to allow students to quickly find specific material. The accompanying Instructor's Manual provides information on general teaching and learning methodology, how to prepare lesson plans, and how to construct an integrated didactic and clinical curriculum. For each chapter of the book, the corresponding chapter in the Instructor's Manual provides specific lesson plans, student exercises, and sample test questions. Also included in the Instructor's Manual are transparency masters for the anatomic illustrations. Slides of the sonograms are available for purchase from Mosby.

Each book chapter contains a list of instructional objectives to encourage the reader to formulate their learning goals before reading the chapter. The "Clinical Problem" section provides an overview of the referring physician's perspective in relation to the clinical management of the patient and the role that sonography plays in providing quality patient care. This section also serves as an introduction to the broader aspects of clinical medicine, which the sonographer uses when obtaining the clinical history. Chapter 1 contains a section on abstracting the patient's chart. This task plays a crucial role in the performance of high-quality examinations. The sections on clinical laboratory tests and related imaging procedures provide important background information that will enhance the reader's comprehension of the clinical history for each specific type of pathology. The pertinent anatomy and normal sonographic patterns are correlated with line illustrations and sonograms to prepare the reader for the task of recognizing these structures under clinical conditions. The "Scanning Protocols and Techniques" section includes a general guide for what the sonographer should image during each specific type of examination. Although individual department protocols vary widely, the sonographer must have an internal checklist and logical system that serves as the framework that can then be modified to fit a required department protocol. With real-time techniques, this framework is based on internal anatomic landmarks.

The application and synthesis levels are covered by the subsections on specific anomalies and pathologic processes. Each disease process section includes a discussion of the pathologic basis, clinical symptoms, laboratory test results, and sonographic patterns. All of this information is included to provide the sonographer with the necessary skills to obtain the clinical history, recognize the pathology during the procedure, and examine other areas to assist the interpreting physician in refining the differential diagnosis.

The field of diagnostic medical sonography requires a highly educated, responsible, and mature professional. The sonographer must demonstrate high levels of initiative and exercise independent judgement. Today's sonographer must readily accept his or her role as an integral and equal member of the health care team. It is my hope that this book makes the learning process easier and helps produce a sonographer who will make important contributions to the continued growth of the profession.

Beth Anderhub

acknowledgments

Special thanks go to Jeanne Rowland, Editor at Mosby, for her support, encouragement, and tenacity throughout the course of this project.

The author wishes to thank the following individuals, whose contributions and support have made this book possible.

Line illustrations: Susan Dodson R.T., R.D.M.S.
Illustrator: Theodore Bolte
Photographic reproductions: Norman L. Hente R. T., Thomas H. Murry, Martin G. Henson R.T.

The following physicians and sonographers generously contributed sonograms:

Anderson Hospital, Maryville, Illinois, Thomas E. Hill, MD, Beth A. Shane, RT, RDMS, Diane Hader, RDCS

Barnes–St. Peter's Hospital, St. Peters, Missouri, Phillip Trotta, MD, Susan Hobson, RT, RDMS

Belleville Memorial Hospital, Belleville, Illinois, Robert Auffenberg, MD, Mary Rohr, RT, RDMS, Donna Friedman, RT, Kim Kirkpatrick, RT

Deaconess Hospital–West Campus, St. Louis, Missouri, Masoud Mehranfar, RT, RDMS, RVT, Kim Palmer, RT, RDMS

Deaconess Hospital–Central Campus, St. Louis, Missouri, Julian N. Verde, MD, Guillermo Geisse, MD, Richard Schulz, MD, Cliff Pyles, RT, RDMS, Katie Secks, RT, RDMS, Linda Lotte, RT, RDMS, Prafulla Nagaraja, RDMS, Pam Sieve, RT, RDMS, Barbara Macke, RT, RDMS

Diasonics Corporation, Mark Muilenburg, RT (N), RDMS, Applications Specialist

Jefferson Memorial Hospital, Festus, Missouri, Alfred D. Shaplin, MD, Anthony M. Raia, RT, RDMS, Kathy Reynolds, RT, RDMS, Kathy House, RT, RDMS

Jewish Hospital–Radiology Department, St. Louis, Missouri, Michael Lind, RT, RDMS, Roger Scott, RT, RDMS

Jewish Hospital–Perinatal Ultrasound, St. Louis, Missouri, James P. Crane, MD, Diana L. Gray, MD, Mazie Havens, RDMS, Teresa Suessen, RT, RDMS, Cindi Ade, RDMS, Renee Winborn, RT, RDMS, Jean Schoenborn, RT, RDMS, Michelle Moennig, RT, RDMS, Marilou Bradley, RDMS, Debbie Timmons, RT, RDMS, Sherri Buchmeier, RT, RDMS

Missouri Baptist Medical Center, St. Louis, Missouri, Dale Fletcher, MD, Alan Arseneau, RT, RDMS, Susan Urban, RT, RDMS, Judy Lopez, RDMS

St. Anthony's Hospital, Alton, Illinois, John Zabrowski, MD, Becky Russell, RT, RDMS, Roger Carroll, RT, RDMS, RVT, Karen Lucker, RT, RDMS, Nancy Brunner, RT, RDMS

St. Anthony's Medical Center, St. Louis, Missouri, Robert W. Smith, MD, Lisa Royle, RT, RDMS, Sandy Barry, RT, RDMS, Linda Poertner, RT, RDMS, Laura Gray, RT, RDMS
St. Elizabeth Medical Center, Granite City, Illinois, Geoffrey Miller, MD, Becky Bierbaum, RT, RDMS, Diane McClary, RT, RDMS, Marianne Mazzola, RT, RDMS
St. Louis Regional Medical Center–Radiology Department, St. Louis, Missouri, Vik Dogra, MD, RDMS, Lela Flumenbaum, RT
St. Louis Regional Medical Center–Antenatal Testing, St. Louis, Missouri, James Smeltzer, MD, Connie Cornell, RT, RDMS, Pauline Chestnut, LPN, Ron Pipes, RT, RDMS
St. Luke's Hospital St. Louis, Missouri, Patrick Dallman, RT, RDMS, Marsha Chavez, RDMS, Susan Dodson, RT, RDMS, Mary Helfrich, RT, RDMS, Krista Guker, RT, RDMS
St. Louis University Medical Center, St. Louis, Missouri, Michael Wolverson, MD, Bernadine Pollihan, RT, RDMS, Linda Schroeder, RT, RDMS, Nicole Madison, RT
St. Mary's Health Center, St. Louis, Missouri, Robert Berg, RT, RDMS, Donald Woodson, RT, RDMS, Herman Celestine, RT, RDMS

REVIEWERS

The following professionals served as reviewers for this project and provided a wealth of valuable comments:

Mary Jane Baker, RT, RDMS
St. Louis Community College–Forest Park
St. Louis, Missouri

Kathy Brewer, RDMS
Audubon Regional Medical Center
Louisville, Kentucky

Jan Bryant, MS, RT, RDMS
El Centro College
Dallas, Texas

Roberta Gunderson, BSRT, RDMS
Wright College
Chicago, Illinois

Lyn Marie Jacobson, RT, RDMS
Pitt Community College
Greenville, North Carolina

Jerry Pearson, MHA, RDMS
Oregon Health Sciences University
Portland, Oregon

Lynne Schreiber, BS, RT, RDMS
Jackson Community College
Jackson, Michigan

Thomas Walsh, MA, RT, RDMS
Middlesex Community College
Bedford, Massachusetts

Kerry Weinberg
New York University Medical Center
New York, New York

contents

detailed contents

10 Scrotum and prostate 176

11 Breast 195

12 Gynecologic anatomy and physiology 203

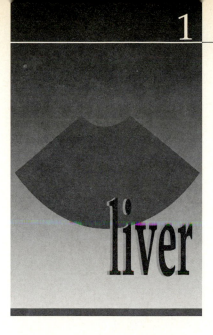

1

INSTRUCTIONAL OBJECTIVES

At the completion of this chapter, the reader will be able to:

1. Describe the clinical problems that are typical reasons for liver sonography.
2. Identify the basic subsections of the patient's medical chart and describe the type of clinical information found in each section.
3. Identify on illustrations and sonograms the major body planes, including coronal, transverse, and longitudinal, and explain the scan plane orientation and anatomic relationships in directional terms.
4. Identify on transverse and longitudinal illustrations and sonograms the major anatomic structures of the liver, including the lobes and their segments, ligaments and fissures, the major tributaries of the portal system, hepatic venous and arterial systems, and the intrahepatic biliary system.
5. Describe the basic scanning protocol for hepatic sonography as defined by national professional organizations.
6. Describe the clinical laboratory tests used for evaluating liver function, including serum glutamic pyruvic transaminase (SGPT) or alanine aminotransferase (ALT), serum glutamic oxaloacetic transaminase (SGOT) or aspartate amine-transferase (AST), alkaline phosphatase (ALP), bilirubin, prothrombin time (PT, PTT), lactic acid dehydrogenase (LDH), and alpha-fetoprotein (AFP), and discuss the specific disease processes they evaluate.
7. Identify the normal sonographic pattern of the liver parenchyma and associated vascular and ligamentous structures.
8. Describe the clinical symptoms and pathologic basis for the disease processes of the liver, including cysts, hepatocellular carcinoma, metastatic disease, abscesses, hematoma, hepatitis, congestive heart failure, fatty infiltration, cirrhosis, portal hypertension, hemangioma, adenoma, and focal nodular hyperplasia.
9. Identify on sectional sonograms the above-mentioned disease processes of the liver based on the sonographic pattern, the clinical history, and the results of other diagnostic procedures.
10. List at least two technical pitfalls associated with liver sonography.

THE CLINICAL PROBLEM

Since normal liver function plays a crucial role in many metabolic processes, liver dysfunction must be considered in patients with general symptoms of numerous metabolic disorders. Therefore abnormal liver function tests play a crucial role in narrowing the clinical diagnosis to the liver. A discussion of these tests appears later in this chapter. Other clinical signs pointing to possible liver involvement include hepatomegaly, right upper quadrant pain, nausea, vomiting, and fatigue. Since pathologic processes involving other organs can also cause these symptoms, the referring physician generally formulates a clinical differential diagnosis and orders further diagnostic procedures to narrow this differential and establish the clinical diagnosis.

Because of its noninvasive nature and low cost, hepatic sonography is an integral diagnostic procedure to establish whether a pathologic disorder of the liver exists. The procedure also provides a differential diagnosis for any abnormal sonographic pattern and assists in determining the necessity of other diagnostic procedures. Since many of the abnormal sonographic patterns are not specific for one type of pathology, the sonographer must gather as much clinical information as possible, including the patient's symptoms and history and the results of clinical laboratory tests and related diagnostic procedures. This information should be obtained before the sonographic examination, since it assists the sonographer in determining the area of sonographic interest, as well as what types of pathology are suspected.

OBTAINING THE CLINICAL HISTORY

The sonographer must gather the pertinent clinical data, laboratory test results, and related diagnostic imaging findings to understand the total medical picture of the patient before the ultrasound examination. To provide an accurate diagnosis, this information is vital to the interpreting physician.

In some departments the interpreting physician abstracts the patient's medical chart and identifies the area of sonographic interest to the sonographer. In other departments the chart is never reviewed. It should be a standard practice in every department to review the medical chart or obtain the clinical history from the patient for every ultrasound examination. Often it is the sonographer's responsibility to review the patient's chart or obtain the clinical history. Many departments have developed a standard form for recording the clinical findings. Examples of subheadings include: clinical symptoms, clinical laboratory tests, surgical history, and the results of other diagnostic imaging procedures. The following sections describe the main divisions of the patient's medical chart.

Physician's Order Sheets

The first task should be to ensure that the correct examination is ordered. For example, the referring physician may have ordered an ultrasound examination of the liver, but the unit secretary orders a computed tomography (CT) examination of the liver. Often the physician expands on the order and notes a specific disease process derived from the clinical findings. An example is "Liver ultrasound—rule out abscess." Another item to check for is whether other diagnostic examinations are ordered for the same day. These procedures should be coordinated to maintain the proper preparation for each procedure and to minimize the amount of time that the patient must spend waiting for the various examinations.

Patient History Section

The patient history section contains the patient's medical history and the results of the physical examination performed during admission to the hospital. The sonographer should note any systemic diseases, such as diabetes and hypertension, heart disease, or a history of malignancy. Other information obtained from this section include previous surgical procedures, alcohol abuse, renal failure, or other processes that may affect the sonographic appearance of the area of interest. Probably every sonographer has had the experience of looking for the gallbladder in a patient who has had a cholecystectomy! With the widespread use of laparoscopic cholecystectomy, the small incisions are often difficult to see on the patient's abdomen.

The physical examination provides information on palpable abdominal masses, on the presence of jaundice or ascites, and on organomegaly and other physical signs of disease processes. At the end of the examination report, the physician often summarizes and discusses the findings, specifies a preliminary clinical diagnosis, and recommends the diagnostic tests to confirm the diagnosis.

Vital Signs Graph

The vital signs graph is the responsibility of the nursing staff. The patient's blood pressure, pulse rate, respirations, and temperature are recorded both numerically and in graph form so that the reader can quickly ascertain the presence of spiking temperatures, hypertension, and other abnormalities. The patient's nutritional input and waste output are also recorded along with instructions for examination preparations that affect these variables. For example, the sonographer can verify that the patient received no meals before a gallbladder examination.

Clinical Laboratory Test Results

The sonographer will find the results of the clinical laboratory tests invaluable in narrowing the site of sonographic interest and specifying the sonographic differential diagnosis. The range of clinical tests is quite extensive and includes tests for evaluating the function of the heart, liver, biliary system, kidneys, pancreas, and many other organs and metabolic processes. Pertinent laboratory tests are discussed in detail in each chapter.

Radiology and Nuclear Medicine Reports

The results of other diagnostic imaging procedures can offer valuable information to the sonographer. Often ultrasound examinations are ordered to gain additional information and correlation with abnormal findings reported from other procedures. For example, an intravenous pyelogram may have demonstrated a mass effect in the kidney, and a sonographic examination is ordered to verify the presence and nature of the mass. The sonographer can shorten the examination time and decrease the risk of missing pathology by checking the report for the exact location of the mass or abnormal area. Other examples of related findings that are typical reasons for sonographic correlation include the following: a nuclear medicine liver scan that reveals an area of decreased radioactive uptake, an upper gastrointestinal series that demonstrates a widened duodenal loop, or abnormal calcifications seen on a plain film radiograph of the abdomen. Each chapter contains specific information on related imaging procedures to sharpen the eye and improve the differential diagnostic skills of the sonographer.

Nurses' Notes

Although sometimes overlooked, the nurses' notes are often a good source for more clinical data about the patient. Usually written at least once every nursing shift, these notes contain information on clinical symptoms, eating patterns and waste elimination, mental status, and vital signs. Nurses are the primary care providers to the patient and often note problems or irregularities before the physician comes for the daily rounds. The nurses' notes are often the only source of information on the recently admitted patient where the physician has not yet written the results of the initial physical examintation or progress notes. The admitting diagnosis, usually listed on the patient's admission papers, can also provide useful information as long as the sonographer remembers that the diagnosis is preliminary and may change during the course of hospitalization.

NORMAL ANATOMY

Standard Body Planes

Before the establishment of sonography, CT, and magnetic resonance imaging, the common plane of anatomic view in diagnostic radiology was the coronal plane. This plane divides the human body or body part into anterior and posterior sections. With the advent of other imaging modalities, two other planes are now in standard use. The **transverse plane** divides the body or body part into superior and inferior sections. The **mid-longitudinal plane** divides the body or body part into equal left and right halves. On either side of midline, the longitudinal plane divides the body or organ into medial and lateral sections. Fig. 1-1 illustrates these three standard body planes. Note the use of transparent sheets of material to demonstrate these planes. In sonography these "sheets" can be compared with the ultrasonic field. The ultrasound beam, which is a specific thickness or width, varies with the crystal diameter and the focusing characteristics of the transducer. As an examination is performed, the sonographer obtains sectional sonograms of a specific thickness and moves the transducer to collect a sequential series of sections through the organ or area of interest. This process can be compared with taking one slice of bread from a loaf, examining it, and then removing the next slice of bread and repeating the process. By mentally recombining the images of all the slices or sections, the sonographer forms a mental image of the entire organ or anatomic area.

The sonographer must orient the plane of section in directional terms. In the coronal imaging plane, the transducer is placed on the lateral aspect of the patient. Therefore the lateral structures are located at the top of the image, adjacent to the transducer; medial structures are located deep in the image; superior areas are toward the sonographer's left on the viewing screen; and inferior structures are on the right of the image. In the transverse plane with the patient supine, anterior areas are located at the top of the image, posterior structures are located at the bottom of the image, the patient's right is on the left side of the image, and the patient's left is on the right side of the image. In supine longitudinal scans, anterior structures are at the top of the image, posterior areas are at the bottom of the image, superior areas are on the left side of the image, and inferior areas are toward the right side of the image.

Anatomic Divisions and Landmarks

The liver is the largest gland of the body and occupies the right upper quadrant, epigastric, and a portion of the left upper quadrant. Fig. 1-2 illustrates the superficial landmarks of the liver in the anterior coronal view. The **falciform ligament** attaches to the anterior surface of the liver slightly to the right of midline and merges with the parietal peritoneum. The inferior portion of the falciform ligament has a

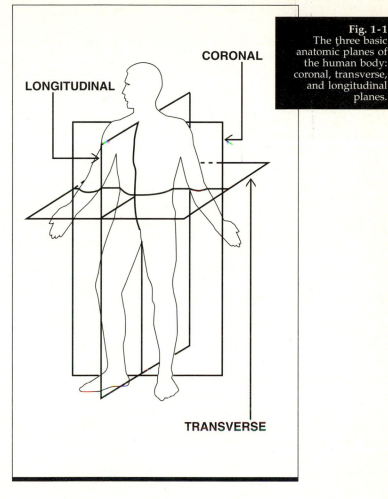

Fig. 1-1 The three basic anatomic planes of the human body: coronal, transverse, and longitudinal planes.

free border that contains the **ligamentum teres** (round ligament), a remnant of the fetal umbilical vein. This ligament passes from the free edge of the falciform ligament through a fissure on the posteroinferior surface of the liver and ascends to the porta hepatis where it fuses with the left branch of the portal vein. The falciform ligament is not routinely seen sonographically, since it forms a thin, flat layer on the anterior surface of the liver. In the presence of ascitic fluid, this ligament may be visualized as a thin hyperechoic structure coursing between the liver and anterior abdominal wall. However, the ligamentum teres is more often seen on transverse images as a hyperechoic, rather round mass in the liver, inferior to the left portal vein. This typical appearance of the round ligament must not be mistaken for a pathologic mass.

The posterior view of the liver (Fig. 1-3) demonstrates the three fossae of the right lobe: the gallbladder, inferior vena cava, and porta hepatis. The **porta hepatis,** located medially in the hilum of the liver, contains the primary vascular and ductal structures that enter and exit the liver, including the main portal vein, proper hepatic artery, and common hepatic bile duct. This region also contains a series of lymph nodes that can cause obstructive jaundice when they enlarge. The common hepatic duct is located to the right of the proper hepatic artery (both are located anterior to the portal vein). This view also depicts the lobes of the liver. In traditional anatomy the liver is divided into four lobes: right, left, caudate, and quadrate. The right and left lobes are divided by the falciform ligament, the caudate lobe lies on the posterosuperior aspect of the left lobe, and the quadrate lobe is situated on the posterior aspect of the right lobe. In sonography, **segmental liver anatomy** has replaced this traditional system. The liver is divided into segments based on the branches of

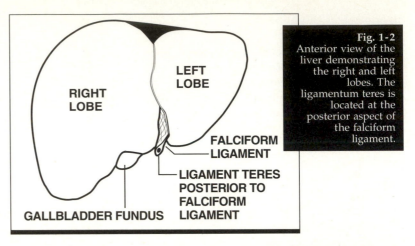

Fig. 1-2
Anterior view of the liver demonstrating the right and left lobes. The ligamentum teres is located at the posterior aspect of the falciform ligament.

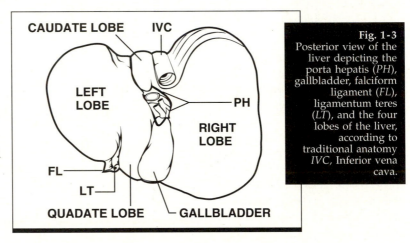

Fig. 1-3
Posterior view of the liver depicting the porta hepatis *(PH)*, gallbladder, falciform ligament *(FL)*, ligamentum teres *(LT)*, and the four lobes of the liver, according to traditional anatomy *IVC*, Inferior vena cava.

the portal vein, hepatic arteries and veins, and the clefts through which these vessels course. Thus the liver contains three lobes: the right, left, and caudate. The quadrate lobe becomes the medial segment of the left lobe. The caudate lobe is considered a separate lobe, since it receives its arterial and venous supply from both the right and left lobes. The **main lobar fissure** divides the liver into its true anatomic right and left lobes by coursing obliquely from the fossa for the inferior vena cava, through the middle hepatic vein, to the gallbladder fossa inferiorly (Fig. 1-4).

On superior transverse scans of the liver, the hepatic veins serve as division points between the various lobes (intrasegmental) and segments (intersegmental). The middle hepatic vein divides the right and left lobes, the right hepatic vein divides the anterior and posterior segments of the right lobe, and the left hepatic vein bisects the medial and lateral segments of the left lobe (Fig. 1-5). The branches of the portal system also serve as sonographic landmarks. The anterior branch of the right portal vein courses through the central portion of the anterior segment of the right lobe, whereas the posterior branch courses through the posterior segment (Fig. 1-6). The initial segment of the left portal vein divides the caudate lobe from the lateral segment of the left lobe. An additional landmark is the ligamentum venosum, which separates the caudate lobe from the left lobe of the liver (Fig. 1-7). The ascending portion of the left portal vein divides the left lobe into medial and lateral segments. The lateral branch of the left portal vein courses through the lateral segment, and the medial branch courses through the medial segment (Fig. 1-8).

Hepatic Vessels

The main vessels in the liver are the hepatic arteries and veins, portal veins, and biliary tributaries. The **common hepatic artery** arises from the celiac trunk of

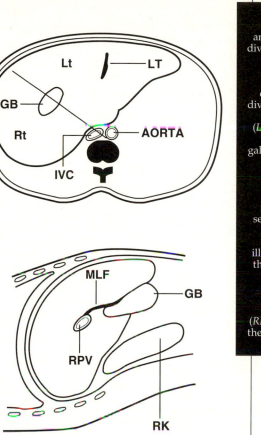

Fig. 1-4 Segmental anatomy—anatomic divisions of the right and left lobes. **A** Transverse illustration demonstrating the division between the right (*Rt*) and left (*Lt*) lobes, using the midpoint of the gallbladder (*GB*) and the inferior vena cava (*IVC*). The ligamentum teres (*LT*) divides the medial and lateral segments of the left lobe. **B** Longitudinal illustration showing the normal position of the main lobar fissure (*MLF*) coursing from the right portal vein (*RPV*) to the neck of the gallbladder (*GB*). *RK*, Right kidney.

the abdominal aorta, courses transversely to the right of midline, and becomes the proper hepatic artery at the level of the origin of the gastroduodenal artery (Fig. 1-9). The **proper hepatic artery** ascends and enters the liver, via the porta hepatis, where it divides into three main branches: right, middle, and left. These branches divide into numerous small tributaries that travel to the hepatic cells. In many cases the middle hepatic artery arises off the left hepatic artery. The **hepatic veins** transport deoxygenated blood from the liver cells to the inferior vena cava. Smaller tributaries converge throughout the liver parenchyma to form the right, middle, and left hepatic veins, which empty into the inferior vena cava in close proximity to the diaphragm. The **portal system** transports nutrient-rich blood from the digestive tract to the liver cells for metabolic processing and storage. The portal system is formed by the merger of the splenic and superior mesenteric veins. The inferior mesenteric vein enters the splenic vein. The **main portal vein** enters the porta hepatis and bifurcates into the left and right branches (Fig. 1-10). The left portal vein further divides into medial and lateral branches, and the right portal vein gives rise to the anterior and posterior branches. The numerous small bile duct tributaries merge to form the right and left hepatic ducts, which merge to form the common hepatic duct. Throughout the liver, the portal vein, hepatic artery, and bile duct tributaries course parallel to one another, providing the primary sonographic evidence in cases of obstructive jaundice. This relationship is often referred to as the "portal triad."

CLINICAL LABORATORY TESTS

Serum Glutamic Oxaloacetic Transaminase

Serum glutamic oxaloacetic transaminase (SGOT), or aspartate amine transferase (AST), is an enzyme present in tissues with a high rate of metabolic activity, including the liver. It is released into the bloodstream in abnormally high levels as a result of death or injury to the producing cells. Hence any disease that causes injury to the cells causes a rise in SGOT levels proportional to the amount of damage and the time between the injury and the test.

Because this enzyme is produced in many types of tissue, elevated levels do not always indicate injury specifically to the liver cells. However, increased levels are associated with active cirrhosis, acute hepatitis, hepatic necrosis, and infectious mononucleosis with acute hepatitis.

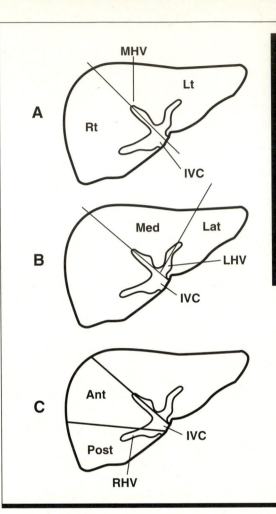

Fig. 1-5
Segmental anatomy based on the hepatic veins—transverse plane.
A The middle hepatic vein (*MHV*) divides the right (*Rt*) and left (*Lt*) lobes.
B The left hepatic vein (*LHV*) divides the medial (*Med*) and lateral (*Lat*) segments of the left lobe.
C The right hepatic vein (*RHV*) divides the anterior (*Ant*) and posterior (*Post*) segments of the right lobe. *IVC,* Inferior vena cava.

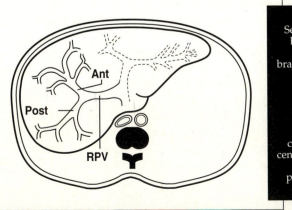

Fig. 1-6
Segmental anatomy based on the right portal vein branches—transverse view. The right portal vein (*RPV*) divides into the anterior (*Ant*) and posterior (*Post*) branches, which course through the central portion of the anterior and posterior segments, respectively.

Serum Glutamic Pyruvic Transaminase

Serum glutamic pyruvic transaminase (SGPT), or alanine aminotransferase (ALT), is more specific than SGOT for evaluating liver function. High concentrations of this enzyme occur in the liver, and relatively low concentrations are found in the heart, muscle, and kidneys. SGPT/ALT is also used to monitor the course of treatment for hepatitis, the effects of drug treatments that are toxic to the liver, and other diffuse medical diseases of the liver. Again, the magnitude of the increase corresponds to the severity of the injury to the hepatic cells and the duration between onset and the performance of the test. Increased levels are associated with hepatocellular diseases, active cirrhosis, metastatic liver disease, and biliary obstruction. A mild increase in the level of SGPT is associated with pancreatitis.

Alkaline Phosphatase

Alkaline phosphatase (ALP) is an enzyme produced primarily by the liver and bones, as well as by the placenta during pregnancy. Hepatocellular diseases cause a mild to moderate increase of ALP, depending on the extent of injury. Since ALP is excreted via the bile ducts, obstructive jaundice typically causes marked elevation.

Lactic Acid Dehydrogenase

Lactic acid dehydrogenase (LDH) is an intracellular enzyme widely distributed in body tissues: kidney, heart, skeletal muscle, liver,

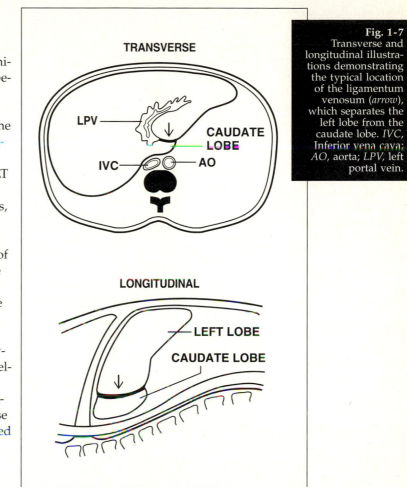

Fig. 1-7 Transverse and longitudinal illustrations demonstrating the typical location of the ligamentum venosum (*arrow*), which separates the left lobe from the caudate lobe. *IVC,* Inferior vena cava; *AO,* aorta; *LPV,* left portal vein.

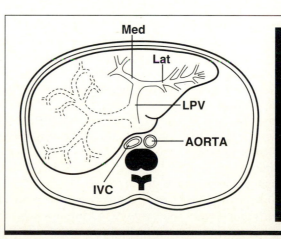

Fig. 1-8 Segmental anatomy of the left portal vein branches—transverse view. The ascending portion of the left portal vein (*LPV*) divides the medial from the lateral segments of the left lobe. The medial (*Med*) and lateral (*Lat*) branches course through the central portion of their respective segments.

brain, and lung. Increased levels typically indicate cellular death and leakage of the enzyme from the cell. This test is not specific for hepatic function and is usually correlated with the results of other tests to verify the presence of myocardial or pulmonary infarction. LDH may be broken down into five isoenzymes, which may provide more specific findings for hepatocellular disease. LDH levels may be moderately increased in cases of infectious mononucleosis and mildly elevated in hepatitis, cirrhosis, and obstructive jaundice.

Bilirubin

Bilirubin is the product resulting from the breakdown of hemoglobin in old red blood cells in the spleen. It is transported to the liver via the portal system, where the liver cells convert these by-products into bile pigments that, along with lecithin, cholesterol, and inorganic salts, are secreted as bile by the liver cells into the bile ducts. Three methods may disrupt this production cycle. **Hemolytic jaun-**

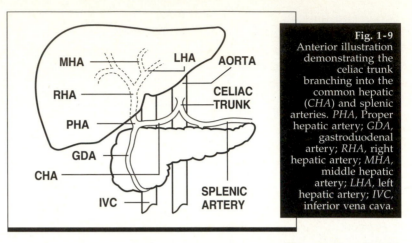

Fig. 1-9 Anterior illustration demonstrating the celiac trunk branching into the common hepatic (*CHA*) and splenic arteries. *PHA*, Proper hepatic artery; *GDA*, gastroduodenal artery; *RHA*, right hepatic artery; *MHA*, middle hepatic artery; *LHA*, left hepatic artery; *IVC*, inferior vena cava.

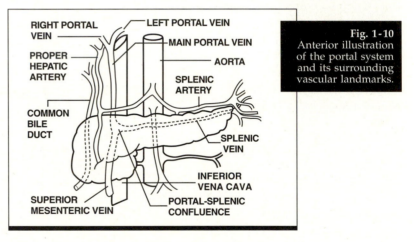

Fig. 1-10 Anterior illustration of the portal system and its surrounding vascular landmarks.

dice consists of an excessive amount of red blood cell destruction. A malfunction of the liver cells causes **medical jaundice.** A blockage of the bile ducts causes **obstructive jaundice.** These disruptions cause an increase in serum bilirubin, that eventually leaks into the tissues, giving a yellow cast to the skin. The clinical term for this condition is jaundice.

The screening procedure for elevated bilirubin levels is the **total bilirubin** assay. An elevated total bilirubin level is a nonspecific finding, since any of the three disruptive processes mentioned above could be the cause of the abnormality. There are two additional tests to help specify the cause of the clinical jaundice.

Indirect bilirubin, or unconjugated bilirubin, is protein bound in the serum. Elevated levels are frequently seen with hemolytic jaundice caused by hemolytic anemias or hemorrhagic pulmonary infarcts.

Direct bilirubin, or conjugated bilirubin, circulates freely in the blood, reaches the liver, is conjugated with glucuronide, and is excreted into the bile. Typically, obstructive jaundice without biliary cirrhosis causes an elevation of only the direct bilirubin.

Medical jaundice, a result of hepatocellular dysfunction, typically causes an increase of both the direct and indirect bilirubin, with a larger increase of the direct bilirubin. Examples include hepatic metastases, hepatitis, cholestasis secondary to drugs, and cirrhosis.

Alpha-fetoprotein

Alpha-fetoprotein (AFP) is a liver enzyme normally secreted by the immature liver cells in the embryo and fetus. Shortly after birth normal liver cell maturation eliminates the secretion of this enzyme. In the adult the presence of AFP in the serum is abnormal and raises the suspicion of malignancy involving the liver.

Prothrombin Time

Prothrombin (PT, PTT), an enzyme produced by the liver, plays a crucial role in the blood clotting mechanism. The production of prothrombin depends on an adequate intake and utilization of vitamin K. The prothrombin time is increased in the presence of liver disease with accompanying cellular damage and dysfunction. Examples include cirrhosis and metastatic disease.

• • •

Interpreted individually, none of these tests offers as high a level of specificity compared with an integrated interpretation of multiple clinical laboratory tests. This approach, coupled with the clinical history and the results of a sonographic examination, allows a higher probability of providing a specific clinical diagnosis.

RELATED IMAGING PROCEDURES

Radiographic Plain Film of the Abdomen

A plain-film radiograph of the abdomen is obtained with the patient supine, without injection of any contrast medium. The image includes the anatomy from the diaphragm to the pubic symphysis. With this simple procedure, the radiologist can often determine the presence of ascites, biliary air, organomegaly, calcifications, and mass effects.

Arteriography

Arteriography involves the injection of iodinated contrast medium into the arterial system of the liver to determine the vascular supply of an abnormal mass. Malignant tumors may demonstrate an increased vascular supply transported by numerous abnormal vessels. Usually, benign cysts and neoplasms only distort the position of the normal vessels. Because this procedure is invasive, it carries some risk of injury and mortality that must be weighed against the benefits of the procedure. Computed tomography with contrast injection offers an alternative to this procedure for some types of pathology.

Computed Tomography

The computed tomography (CT) examination is a computerized radiographic procedure that produces sectional images based on the radiographic densities of human tissues. This procedure often involves a venous injection of iodinated contrast media that provides more information regarding the vascular supply of discrete liver masses.

Current systems are quite sensitive to small density changes, although a lack of body fat surrounding the organs may degrade resolution. In cases where the CT examination cannot ascertain the consistency of a hepatic mass, sonography may provide a more definitive diagnosis.

Nuclear Medicine Imaging

Nuclear medicine procedures demonstrate the physiological function of various organs. A small amount of a radioactive tracer element is bound to an organic compound that is normally acted on by the cells of the target organ. A radioactive detection device, a gamma camera, amplifies and processes the radiation emitted by the target organ and displays this information on a display monitor.

To evaluate the function of hepatic cells, a tracer amount of ^{99m}Tc is bound to sulfur colloid particles that are normally trapped and processed by the hepatic cells. In the presence of hepatocellular disease or malignant cells, cellular function decreases with a resulting loss of trapping ability. Therefore abnormal hepatic cells contain only a small amount of radioactive tracer and display as areas of decreased radioactive uptake, or "cold spots." A primary limitation of this procedure is difficulty in differentiating benign from malignant processes, since both can produce similar patterns.

SCANNING PROTOCOLS AND TECHNIQUES

Several professional organizations have published scanning guidelines for the various sonographic examinations.[1,2] From a legal standpoint, the sonographer must ensure that their examinations meet these national standards of practice. These standards are minimum guidelines that specify the basic anatomy that should be documented. The sonographer, in conjunction with the interpreting physician, should expand on these guidelines and adapt them to their unique requirements. Any liver examination should include both longitudinal and transverse views with specific anatomic structures to localize the region of the liver represented on that view. The vascular structures in the liver serve as the primary tool in this identification process.

Transverse Scans
From superior to inferior:
- Hepatic veins merging with inferior vena cava
- Left portal vein, ligamentum venosum
- Right portal vein
- Liver, gallbladder interface
- Liver, right kidney interface

Longitudinal Scans
From midline to right:
- Liver, inferior vena cava, left portal vein origin
- Liver, gallbladder, right portal vein
- Liver, diaphragm
- Liver, kidney
- Lateral aspect liver

From midline to left:
- Liver, ligamentum venosum, aorta
- Liver, diaphragm
- Lateral aspect, left lobe

Another very important but often neglected consideration is that all images should be recorded in sequence, that is, from superior to inferior on transverse scans (or vice versa), and medial to lateral on longitudinal scans. Again, this protocol allows the interpreting physician to gain rapid orientation to the depicted anatomy and allows more specific localization of any pathology. A sample protocol based on anatomic landmarks and performed in sequence is presented in the box on the previous page.

This list comprises the anatomy visualized in the optimal sonographic evaluation of the liver. Figs. 1-11 through 1-20 illustrate the normal anatomy depicted in this protocol. The patient's condition and body habitus may interfere with adequate documentation of such detailed anatomy. However, the sonographer should still scan in sequence and include as many anatomic landmarks as possible in each image.

The scanning technique will vary depending on the patient's condition and body habitus, and on the type of pathology present. The subcostal approach requires the patient to maintain deep inspiration while obtaining the scan. The intercostal approach often works best with uncooperative patients, patients with excessive bowel gas, or patients with a large body habitus. Raising the patient's right arm will enlarge the intercostal space, as well as minimize the thickness of adipose tissue in obese patients. The patient should stop

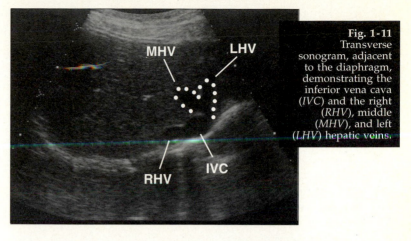

Fig. 1-11 Transverse sonogram, adjacent to the diaphragm, demonstrating the inferior vena cava (*IVC*) and the right (*RHV*), middle (*MHV*), and left (*LHV*) hepatic veins.

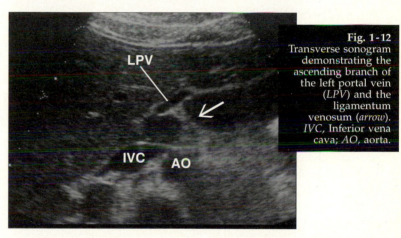

Fig. 1-12 Transverse sonogram demonstrating the ascending branch of the left portal vein (*LPV*) and the ligamentum venosum (*arrow*). *IVC,* Inferior vena cava; *AO,* aorta.

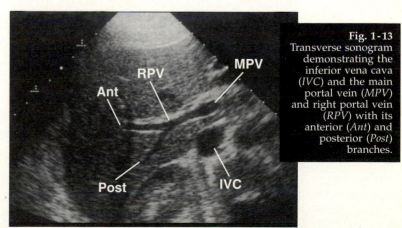

Fig. 1-13 Transverse sonogram demonstrating the inferior vena cava (*IVC*) and the main portal vein (*MPV*) and right portal vein (*RPV*) with its anterior (*Ant*) and posterior (*Post*) branches.

breathing while the image is obtained. The sonographer can place the area of interest in the scanning window, remembering that abdominal structures move inferiorly on inspiration and superiorly on expiration. Typically the patient is supine for the examination. However, having the patient roll partially on the left side, forming a 45-degree angle to the cart, can result in better visualization of the lateral and posterior aspects of the liver and can displace surrounding bowel gas from the liver.

The sonographer must pay attention to a number of technical factors. Transducer selection is very important. The transducer should provide adequate penetration with optimum resolution. A selection of 3.5 MHz fulfills these criteria for the normal patient. A 5.0 MHz may be an optimum selection for thin patients, whereas selecting 2.25 MHz may be necessary for large patients. The area of sonographic interest should be placed within the focal zone of the transducer. With electronic focusing, dynamic focusing throughout the depth of the liver will provide the best overall resolution. However, the frame rate usually decreases with dynamic focusing, which could degrade resolution if the patient cannot hold his or her breath. In these instances the sonographer may want to place the focal zone in the posterior aspect of the liver for a general survey scan, since lateral resolution is typically worse in this region compared with more superficial areas in

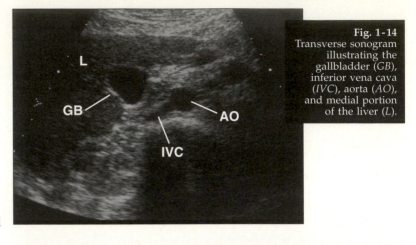

Fig. 1-14
Transverse sonogram illustrating the gallbladder (*GB*), inferior vena cava (*IVC*), aorta (*AO*), and medial portion of the liver (*L*).

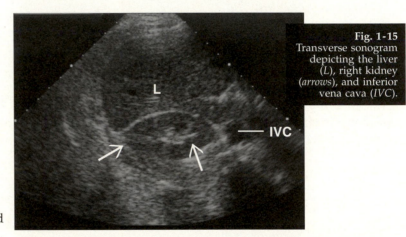

Fig. 1-15
Transverse sonogram depicting the liver (*L*), right kidney (*arrows*), and inferior vena cava (*IVC*).

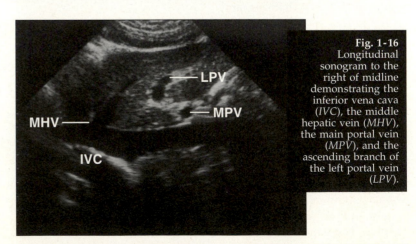

Fig. 1-16
Longitudinal sonogram to the right of midline demonstrating the inferior vena cava (*IVC*), the middle hepatic vein (*MHV*), the main portal vein (*MPV*), and the ascending branch of the left portal vein (*LPV*).

the scan. If abnormal areas are found, the focal zone should be positioned to correspond to the depth of the abnormality.

The manipulation of the ultrasound unit's gain and acoustic power controls poses problems for many sonographers. The acoustic power control determines the intensity and amplitude of the emitted ultrasonic field. Therefore this control directly determines the patient's ultrasound exposure. To minimize the patient's exposure, the acoustic power should be set at the minimum level to allow adequate penetration. The system gain control increases the amplitude of the echo signal in the ultrasound unit and has no effect on ultrasonic exposure. Therefore the sonographer should always increase the gain controls first if the displayed echoes are not strong enough. The acoustic power should be increased only if increasing the gain does not produce a diagnostic image.

NORMAL SONOGRAPHIC PATTERNS

The normal liver parenchyma should display a diffusely homogeneous, moderately echogenic pattern that is hypoechoic to the normal walls of the right and left portal veins. Other organs serve as additional parameters to verify the liver pattern. The normal renal cortex is hypoechoic to the normal liver, and the pancreas in younger patients is isoechoic to the normal liver parenchyma. In the elderly the normal pancreatic pattern may be hyperechoic in comparison with the normal liver pattern because of

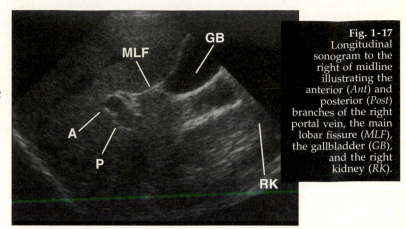

Fig. 1-17 Longitudinal sonogram to the right of midline illustrating the anterior (*Ant*) and posterior (*Post*) branches of the right portal vein, the main lobar fissure (*MLF*), the gallbladder (*GB*), and the right kidney (*RK*).

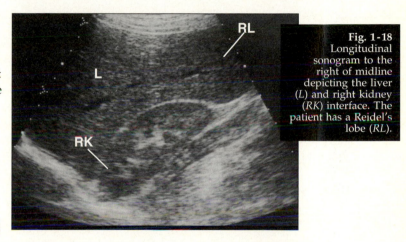

Fig. 1-18 Longitudinal sonogram to the right of midline depicting the liver (*L*) and right kidney (*RK*) interface. The patient has a Reidel's lobe (*RL*).

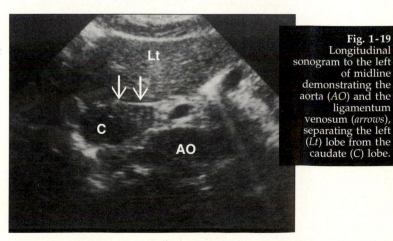

Fig. 1-19 Longitudinal sonogram to the left of midline demonstrating the aorta (*AO*) and the ligamentum venosum (*arrows*), separating the left (*Lt*) lobe from the caudate (C) lobe.

increased fatty deposition. In comparing these organs, the sonographer must verify the patient's clinical history to avoid erroneous pattern classifications resulting from disease processes such as chronic renal failure or pancreatitis.

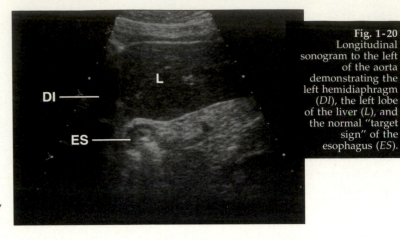

Fig. 1-20 Longitudinal sonogram to the left of the aorta demonstrating the left hemidiaphragm (*DI*), the left lobe of the liver (*L*), and the normal "target sign" of the esophagus (*ES*).

CONGENITAL ANOMALIES

Body Habitus

The anatomy described in this text corresponds to the "normal" anatomy for the "average" body habitus found in approximately 50% of the population. This type of body habitus, or build, is called the **sthenic** body habitus.[7] The other body habitus types are the hypersthenic, hyposthenic, and asthenic builds (Fig. 1-21).

The **hypersthenic** individual is usually tall and/or obese. The chest is broad, deep, and short, with the ribs assuming an almost horizontal plane. The diaphragm is high, producing a long abdominal cavity that is broad in its upper regions and narrow in its lower areas. Sonographically, the liver is high and most accessible with an intercostal approach. The left lobe may appear small in comparison with the sthenic build.

The **asthenic** build is found in the small, slender individual. The chest is long and narrow with the rib cage sloping downward at a sharp angle. The diaphragm is lower, so that the abdominal cavity is shorter and broader in its lower portion than in the sthenic build. The liver tends to be longer, so that the subcostal approach is easier. The intercostal spaces are often small, making intercostal scanning a challenge.

The **hyposthenic** build falls in between the extreme asthenic and sthenic types. The abdominal organs are not quite as low lying as in the asthenic individual.

Riedel's Lobe

Riedel's lobe is a congenital anomaly that produces a prominent extension of normal liver parenchyma. This anomaly primarily affects the right lobe, although it may occur on the left lobe as well. Clinically, it may present as hepatomegaly or produce an area of decreased uptake on a nuclear medicine scan of the liver. With sonography the parenchymal pattern of the Riedel's lobe should be isoechoic to the rest of the liver parenchyma.

PATHOLOGIC PROCESSES OF THE LIVER

Hepatic Cysts

Hepatic cysts are congenital structures thought to form from an obstruction of biliary ductules, although they may be acquired later in life. These cysts may occur singly or in groups and may vary in size from small to quite large. Since the widespread use of ultrasound, simple cysts have become a common incidental finding. These cysts can become infected or undergo hemorrhage. In cases of multiple hepatic cysts the sonographer should examine the kidneys to rule out polycystic disease.

Most hepatic cysts are asymptomatic, although patients may have a palpable mass or hepatomegaly. The laboratory liver function tests are usually normal unless the cyst is quite large and interferes with the function of adjacent liver parenchyma. If a cyst has become infected, the patient may have a fever and elevated white blood cell count and may complain of localized pain. If hemorrhage has occurred, the patient may rarely have a decreased red blood cell count and may also complain of pain.

These round to oval-shaped hepatic cysts should demonstrate all the ultrasonic signs of a cyst: smooth walled, anechoic interior, and exhibit acoustic enhancement distal to the cyst (Fig. 1-22). Benign cysts may contain septa but should meet all other cystic criteria to be classified as a benign cyst. Cysts with irregular walls or containing debris may indicate an infected or hemorrhagic cyst or, more rarely, a malignancy.[8] If a malignancy is suspected, the liver should be carefully scanned for the presence of any solid masses, and the retroperitoneal nodes checked for signs of metastases. Obtaining a complete clinical history is crucial to the interpreting physician in order to narrow the differential diagnosis.

Echinococcal Cyst

The echinococcal cyst, or hydatid disease, results from the acquisition of the parasite **echinococcus granulosis,** which is excreted in the feces of contaminated ani-

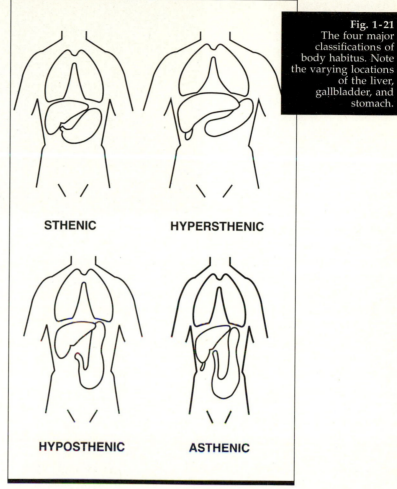

STHENIC   HYPERSTHENIC

HYPOSTHENIC   ASTHENIC

Fig. 1-21 The four major classifications of body habitus. Note the varying locations of the liver, gallbladder, and stomach.

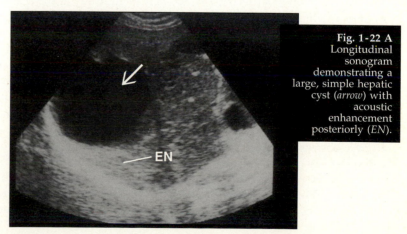

Fig. 1-22 A Longitudinal sonogram demonstrating a large, simple hepatic cyst (*arrow*) with acoustic enhancement posteriorly (*EN*).

mals such as cows, dogs, cattle, and humans. The patient ingests the eggs of the worm, which later enter the circulatory system and contaminate various organs. The primary result of this disease is the formation of cysts, with over a 50% incidence in the liver. The cyst formation is quite slow, typically taking several years to gain an appreciable size.

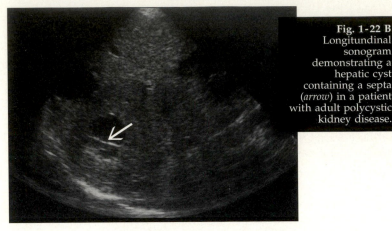

Fig. 1-22 B Longitundinal sonogram demonstrating a hepatic cyst containing a septa (*arrow*) in a patient with adult polycystic kidney disease.

The typical population susceptible to this disease includes immigrants and tourists who have visited underdeveloped countries. Because this disease may stay asymptomatic for years, the sonographer must extend the time period to obtain the pertinent clinical history. The patient may demonstrate signs of infection, such as a fever and elevated white blood cell count, and may complain of pain. If the cysts are large, the patient may have hepatomegaly or a palpable mass.

The various sonographic patterns include multiple thick-walled cysts (with or without calcified walls), septated cysts, the presence of daughter cysts (cysts within cysts), and cysts with an echogenic interior.[4] The sonographer should check for a contributing clinical history whenever multiple, septated, and/or complex cysts are demonstrated in the liver.

Hepatocellular Carcinoma

The hepatocellular carcinoma, also known by the misnomer hepatoma, has the highest incidence in patients with cirrhosis.[3] This primary malignancy has a marked tendency to metastasize into the hepatic and portal veins, which may lead to thrombosis. The tumor may present as a discrete single mass, multiple masses, or a diffuse disruption of the liver parenchyma.

The clinical signs of this malignancy may include any of the following: hepatomegaly, palpable mass, jaundice, weight loss, and splenomegaly. Because of the typical presence of cirrhosis, elevation of liver function tests may be difficult to interpret. AFP, which is not usually present in adults, is found in 50% to 70% of patients with hepatocellular carcinoma.[12]

The sonographic pattern is variable, including single or multiple hypoechoic to hyperechoic masses (Fig. 1-23). This entity may also present as a diffuse infiltrative process. The sonographer should carefully scan the hepatic veins for the presence of thrombus and **Budd-Chiari syndrome.** This syndrome occurs when the pathologic condition obstructs the hepatic veins, causing decreased flow and collapsed veins distal to the site of obstruction.[5] The portal veins should be evaluated for evidence of tumor thrombus. The sonographic pattern of thrombus is typically a hypoechoic mass in the lumen (Fig. 1-24). Color Doppler will verify the decrease or absence of blood flow in the vessel and is very important when the sonographic pattern of the thrombus is not readily demonstrated.[15] Patients with portal vein thrombosis may also develop portal hypertension.

Metastatic Carcinoma

Metastasis refers to the occurrence of secondary malignant tumors at sites distant from the primary carcinoma. The malignant cells travel through the blood or lymph vessels or transfer directly from an adjacent organ or structure. The highest incidence of liver metastasis is associated with carcinoma of the colon, breast, lung, pancreas, and gallbladder.

The clinical symptoms include hepatomegaly, palpable mass, jaundice, and/or an unexplained weight loss. Typically, there is hepatocellular dysfunction leading to increased SGOT/SGPT levels, as well as ALP. The more diffuse the metastatic involvement, the more hepatic cellular dysfunction will be indicated by these tests. When located in or adjacent to the porta hepatis, metastasis may cause obstructive jaundice.

There are three patterns associated with hepatic metastasis. Hypoechoic or hyperechoic discrete masses and a diffuse disruption of the parenchymal pattern are common. Other, more rare patterns include cystic.[17]

Many researchers have tried to find a tissue characterization pattern to determine the exact etiology of liver metastasis. Although promising, only a few generalities can be inferred related to specific sonographic patterns for specific carcinomas.

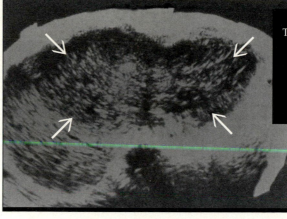

Fig. 1-23 A Transverse sonogram depicting a hepatocellular carcinoma (*arrows*), occupying the anterior portion of the right and left lobes.

Fig. 1-23 B Nuclear medicine examination using [99mTc] sulphur colloid illustrating the huge area of decreased radioactive uptake corresponding to the malignancy.

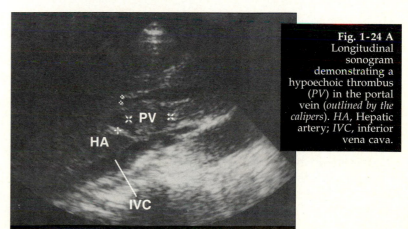

Fig. 1-24 A Longitudinal sonogram demonstrating a hypoechoic thrombus (*PV*) in the portal vein (*outlined by the calipers*). *HA*, Hepatic artery; *IVC*, inferior vena cava.

Most hyperechoic lesions are from primary adenocarcinomas, most typically from the colon. These may also present as a "bull's eye" pattern that consists of a hyperechoic central core surrounded by a hypoechoic halo (Fig. 1-25). Lymphomatous invasion of the liver, as well as primary ovarian tumors, tend to produce hypoechoic masses.[16] Typically, the diffuse pattern occurs with widespread dissemination throughout the liver, producing a distortion of the normal parenchymal pattern (Fig. 1-26). Since discrete masses may not be apparent, the sonographer should check for contour abnormalities, hepatomegaly, and distorted relationships to adjacent structures. Acoustic power and gain settings play important roles in detecting these subtle masses, since excessive settings may mask their appearance.

It is important to remember that none of these patterns is totally specific. In fact, hypoechoic and hyperechoic masses are often found together. Larger masses may contain a central area of necrosis secondary to outstripping their vascular supply. Patients receiving chemotherapy may have a similar pattern that indicates that the agent is causing necrosis. Metastatic deposits may contain areas of calcification. The amount of vascularity varies, so that pulsed Doppler and color flow do not offer signs specific enough to definitively diagnose malignancy.[14] Doppler plays an adjunct role and requires correlation with the sonographic appearance and the patient's clinical his-

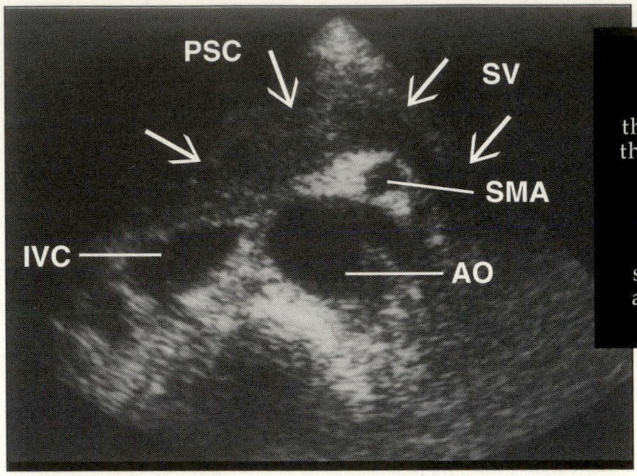

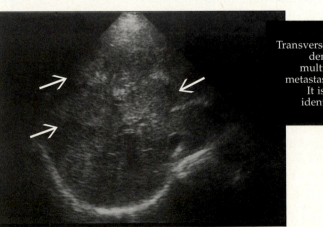

Fig. 1-24 B Transverse image demonstrating the thrombus (*arrows*) in the splenic vein (*SV*) and the portal-splenic confluence (*PSC*). *AO*, aorta; *SMA*, superior mesenteric artery; *IVC*, inferior vena cava.

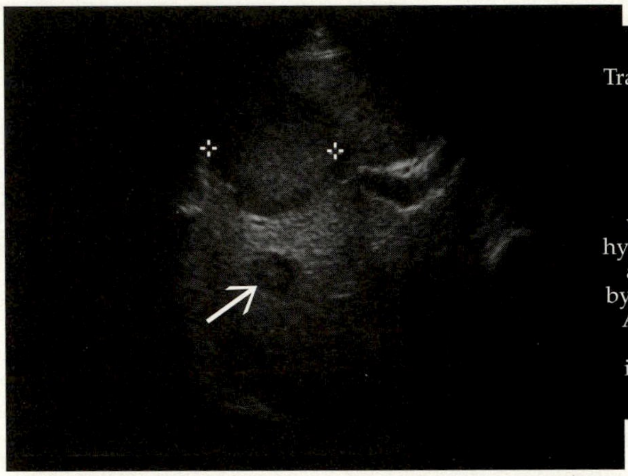

Fig. 1-25 Transverse sonogram depicting a large liver metastases (*calipers*) that demonstrates the "bull's eye" sign, which consists of a hyperechoic center of a mass surrounded by a hypoechoic rim. A smaller, posterior mass (*arrow*) illustrates the same pattern.

Fig. 1-26 A Transverse sonogram demonstrating multiple, diffuse metastases (*arrows*). It is difficult to identify discrete masses.

tory. The sonographer should also scan the retroperitoneal lymph nodes and the spleen to check for signs of further metastasis.

Abscesses

An abscess is a necrotic cavity in soft tissue or a collection of purulent material. There are five major pathways by which bacteria can enter the liver and cause abscess formation: (1) through the portal system, (2) by way of ascending cholangitis of the common bile duct, (3) via the hepatic artery secondary to bacteremia, (4) by direct extension from adjacent structures, and (5) by implantation of bacteria after trauma to the abdominal wall (6). In the United States, ascending cholangitis is the most common cause of a hepatic abscess.[16]

Patients with a hepatic abscess may have several symptoms: fever (often spiking), chills, and right upper quadrant pain. The liver function tests are typically normal, but the white blood cell count is often elevated.

The sonographic appearance of abscesses varies and may depend on the evolutionary stage at the time of the sonographic examination. Abscesses begin as localized areas of inflammation characterized by edema and sonographically may appear as a solid, hypoechoic area. Later they undergo cystic changes with the production of pus. The more typical pattern of a formed abscess is predominantly fluid filled with irregular borders (Fig. 1-27). However, they may con-

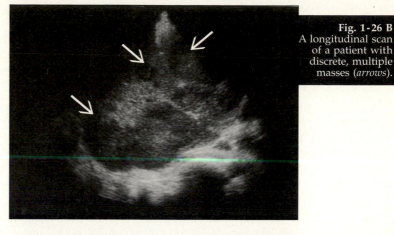

Fig. 1-26 B
A longitudinal scan of a patient with discrete, multiple masses (*arrows*).

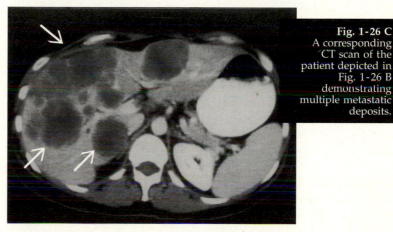

Fig. 1-26 C
A corresponding CT scan of the patient depicted in Fig. 1-26 B demonstrating multiple metastatic deposits.

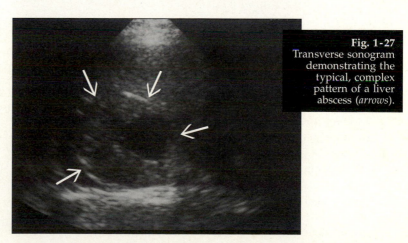

Fig. 1-27
Transverse sonogram demonstrating the typical, complex pattern of a liver abscess (*arrows*).

tain debris and occasional septa. The sonographer should carefully scan the rest of the liver to ensure the absence of other abscesses. In addition, the potentional peritoneal spaces, including the subphrenic and subhepatic areas, should be examined for further spread of the infection. Because of the variable sonographic patterns, the diagnosis of abscess relies on the correlation with clinical symptoms and laboratory test values.

Hematoma

A hematoma is a localized collection of extravasated blood that is confined in an organ, tissue, or potential space. It can occur postoperatively, after abdominal trauma, in conjunction with anticoagulation therapy, or for unknown reasons. The hematoma may contain unclotted blood if actively bleeding, or partially or completely coagulated blood. The degree of coagulation is related to the length of time that has elapsed since the initial injury.

The clinical symptoms range from asymptomatic for very small hematomas to localized pain and shock. Depending on the size of the hematoma and the amount of active bleeding, the red blood cell count may be decreased. If the hematoma is not completely walled off and becomes infected, signs of general peritonitis may be present.

Because of the variability of coagulation stages, hematomas have a variety of sonographic patterns. Fresh or actively bleeding hematomas may appear to have a homogeneous solid pattern, but exhibit acoustic enhancement. Another pattern consists of a mass displaying both cystic and solid components (Fig. 1-28). As the amount of time increases after the initial injury, general lysis occurs, producing a more cystic pattern. As in the case of an abscess, the diagnosis of a hematoma cannot be made on the basis of the sonographic pattern alone. The patient's symptoms and the sonographic appearance may allow a specific diagnosis of a hematoma.

Congestive Heart Failure

Congestive heart failure is a progressive loss of cardiac function that has widespread effects on the general circulatory system. One specific type of congestive heart failure is termed right ventricular failure, which raises the pressure in the venous circulatory system.

The symptoms for right ventricular failure are elevated venous pressure, hepatomegaly, and edema of the extremities. The liver function tests may be normal or slightly increased. As the disease progresses, other body systems and organs may be affected. Examples include the development of pleural effusions, ascites, and chronic renal failure.

Because of the rise in venous pressure in right heart failure, the primary sonographic sign

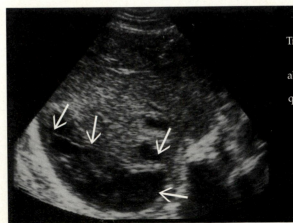

Fig. 1-28 Transverse sonogram of a patient with a history of blunt abdominal trauma to the right upper quadrant. A complex hematoma (*arrows*) developed in the posterior aspect of the liver. The liver capsule was intact.

consists of dilated hepatic veins and inferior vena cava (Fig. 1-29). With normal venous pressure, the size of the inferior vena cava varies with respiration and achieves its largest diameter with deep inspiration and by use of the Valsalva maneuver. The Valsalva maneuver consists of taking a deep inspiration and simultaneously bearing down, as in defecation. The liver parenchyma is typically normal in the absence of hepatocellular dysfunction. The sonographer should also check for the presence of pleural effusions (Fig. 1-30), ascites, and portal hypertension. The kidneys should be checked for signs of renal failure.

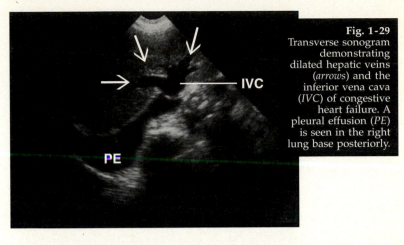

Fig. 1-29 Transverse sonogram demonstrating dilated hepatic veins (*arrows*) and the inferior vena cava (*IVC*) of congestive heart failure. A pleural effusion (*PE*) is seen in the right lung base posteriorly.

Hepatitis

Infectious hepatitis (type A) is a viral infection of the liver that is transmitted by the fecal-oral route. Hepatitis B, or serum hepatitis, is also a viral infection of the liver that is transmitted by inoculation of infected blood or blood products. Type B has an incubation period of 6 weeks to 6 months; type A has a much shorter period of 30 to 40 days. Infectious mononucleosis is also a viral infection that may cause hepatitis in severe cases. Gloves and other precautions should be used for patients suspected to have hepatitis. Since the sonographer may not know the suspected diagnosis at the time of the examination, the best safeguard against hepatitis and other infectious diseases is to wear gloves during all sonographic examinations.

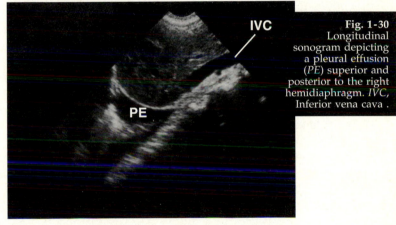

Fig. 1-30 Longitudinal sonogram depicting a pleural effusion (*PE*) superior and posterior to the right hemidiaphragm. *IVC*, Inferior vena cava.

The clinical symptoms vary depending on the severity and stage of disease. The symptoms range from fatigue, loss of appetite, and nausea to jaundice, fever, and chills. The liver function tests usually demonstrate markedly increased SGOT/SGPT levels, especially in the acute stages of the disease. If the patient is jaundiced, both the direct and indirect bilirubin levels are increased, indicating medical jaundice.

The sonographic appearance depends on the stage and severity of the disease. Since the sonographic examination is often requested before the results of the hepatitis tests are obtained, the clinician often needs to differentiate medical from obstructive jaundice. In mild or less acute cases, the parenchymal pattern may be normal. In more severe cases or in the acute stage, the liver parenchyma may be diffusely hypoechoic secondary to edema. This change will typically cause prominence of the portal vein walls, including the appearance of small peripheral tributaries not normally demonstrated (Fig. 1-31). It has been noted that in some acute cases the gallbladder cannot be identified, but on follow-up examination a normal gallbladder is demonstrated. Perhaps this is related to dysfunction of the biliary ductules or some part of the bile production process in the acute stages. The sonographer should examine the spleen for signs of splenomegaly.

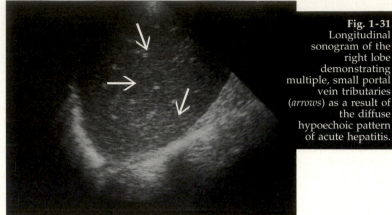

Fig. 1-31 Longitudinal sonogram of the right lobe demonstrating multiple, small portal vein tributaries (*arrows*) as a result of the diffuse hypoechoic pattern of acute hepatitis.

Fatty Infiltration

Fatty infiltration is the term used to describe the extra deposition of fat that occurs with a number of physiologic and pathologic entities. These processes can range from simple obesity to metabolic disorders, such as glycogen storage disease, to diabetes mellitis, cirrhosis, ulcerative collitis, and severe hepatitis.[10] Because of the diversity of causes, the sonographer should obtain as complete a clinical history as possible.

Excessive fat deposition can lead to hepatic dysfunction, indicated by increased SGOT/SGPT levels. Other clinical symptoms may point to the underlying cause of the fatty infiltration.

The sonographic pattern in mild cases is often normal. In more advanced cases the excessive fat deposition leads to a typical hyperechoic, fine parenchymal pattern with increased attenuation.[13] As the liver parenchyma becomes more hyperechoic, comparison with the normal, hyperechoic portal vein walls allows the sonographer to verify that the abnormality relates to a diffuse parenchymal disease. As the liver pattern becomes more hyperechoic, the portal vein walls appear less prominent. This sonographic pattern is called portal vein wall masking (Fig. 1-32). Generally, the more severe the fatty infiltration, the harder it is to distinguish the portal vein walls from the liver parenchyma. The proper adjustment of the acoustic power and gain controls is very important, since the sonographer must know when the increased attenuation causes an increase in the time gain compensation (TGC) rate and acoustic power level. The sonographer may need to scan other organs and areas, depending on the underlying cause of the fatty infiltration. In the case of alcohol abuse, the spleen should be checked for splenomegaly, the portal vein for signs of portal hypertension, and the peritoneal spaces for indications of ascites. In some patients the fatty deposits may appear as discrete masses, which may be difficult to differentiate from malignant entities. In these cases CT plays a role in establishing the diagnosis.

Portal Hypertension

Portal hypertension, an increase in the venous pressure of the portal system, occurs most frequently with cirrhosis of the liver. Because of the progressive destruction of the hepatic cells, the portal blood can no longer flow through the cells at the normal rate, causing a progressive dilatation of the portal system. Systemic diseases, such as congestive heart failure, may also cause the development of portal hypertension. As this disease progresses, collateral flow may develop as the portal system tries to relieve the pressure. Sites for the development of collaterals include renal, splenic, gastroesophageal, and intestinal, as well as patent umbilical vein.

Since portal hypertension is typically associated with cirrhosis, the clinical symptoms include a history of alcohol abuse, hepatic dysfunction, and hepatosplenomegaly. A later symptom is ascites.

The sonographic pattern of portal hypertension is an enlarged main portal vein with a diameter exceeding 1.3 cm[6] (Fig. 1-33 A). The sonographer should check to ensure that the flow is hepatopetal flow (flow toward the liver) and varies with respiration. There is decreased portal vein flow during inspiration and increased flow during expiration. Hepatofugal flow (flow away from the liver) is a definitive diagnostic sign of portal hypertension. The sonographer should also scan the splenic and superior mesenteric veins, checking for enlargement, as well as checking normal or abnormal flow patterns. If the findings are suggestive of portal hypertension, the sonographer should check for collaterals (Fig. 1-33 B). The protocol should include the gastroe-

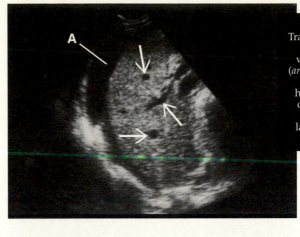

Fig. 1-32
Transverse sonogram illustrating "portal vein wall masking" (*arrows*) as a result of the diffuse hyperechoic pattern of cirrhosis. Ascites (*A*) is seen at the lateral aspect of the liver.

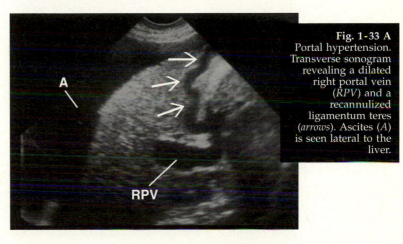

Fig. 1-33 A
Portal hypertension. Transverse sonogram revealing a dilated right portal vein (*RPV*) and a recannulized ligamentum teres (*arrows*). Ascites (*A*) is seen lateral to the liver.

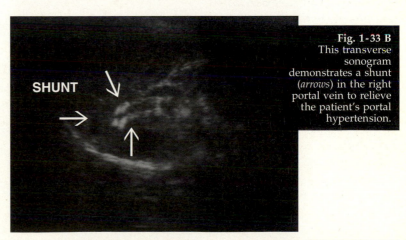

Fig. 1-33 B
This transverse sonogram demonstrates a shunt (*arrows*) in the right portal vein to relieve the patient's portal hypertension.

sophageal area located anterior to the proximal abdominal aorta, the splenic hilum, renal hilum, and general abdomen for signs of intestinal collaterals. Although only a small percentage of patients develop a patent umbilical vein, the course of the falciform ligament should be followed for evidence of a recannulated lumen, and Doppler should be used to detect the presence and direction of flow.

Cirrhosis

Cirrhosis is a progressive disease of the liver characterized by diffuse damage to the hepatic parenchymal cells resulting in nodular regeneration, fibrosis, and disturbance of the normal hepatic architecture. The main cause of cirrhosis is alcohol abuse, although other toxic substances and chronic biliary obstruction can also cause this disease. In more advanced cases, the cellular damage results in medical jaundice, ascites, and portal hypertension, all of which are poor prognostic signs.

The clinical signs of cirrhosis range from jaundice, spider angiomas of the face, and palmar erythema to ascites, gastrointestinal bleeding, and esophageal varices. Laboratory tests demonstrate increased levels of SGOT/SGPT and LDH. If the patient is jaundiced, both the direct and indirect bilirubin levels are elevated, indicating medical jaundice.

The sonographic pattern varies with the stage of the disease. Mild cases may show a normal parenchymal pattern. As the disease progresses, the liver pattern may become more hyperechoic with increased attenuation and regenerative nodules may appear. In advanced stages a small, hyperechoic liver surrounded by ascitic fluid may be seen, usually accompanied by splenomegaly (Fig. 1-34). An incidental finding of a thick-walled gallbladder may be noted and is attributable to the ascitic fluid and not necessarily a result of a pathologic process of the biliary system. The sonographer should also check for signs of portal hypertension and any associated collaterals.

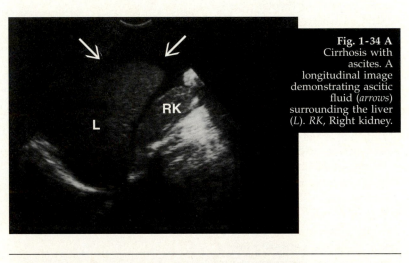

Fig. 1-34 A Cirrhosis with ascites. A longitudinal image demonstrating ascitic fluid (*arrows*) surrounding the liver (*L*). *RK*, Right kidney.

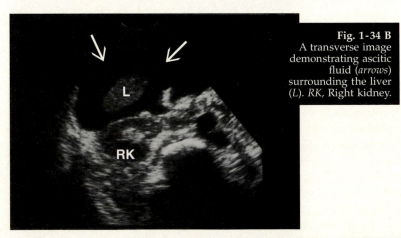

Fig. 1-34 B A transverse image demonstrating ascitic fluid (*arrows*) surrounding the liver (*L*). *RK*, Right kidney.

Hemangioma

The hemangioma is the most common benign hepatic neoplasm. This is usually an arteriovenous malformation that results in the formation of blood-filled spaces, apparently due to dilatation and thickening of capillary walls. These entities are more common in women and in patients with advancing age.

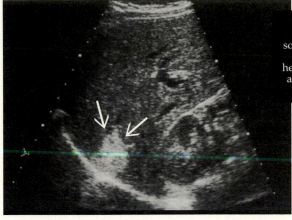

Hemangiomas are generally asymptomatic, and hence the sonographic findings are incidental. Occasionally they may present as palpable masses, cause pain, or result in an elevation of SGOT/SGPT and LDH levels on the clinical laboratory liver function tests.

The typical pattern of a hemangioma is a hyperechoic, discrete mass measuring less than 3 cm (Fig. 1-35). They may present as multiple masses. Several studies have demonstrated an increased blood flow when posterior enhancement is present.[11] As the size of the mass increases, the sonographic appearance becomes variable, including hypoechoic and complex patterns. For these cases, a CT examination will often reveal the characteristic appearance of the hemangioma after contrast injection. This pattern consists of the initial opacification of the outer portion of the hematoma followed by the central portion of the mass absorbing the contrast media.

Liver Cell Adenoma

The adenoma is a rare benign lesion of the liver. The incidence is higher in females, and several studies have demonstrated a link with the use of oral contraceptives.[13] Typically, patients have a single mass with the formation of a capsule. The adenoma has an increased risk of rupture with bleeding into the perioneal cavity.

The typical clinical symptoms include a palpable mass and right upper quadrant pain, usually related to bleeding. Occasionally, adenomas may cause abnormal liver function tests, particularly if they become large or occur in multiples. The sonographer should check for the use of oral contraceptives in all female patients where the adenoma is suspected.

The sonographic pattern depends on the absence or presence of bleeding. The sonographic pattern ranges from hyperechoic to hypoechoic to complex.

Focal Nodular Hyperplasia

Focal nodular hyperplasia is another benign hepatic disease that is also more common in female patients and in patients who have used oral contraceptives. They are usually asymptomatic, and hence the sonographic findings are incidental. Liver function tests are usually in the normal range. The typical sonographic pattern includes a discrete, lobulated hyperechoic mass located adjacent to the liver capsule. Other patterns may be hypoechoic and isoechoic to the normal liver parenchyma. An additional pattern is a hyperechoic, star-shaped area in the central portion of the tumor.[9]

TECHNICAL PITFALLS

There are several pitfalls related to hepatic sonography. The sonographer must remember that the identification of an abnormality is based on its deviance from the normal sonographic pattern. One must guard against overcompensating or undercompensating by manipulating the gain controls from the normal TGC curve. This may result in the identification of pseudomasses. Careful inspection of the image will often demonstrate that the "mass" involves the entire image area at a constant depth corresponding to the maladjusted TGC controls. Using excessive overall gain or acoustic power can alter the sonographic characteristics of masses or cause them to be missed entirely.

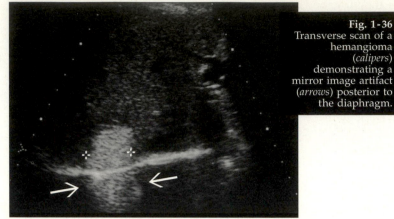

Fig. 1-36 Transverse scan of a hemangioma (*calipers*) demonstrating a mirror image artifact (*arrows*) posterior to the diaphragm.

Transducer selection is also important. The patient should be positioned so that the area of interest is placed within the focal zone of the transducer with adequate penetration at optimum resolution. In large or obese patients intercostal scanning may improve the appearance of the parenchymal pattern.

The sonographer must check all suspected abnormal areas in at least two scanning planes to verify that it is not an artifact and to determine the organ of origin. There is another pitfall when imaging pathologic conditions adjacent to the diaphragm. Because the diaphragm is a specular reflector and therefore angle-dependent, it can act like a mirror during scanning and create a double image of a hepatic mass superior to the diaphragm (Fig. 1-36). This could result in the sonographer's judging the mass to be twice its true size or falsely indicating that the mass extends above the diaphragm. This artifact disappears if the scanning angle is changed.

SUMMARY

The diagnosis of many hepatic pathologic processes cannot be made on the sonographic pattern alone. The clinical history, laboratory test results, and the results of other diagnostic imaging procedures allows a more definitive diagnosis. The sonographer should ensure that this information is available to the interpreting physician. Also, this information assists the sonographer in determining what abnormal sonographic patterns to expect during the performance of the examination. As a review, Table 1-1 summarizes the clinical laboratory test data associated with specific liver pathology.

REFERENCES

1. American College of Radiology: *Sonographic examination guidelines,* Washington, 1992, The College.
2. American Institute of Ultrasound in Medicine: *Sonographic examination guidelines,* Bethesda, MD, 1991, The Institute.
3. Cottone M, Marcenu MP, et al: Ultrasound in the diagnosis of hepatocellular carcinoma associated with cirrhosis, *Radiology* 147:517, 1983.

TABLE 1-1 CLINICAL LABORATORY TEST VALUES – LIVER							
	SGOT	SGPT	ALP	DIR BR	IND BR	AFP	Other Tests
METASTASES*	Increase	Increase	Mild Increase	Increase[†]	Increase		Increased PTT
CIRRHOSIS*	Increase	Increase	Mild Increase	Increase[†]	Increase		Increased LDH and PTT
ACUTE HEPATITIS*	High Increase	High Increase	Increase	Increase[†]	Increase		Increased LDH
HEPATOMA	Increase	Increase	Mild Increase	Increase[†]	Increase	Increase	
ABSCESS	Normal	Normal	Normal	Normal	Normal		Increased WBC
HEMANGIOMA	Normal	Normal	Normal	Normal	Normal		
HEMATOMA	Normal	Normal	Normal	Normal	Normal		Decreased RBC and HCT
ADENOMA	Normal	Normal	Normal	Normal	Normal		

*The size of the abnormal elevation depends on the severity of cellular dysfunction.

[†]In medical jaundice, both the direct and indirect bilirubin levels increase, typically with a higher level for the direct bilirubin.

SGOT, Serum glutamic oxaloacetic transaminase; SGPT, serum glutamic pyruvic transaminase; ALP, alkaline phosphatase; DIR DR, direct bilirubin; IND BR, indirect bilirubin; AFP, alpha feto-protein; PTT, prothrombin time; LDH, lactic acid dehydragenase; HCT, hematocrit; WBC, white blood cells; RBC, red blood cells.

4. Esfahani F, Rooholamini SA, Vessal K: Ultrasonography of hepatic hydatid cysts: new diagnostic signs, J Ultrasound Med 7:443, 1988.
5. Grant EG, Perrella RR, et al: Budd-Chiari Syndrome: the results of duplex and color Doppler imaging, AJR 152:377, 1989.
6. Kane RA, Katz SG: The spectrum of sonographic findings in portal hypertension: a subject review and new observations, Radiology 142:453, 1982.
7. Merrill, V: Atlas of roentgenographic positions, ed 4, St Louis, 1967, Mosby Year-Book, pp 542–543.
8. Roemer CE, Ferrucci JT, et al: Hepatic cysts: diagnosis and therapy by sonographic needle aspiration, AJR 136:1065, 1981.
9. Scatarige JC, Fishman EK, Sanders, RC: The sonographic "scar sign" in focal nodular hyperplasia of the liver, J Ultrasound Med 1:275, 1982.
10. Scatarige JC, Scott WW, et al: Fatty infiltration of the liver: ultrasonographic and computed tomographic correlation, J Ultrasound Med 3:9, 1984.
11. Taboury J, Porcel A, et al: Cavernous hemangioma of the liver studied by ultrasound: enhancement posterior to a hyperechoic mass as a sign of hypervascularity, Radiology 149:781, 1983.
12. Tanaka, S., Kitamurat, T, et al: Hepatocellular CA: sonographic and histologic correlation, AJR 140:701, 1983.
13. Tanaka S, Kitamura T, et al: Color Doppler flow imaging of liver tumors, AJR 154:509, 1990.
14. Taylor KJW, Gorelick FS, et al: Ultrasonography of alcoholic liver disease with histological correlation, Radiology 141:157, 1981.
15. Tessler FT, Gehring BJ, et al: Diagnosis of portal vein thrombosis: value of color Doppler imaging, AJR 157:293, 1991.
16. Tierney LM, McPhee St, et al (editors): Current medical diagnosis and treatment, Norwalk, Conn, 1993, Appleton and Lange, p 522 (liver abscess pathways).
17. Viscomi GN, Gonzalez, R et al: Histopathologic correlation of ultrasound appearances of liver metastases, J. Clin Gastroenterol 3:395, 1981.

2

biliary system

INSTRUCTIONAL OBJECTIVES

At the completion of this chapter, the reader will be able to:

1. Describe the clinical problems that are typical reasons for biliary system sonography.
2. Identify on transverse and longitudinal illustrations and sonograms the major anatomic structures of the biliary system, including the divisions of the gallbladder, the intrahepatic biliary system, and the extrahepatic biliary system; and discuss the relationship of the biliary system to surrounding anatomic structures.
3. Describe the basic scanning protocol for sonography of the biliary system as defined by national professional organizations.
4. Describe the clinical laboratory tests used for evaluating the function of the biliary system, including the white blood cell count, bilirubin, and alkaline phosphatase, as well as the specific disease processes that they evaluate.
5. Describe the clinical symptoms and pathologic basis for the disease processes of the biliary system, including medical versus obstructive jaundice, cholelithiasis, acute and chronic cholecystitis, benign diseases of the gallbladder wall, carcinoma of the gallbladder, cholangiocarcinoma, choledocholithiasis, cholangitis, and biliary cirrhosis.
6. Identify on sectional sonograms the above-mentioned disease processes of the biliary system, based on the sonographic appearance, the clinical history, and the results of other diagnostic procedures.
7. List several technical pitfalls associated with sonography of the biliary system.

THE CLINICAL PROBLEM

Diseases of the biliary system affect many Americans each year. Sonography has established a reputation for diagnostic accuracy in determining many of the disease processes of the biliary system. The primary clinical signs that lead the physician to suspect biliary dysfunction include right upper quadrant pain, nausea, and vomiting. An additional important sign is jaundice, although further testing is necessary to determine the specific cause and type of jaundice. Occasionally patients have symptoms more commonly associated with a heart attack, but the biliary system becomes suspect when heart enzyme levels and other diagnostic tests rule out this preliminary clinical diagnosis. The presence of gallstones and other pathologic conditions are also incidental findings during a sonographic examination of the upper abdomen for other clinical reasons. To obtain high diagnostic accuracy, the sonographer must know the anatomy, physiology, pertinent clinical laboratory tests, related diagnostic tests and scanning techniques, and technical pitfalls, as well as recognize the various abnormal sonographic patterns.

NORMAL ANATOMY

The biliary system originates in the liver as a series of small ducts coursing between the liver cells. These ramify, forming larger ducts that merge to form the left and right hepatic ducts, which head toward the porta hepatis. Throughout the liver parenchyma, the bile ducts and hepatic arterial tributaries course parallel to the branches of the portal vein. The **left and right hepatic ducts** merge to form the **common hepatic duct** at the level of the porta hepatis. Fig. 2-1 illustrates all the anatomic structures of the biliary system.

The **gallbladder** is situated in its shallow fossa on the posterior aspect of the right lobe of the liver. The exact location of the gallbladder varies, depending on body habitus. It may be partially or totally embedded in the liver parenchyma (intrahepatic location) or totally suspended in the abdomen (intraperitoneal location). The primary landmark for localization and identification of the gallbladder is the **main lobar** or **intralobar fissure**, which courses from the right portal vein to the neck of the gallbladder (Fig. 2-2). The gallbladder consists of three anatomic areas: fundus, body, and neck (Fig. 2-3). Normally the fundus is the most inferior portion, bordered anteriorly by the abdominal wall and posteriorly by the transverse colon. The body, which is also bordered posteriorly by bowel, forms the main component of this reservoir and continues superiorly into the narrow neck, which usually lies to the right of the porta hepatis and inferior to the right portal vein. In the neck the sonographer may occasionally see a small posterior pouch. This is called **Hartmann's pouch** and is

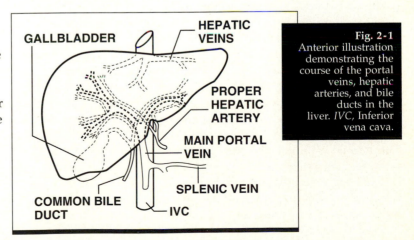

GALLBLADDER

HEPATIC VEINS

PROPER HEPATIC ARTERY

MAIN PORTAL VEIN

SPLENIC VEIN

COMMON BILE DUCT

IVC

Fig. 2-1 Anterior illustration demonstrating the course of the portal veins, hepatic arteries, and bile ducts in the liver. *IVC,* Inferior vena cava.

a prime site for gallstones, since it is often the most dependent portion of the gallbladder. The neck merges superiorly with the **cystic duct,** whose length varies from 2 to 6 cm. The lumen of the cystic duct contains a series of mucous folds, called the **spiral valves of Heister.** These valves prevent the duct from collapsing or overdistending when sudden gravitational pressure changes are caused by the patient's moving from the supine to an upright position.

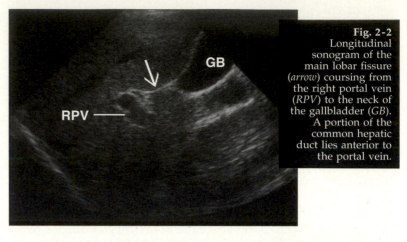

Fig. 2-2 Longitudinal sonogram of the main lobar fissure (*arrow*) coursing from the right portal vein (*RPV*) to the neck of the gallbladder (*GB*). A portion of the common hepatic duct lies anterior to the portal vein.

The cystic duct proceeds from the neck of the gallbladder and travels at a posteroinferior angle toward the midline. At a variable distance inferior to the porta hepatis, it merges with the common hepatic duct to form the **common bile duct.** When the sonographer measures the duct anterior to the right portal vein on a longitudinal oblique scan, usually the measurement is of the common hepatic duct, since this duct is in the porta hepatis. The common bile duct courses inferiorly along the right border of the lesser omentum, anterior to the main portal vein and to the

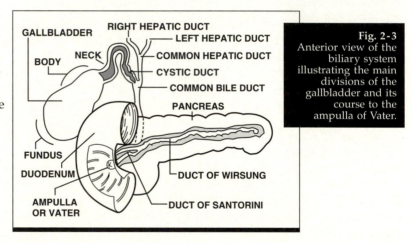

Fig. 2-3 Anterior view of the biliary system illustrating the main divisions of the gallbladder and its course to the ampulla of Vater.

right of the proper hepatic or common hepatic artery (Fig. 2-3). The **lesser omentum** is a peritoneal fold that extends from the lesser curvature of the stomach toward the right to the porta hepatis and inferiorly to the superior portion of the duodenum. The transverse depiction of the main portal vein, common bile duct, and common hepatic artery is called the portal triad, or "mickey mouse" sign (Fig. 2-4). The common bile duct continues its caudal path posterior to the first portion of the duodenum. It then runs in a groove posterior to the lateral border of the head of the pancreas and anterior to the inferior vena cava. In some patients the duct is surrounded by pancreatic tissue. The normal common bile duct narrows as it courses inferiorly, and the pancreatic portion is a prime location for ductal stones. The duct enters the descending portion of the duodenum in its posteromedial aspect. Here it is joined by the pancreatic duct, or the duct of Wirsung, and both empty into the duodenum through the **ampulla of Vater,** which is a protrusion of the mucosal lining into the duodenal lumen caused by the sphinctor of Oddi. The duct of Santorini is an accessory duct that may merge with the duct of Wirsung or may empty into the duodenum through a separate ampulla.

CLINICAL LABORATORY TESTS

Bilirubin

As mentioned in Chapter 1, obstructive jaundice usually causes an elevation only of the direct bilirubin. Longstanding obstructive jaundice can cause biliary cirrhosis, a form of medical jaundice. This parenchymal disease causes an elevation of both the direct and indirect bilirubin levels. The superimposition of both obstructive and medical jaundice can confuse the interpretation of the laboratory tests. Obstructive jaundice caused by a neoplasm, such as carcinoma of the head of the pancreas, typically produces a moderate to marked increase in the direct bilirubin. Usually, common bile duct stones produce a mild to moderate direct bilirubin increase.

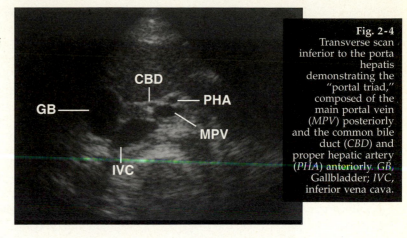

Fig. 2-4 Transverse scan inferior to the porta hepatis demonstrating the "portal triad," composed of the main portal vein (*MPV*) posteriorly and the common bile duct (*CBD*) and proper hepatic artery (*PHA*) anteriorly. *GB*, Gallbladder; *IVC*, inferior vena cava.

Alkaline Phosphatase

Alkaline phosphatase (ALP) is an enzyme produced in the liver and secreted through the bile ducts. With obstructive jaundice, the ALP levels are moderately to markedly increased. The severity relates to the completeness and duration of the obstruction. Gallstones without obstruction usually produce a mild elevation of ALP.

Serum Glutamic Oxaloacetic Transaminase and Serum Glutamic Pyruvic Transaminase

The serum glutamic oxaloacetic transaminase (SGOT) and, more specifically, the serum glutamic pyruvic transaminase (SGPT) values can undergo a mild to moderate increase in cases of obstructive jaundice. The obstruction can cause biliary regurgitation, which, in turn, can cause hepatocellular damage if present for an extended period of time.

RELATED IMAGING PROCEDURES

Plain-Film Radiograph

The plain-film radiograph is obtained with the patient supine and without the use of contrast media. Calcified gallstones, a calcified gallbladder wall, or air in the biliary system can be identified with this examination. Occasionally, mass effects distorting the position of surrounding abdominal organs can be diagnosed with this technique.

Oral Cholecystogram

The oral cholecystogram (OCG) involves the radiographic demonstration of the gallbladder after the oral ingestion of iodinated contrast material. This procedure has been widely replaced with sonography. The OCG has a high rate of accuracy for the detection of pathologic conditions when the contrast material concentrates in the gallbladder. Accuracy declines when the gallbladder poorly opacifies or is not visualized. Pathologic conditions of the gallbladder, such as stones and acute cholecystitis, may cause this problem. Other causes of poor visualization include vomiting after the ingestion of the pills, sensitivity to iodine, malabsorption syndromes, superimposition of bowel gas, and even previous cholecystectomy. Currently a patient with a suboptimal OCG examination is referred for a sonographic evaluation.

Intravenous Cholangiography

Intravenous cholangiography is a radiographic procedure that involves the slow intravenous administration of an iodinated contrast medium. This technique demonstrates the gallbladder and extrahepatic biliary system 1 to 24 hours after injection. Today, intravenous cholangiography is rarely performed because of the availability of other diagnostic procedures, the length of the examination, and the increased risk of contrast media reactions. Also, the visualization rate is low in patients with a moderate elevation of bilirubin.

Percutaneous Transhepatic Cholangiography

Percutaneous transhepatic cholangiography (PTC) is an invasive procedure that opacifies the biliary system with an iodinated contrast media. It is performed by passing a thin, small-gauge needle through the liver and inserting it into the biliary tree. This method accurately determines the site and often the cause of the obstruction. The procedure is very effective for common bile duct abnormalities. The test has a slightly higher morbidity and mortality rate than noninvasive tests, but its accuracy is such that many surgeons order it before performing surgery.

Nuclear Medicine Hepatobiliary Imaging

Within the last decade a new group of radiopharmaceuticals has been used to study the function of the biliary system. These agents are usually derived from iminodiacetic acid (IDA) and are tagged to ^{99m}Tc. This substance is initially processed by the liver cells and excreted through the bile ducts. With normal function, the gallbladder, the major bile ducts, and the activity in the duodenum are visualized within an hour after injection. In cases of acute cholecystitis the gallbladder does not visualize, whereas the ducts and duodenum appear to contain a normal amount of radioactivity. In cases of obstructive jaundice there is delayed or absent excretion into the duodenum, and the general level of obstruction can sometimes be identified. This test is more sensitive for evaluating biliary function than it is for demonstrating anatomic detail.

Computed Tomography

Computed tomography (CT) also provides a valuable tool for the evaluation of the biliary system. CT can demonstrate dilated bile ducts, intrahepatic and extraheptaic masses, and a contracted or distended gallbladder. Small gallstones, particularly common duct stones, are not usually identified. When the obstructive jaundice is the result of carcinoma of the head of the pancreas, CT provides an examination of the retroperitoneal lymph nodes and other sites of distant metastases.

SCANNING PROTOCOLS AND TECHNIQUES

The routine scanning protocol for the biliary system includes transverse and longitudinal views through the neck, body, and fundus of the gallbladder. Additional routine views include a longitudinal section through the common hepatic duct. A sample scanning protocol is presented in the box on this page.

Figs. 2-5 through 2-10 illustrate the routine examination. Images should be obtained in at least two different patient positions. Generally the patient is initially scanned in the supine position and then rolled onto the left side. If gallbladder visualization is suboptimal on supine scans, the patient may be rolled approximately 45 degrees onto the left side. The prone or upright position may work best for some patients. These various patient positions are performed for several reasons. A high-quality examination should display the gallbladder free of any bowel gas superimposition, and it should provide optimum visualization of the gallbladder neck, since this is a prime area for gallstone collection. In addition, small gallstones may layer along the posterior wall in a supine position but collect in the most dependent portion in other patient positions, allowing the identification of stones with good posterior acoustic shadowing. Prone and upright views work well for patients with a hypersthenic body build in which the gallbladder is in a vertical posi-

BASIC SCANNING PROTOCOL

Longitudinal
- Common hepatic duct with measurement
- Common bile duct to the level of the head of the pancreas (when possible)
- Medial aspect of the gallbladder
- Midline axis of the gallbladder demonstrating main lobar fissure, neck, body, and fundus
- Lateral aspect of the gallbladder
- Representative sections through the liver for evidence of intrahepatic ductal dilatation

Transverse
- Gallbladder neck, body, and fundus (Measure the gallbladder wall if it appears to exceed 3 mm.)
- Representative sections through the liver for evidence of intrahepatic ductal dilatation
- Common bile duct at the level of the head of the pancreas

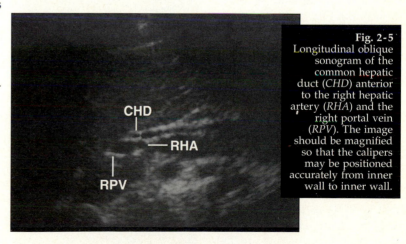

Fig. 2-5 Longitudinal oblique sonogram of the common hepatic duct (*CHD*) anterior to the right hepatic artery (*RHA*) and the right portal vein (*RPV*). The image should be magnified so that the calipers may be positioned accurately from inner wall to inner wall.

tion and located high under the ribs, or if there is a large amount of bowel gas inferior to the gallbladder.

Normal intrahepatic biliary ducts are not visualized sonographically. The left and right hepatic ducts may be demonstrated as 1 to 2 mm tubular structures coursing parallel to the left and right portal veins, respectively. The common hepatic duct courses anterior to the right portal vein and the right hepatic artery. Usually the length of the common hepatic duct is obtained in an oblique longitudinal plane (Fig. 2-11). A routine examination of the biliary system includes a measurement of the common hepatic duct in the area of the porta hepatis. The duct at this level may be visualized in most patients, wheres the more distal common bile duct may be obscured by bowel gas. The sonographer should try to demonstrate as much of the course of the common bile duct as possible. The duct should be measured from inner wall to inner wall, in a plane perpendicular to its course. The walls should lie at different depths in the sound field to ensure that the better axial resolution characteristics are used. The normal range of the common hepatic duct is 4 to 5 mm, although roughly 1 mm per decade of life has been added to the normal range. For example, the upper limits of normal for a 70-year-old patient may be 7 mm.[3] However, all duct measurements must be interpreted along with any other abnormal or normal sonographic

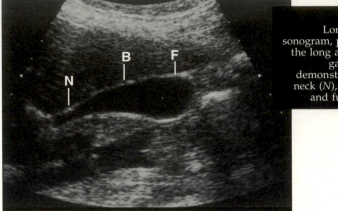

Fig. 2-6 Longitudinal sonogram, parallel to the long axis of the gallbladder, demonstrating the neck (*N*), body (*B*), and fundus (*F*).

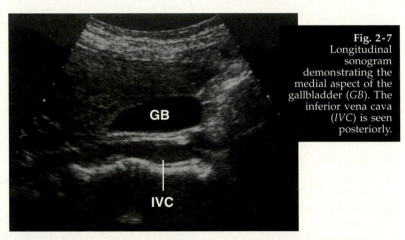

Fig. 2-7 Longitudinal sonogram demonstrating the medial aspect of the gallbladder (*GB*). The inferior vena cava (*IVC*) is seen posteriorly.

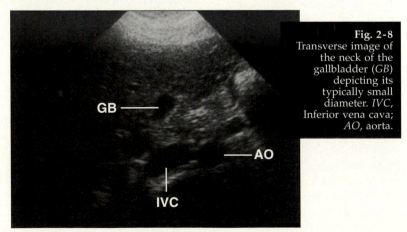

Fig. 2-8 Transverse image of the neck of the gallbladder (*GB*) depicting its typically small diameter. *IVC*, Inferior vena cava; *AO*, aorta.

patterns. A mildly enlarged duct, with no sonographic evidence indicating a pathologic condition, is termed equivocal. The patient may ingest a fatty meal to ascertain normal function of the biliary system. If normal, the gallbladder and duct should reduce in size. If the gallbladder does not contract and if the duct stays the same size or enlarges, further testing for biliary system function may be necessary.[3]

The course of the common bile duct varies among patients. At times it runs in a straight path from the porta hepatis to the duodenum. It may angle sharply at its distal portion, or it may be C-shaped, swinging laterally from the porta hepatis and turning medially at the level of the pancreas. Typically the sonographer will find it easier to identify the common bile duct and its course in the transverse scanning plane, since the surrounding vascular and other anatomic landmarks are more discernable. Once localized on transverse scans, longitudinal scans of the correct obliquity are more readily attained. Placing the patient in the left posterior oblique or left lateral position can help displace the surrounding bowel gas, and either position can use the gallbladder as an acoustic window to demonstrate the entire course of the duct (Fig. 2-12). The upper limits of normal for the common bile duct should not exceed 6 to 7 mm and will normally taper to 1 to 2 mm posterior to the pancreas.

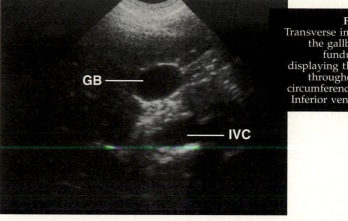

Fig. 2-9 Transverse image of the gallbladder fundus (*GB*) displaying the wall throughout the circumference. *IVC*, Inferior vena cava.

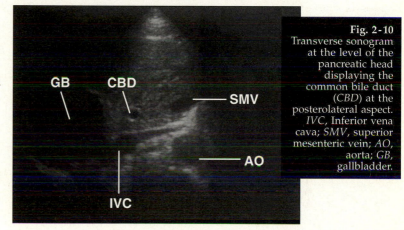

Fig. 2-10 Transverse sonogram at the level of the pancreatic head displaying the common bile duct (*CBD*) at the posterolateral aspect. *IVC*, Inferior vena cava; *SMV*, superior mesenteric vein; *AO*, aorta; *GB*, gallbladder.

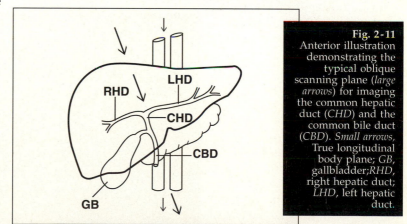

Fig. 2-11 Anterior illustration demonstrating the typical oblique scanning plane (*large arrows*) for imaging the common hepatic duct (*CHD*) and the common bile duct (*CBD*). *Small arrows*, True longitudinal body plane; *GB*, gallbladder; *RHD*, right hepatic duct; *LHD*, left hepatic duct.

NORMAL SONOGRAPHIC PATTERNS

To guarantee a fully distended gallbladder for proper evaluation, the patient should fast for at least 4 hours or, preferably, for 8 hours. Normal bile is anechoic and demonstrates acoustic enhancement. The gallbladder wall visualizes as a thin, smooth hyperechoic rim less than 3 mm thick. A true midline longitudinal scan should demonstrate the right portal vein, the main lobar fissure, and the neck, body, and fundus of the gallbladder. The cystic duct may also appear as a small tubular structure at the posterosuperior aspect of the neck. The distal portion of the cystic duct, close to its union with the common hepatic duct, is more difficult to image. Usually an oblique transverse plane will demonstrate this portion of the cystic duct (Fig. 2-13). The common hepatic duct appears as a small tubular structure anterior to the right portal vein and right hepatic artery. However, in approximately 30% of the population, the right hepatic artery is anterior to the common hepatic duct[19] (Fig. 2-14). The use of color Doppler to ascertain an arterial signal and to trace the course back to the proper hepatic artery will prevent misidentification. Color flow does not discriminate motion in the biliary system. Many department protocols document the common bile duct on a transverse scan through the head of the pancreas. At this level the duct is located at the posterolateral aspect of the head

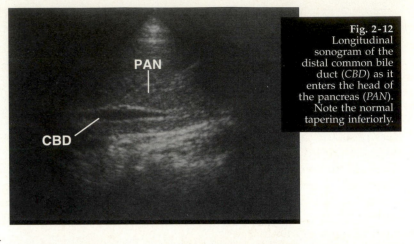

Fig. 2-12
Longitudinal sonogram of the distal common bile duct (*CBD*) as it enters the head of the pancreas (*PAN*). Note the normal tapering inferiorly.

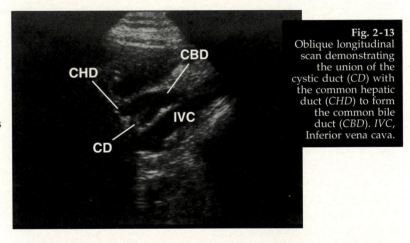

Fig. 2-13
Oblique longitudinal scan demonstrating the union of the cystic duct (*CD*) with the common hepatic duct (*CHD*) to form the common bile duct (*CBD*). *IVC*, Inferior vena cava.

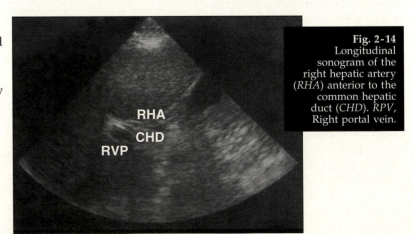

Fig. 2-14
Longitudinal sonogram of the right hepatic artery (*RHA*) anterior to the common hepatic duct (*CHD*). *RPV*, Right portal vein.

of the pancreas, anterior to the inferior vena cava.

CONGENITAL ANOMALIES

There are various congenital anomalies associated with the gallbladder. Agenesis and especially **duplication** of the gallbladder are rare (Fig. 2-15). Varying shapes of the gallbladder are a more common anomaly. A **bilobed gallbladder** contains an internal septum that forms two chambers (Fig. 2-16). A multiseptated gallbladder and diverticula in the lumen are rare. The most common anomaly is the **phrygian cap,** which occurs when the fundus is doubled back over the body of the gallbladder (Fig. 2-17). Another anomaly is the **hourglass gallbladder,** which narrows in the midpoint of its body. Anomalies in position also occur. Peritoneal folds may suspend the gallbladder, so that it is unusually low; it may even be inferior to the right kidney and in the pelvis. Liver parenchyma may partially or totally embed the gallbladder. A **transverse-lie gallbladder** is quite common, especially in obese or tall patients who have a large body habitus. The longitudinal axis of the gallbladder is obtained in the transverse body plane. **Situs inversus** is a rare anomaly in which the position of the body organs is reversed, so that the gallbladder is found in the left upper quadrant.

All of the major bile ducts can vary as to the site of anastomoses and their general course. For example, the cystic duct may course several centimeters below

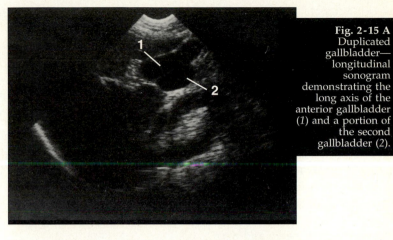

Fig. 2-15 A Duplicated gallbladder—longitudinal sonogram demonstrating the long axis of the anterior gallbladder (1) and a portion of the second gallbladder (2).

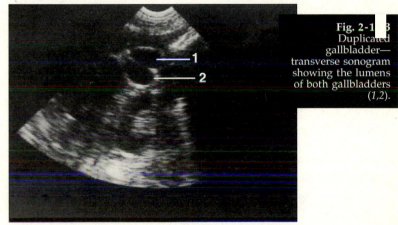

Fig. 2-15 B Duplicated gallbladder—transverse sonogram showing the lumens of both gallbladders (1,2).

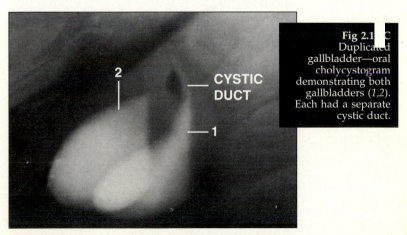

Fig 2-15 C Duplicated gallbladder—oral cholycystogram demonstrating both gallbladders (1,2). Each had a separate cystic duct.

CYSTIC DUCT

the porta hepatis before joining the common hepatic duct, or there may be accessory ducts present. The primary ductal anomaly is the **choledochal cyst.** These cysts are caused by a congenital weakness of the ductal wall with the resultant formation of a cystic structure. The cysts can occur anywhere in the biliary system, but occurrences are more frequently found in the common bile duct. This anomaly occurs four times as frequently in females as in males, and over 50% of the cases are diagnosed during the first 10 years of life.[15] The primary sonographic criteria include a cystic mass medial to the gallbladder and lateral to the pancreatic head with evidence of obstructive jaundice. The sonographer should try to demonstrate the proximal duct entering the mass. The physical symptoms are pain, jaundice, and a palpable epigastric mass. Surgery is usually indicated.

PATHOLOGIC PROCESSES OF THE BILIARY SYSTEM

Cholelithiasis

Cholelithiasis, or gallstones, affects thousands of Americans annually. Gallstones are more common in women and occur more frequently in Caucasians than in African-Americans. The frequency of cholelithiasis is increased in patients with regional enteritis and diabetes mellitus. The incidence of gallstones is slightly increased during pregnancy. Although sometimes asymptomatic, most patients with cholelithiasis experience right upper quadrant pain that

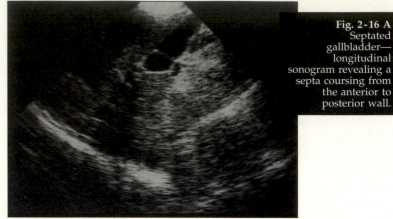

Fig. 2-16 A Septated gallbladder— longitudinal sonogram revealing a septa coursing from the anterior to posterior wall.

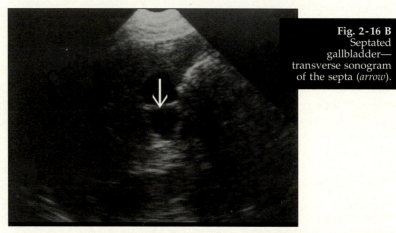

Fig. 2-16 B Septated gallbladder— transverse sonogram of the septa (*arrow*).

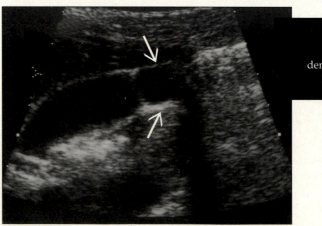

Fig. 2-17 Longitudinal sonogram demonstrating a phrygian cap (*arrows*).

sometimes radiates to the right shoulder or epigastric regions. Patients may experience nausea, vomiting, and an intolerance for fatty foods. Clinical laboratory tests show an elevated ALP and may show elevated SGOT/SGPT levels.

Usually gallstones contain bile pigment, cholesterol, and bile calcium salts. Typically the latter compound causes increased attenuation and the diagnostic acoustic shadow distal to the stone (Fig. 2-18). Although less common, stones with a high cholesterol content appear as rounded, hyperechoic intraluminal masses that do not cause acoustic shadowing[11] (Fig. 2-19). Most stones sink to the bottom of the dependent portion of the gallbladder. However, sometimes the viscocity of the bile is increased and/or the stones are small and light. In this case the stones appear to float in the lumen (Fig. 2-20). The use of iodinated oral contrast agents for the radiographic opacification of the gallbladder can increase bile viscocity and cause this phenomenon.[12] In all instances the sonographer must demonstrate three sonographic signs for gallstones. First, the sonographer must determine that there is a hyperechoic structure in the lumen of the gallbladder. Transverse scans are often best for proving that the "stone" is not a loop of bowel. Second, the sonographer must demonstrate acoustic shadowing distal to the stone. For small stones this often requires a higher frequency transducer with the focal zone

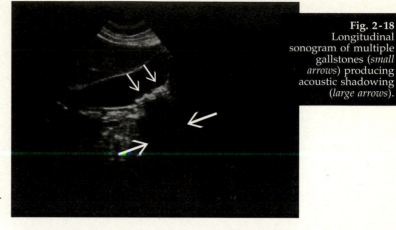

Fig. 2-18 Longitudinal sonogram of multiple gallstones (*small arrows*) producing acoustic shadowing (*large arrows*).

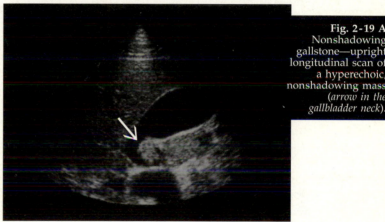

Fig. 2-19 A Nonshadowing gallstone—upright longitudinal scan of a hyperechoic, nonshadowing mass (*arrow in the gallbladder neck*).

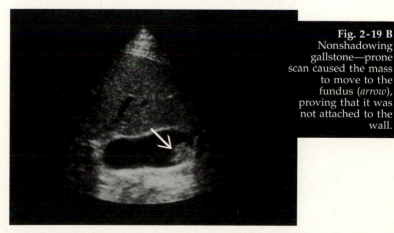

Fig. 2-19 B Nonshadowing gallstone—prone scan caused the mass to move to the fundus (*arrow*), proving that it was not attached to the wall.

placed at the depth of the stone (Fig. 2-21). As the frequency increases, small stones will cause increased attenuation and display a more prominent acoustic shadow. Third, the sonographer must determine if the stone will move. This is particularly important when the stone initially appears in the neck. If the stone cannot be moved from this position, the possibility of obstruction and/or acute cholecystitis must be considered. In the case of a hyperechoic, nonshadowing intraluminal mass, movement allows the diagnosis of a nonshadowing gallstone, whereas a lack of movement indicates a polyp or malignancy, depending on the size, shape, and consistency of the mass.

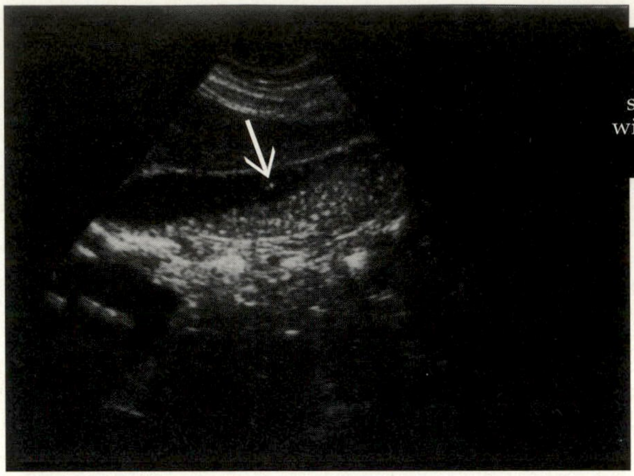

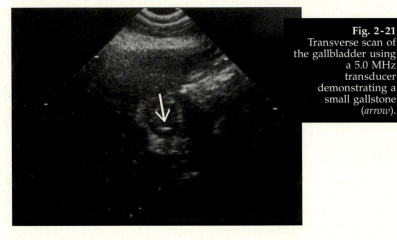

Fig. 2-20
Longitudinal sonogram of sludge with small "floating" gallstones (*arrow*).

Fig. 2-21
Transverse scan of the gallbladder using a 5.0 MHz transducer demonstrating a small gallstone (*arrow*).

Acute Cholecystitis

Acute cholecystitis, or inflammation of the gallbladder, is associated with gallstones in 90% of the cases. It is caused by the impaction of a gallstone in the region of the gallbladder neck or cystic duct, with inflammation occurring distal to the obstruction. If this obstruction is not alleviated, more serious inflammation, such as necrosis, ulceration, and edema, may result. This inflammatory process can produce an enlarged gallbladder, termed **hydrops.** Because the cystic duct or neck of the gallbladder is obstructed, no bile can leave or enter the gallbladder. However, the gallbladder wall normally produces a mucinous secretion. As a result of the obstruction, the secretion collects in the gallbladder and leads to the enlargement. As the hydrops and obstruction progress, pus may collect in the lumen. This condition is called an **empyema** of the gallbladder. Late and more rare complications include the development of gangrene, cholangitis, and perforation of the gallbladder.

Usually a large or fatty meal brings on an attack of biliary colic. The symptoms include steady, severe pain in the right upper quadrant (or epigastrium) that usually subsides over a period of 12 to 18 hours. Nausea and vomiting are seen in 75% of the cases, a palpable gallbladder is present in 15%, and jaundice occurs in 25%.[6] Fever and an elevated white blood cell count are often present. Other disease processes that can be confused with acute cholecystitis are acute pancreatitis, perforated peptic ulcer, liver abscess, and hepatitis.[6]

The clinical laboratory tests may show an elevated ALP and mildly elevated SGOT/SGPT values. In the presence of jaundice the direct bilirubin level is elevated. An elevated white blood cell count indicates the presence of infection and inflammation.

The typical sonographic appearance of acute cholecystitis is a thick, edematous gallbladder wall with a stone in the area of the neck or cystic duct (Fig. 2-22). The gallbladder wall is abnormally thick if it measures greater that 3 mm, but a wall thickness of 5 mm or larger is more specific for acute cholecystitis[18] (Fig. 2-23). There are other causes of gallbladder wall thickening, including benign, non-inflammatory diseases of the wall, a partially contracted gallbladder in a nonfasting patient, and the presence of cirrhosis or ascites (Fig. 2-24). An additional physical sign that the sonographer should always check for is **Murphy's sign.** This sign is present when the patient complains of tenderness or pain as the sonographer gently presses the transducer directly over the gallbladder. The most specific sign for acute cholecystitis is the presence of fluid in the gallbladder bed, or pericholecystic fluid[1] (Fig. 2-25). As is often the case, if the sonographer demonstrates more than one of the signs and criteria discussed, the diagnosis is more confident. When the sonographic examination is equivocal, the

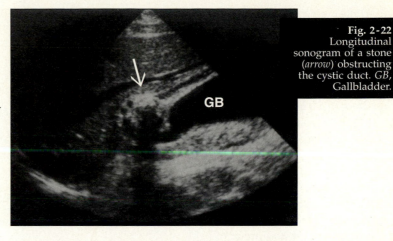

Fig. 2-22
Longitudinal sonogram of a stone (*arrow*) obstructing the cystic duct. *GB*, Gallbladder.

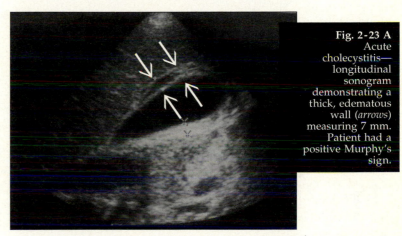

Fig. 2-23 A
Acute cholecystitis—longitudinal sonogram demonstrating a thick, edematous wall (*arrows*) measuring 7 mm. Patient had a positive Murphy's sign.

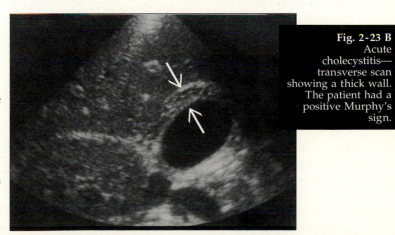

Fig. 2-23 B
Acute cholecystitis—transverse scan showing a thick wall. The patient had a positive Murphy's sign.

patient may undergo a nuclear hepatobiliary imaging procedure, which has a better sensitivity and specificity for diagnosing acute cholecystitis.[17]

Chronic Cholecystitis

Usually, chronic cholecystitis occurs in the presence of gallstones. Generally, acute attacks precede this condition, which is characterized by fibrosis of the wall. A stone that causes obstruction in the area of the cystic duct or gallbladder neck can occur with the same ramifications as in acute cholecystitis. The patient usually experiences moderate, intermittent pain in the right upper quadrant and epigastrium, which occasionally radiates to the right scapula. Usually the patient has a history of fatty or fried food intolerance and may have experienced intermittent nausea and vomiting. The ALP level may be elevated, and the SGOT/SGPT levels may be mildly elevated. The direct bilirubin level is elevated in the presence of jaundice.

In the absence of an acute episode, chronic cholecystitis is recognized sonographically as a contracted gallbladder lumen with a thick, hyperechoic wall containing stones (Fig. 2-26). In advanced cases the gallbladder loses its ability to function and thus is not visualized on the oral cholecystogram. In the case of a recent acute attack, the gallbladder wall may appear edematous and present other sonographic criteria of acute cholecystitis. The presence of a positive Murphy's sign is an important adjunct to

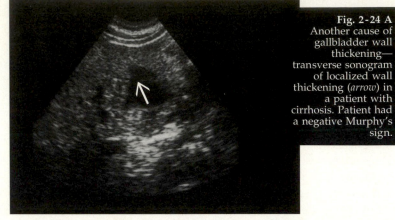

Fig. 2-24 A Another cause of gallbladder wall thickening—transverse sonogram of localized wall thickening (*arrow*) in a patient with cirrhosis. Patient had a negative Murphy's sign.

Fig. 2-24 B Another cause of gallbladder wall thickening—longitudinal sonogram of diffuse wall thickening (*calipers*) caused by acute liver failure. Patient had a negative Murphy's sign.

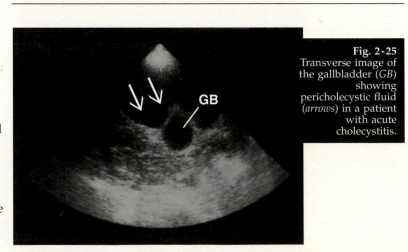

Fig. 2-25 Transverse image of the gallbladder (*GB*) showing pericholecystic fluid (*arrows*) in a patient with acute cholecystitis.

this diagnosis. If the gallbladder is severely contracted, the sonographer should demonstrate the main lobar fissure leading to the area of acoustic shadowing and use a high-frequency transducer to differentiate the gallbladder wall from the stone.

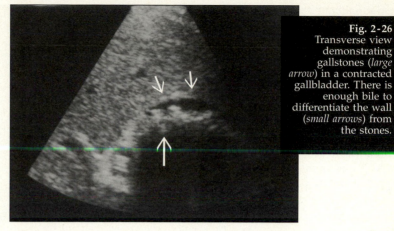

Fig. 2-26
Transverse view demonstrating gallstones (*large arrow*) in a contracted gallbladder. There is enough bile to differentiate the wall (*small arrows*) from the stones.

Biliary Sludge

Biliary sludge occurs when the viscocity of the bile is increased because of the precipitation of some of the solid components of bile. Recent literature has pointed out that biliary sludge is not always the precursor to gallstones (nor, in fact, are very small stones) and should be labeled viscous bile in the absence of any other sonographic signs indicating a pathologic process.[11] Biliary sludge can occur in normal fasting patients or in those who have been on a diet of total intravenous fluids for extended periods of time. Sludge can also occur in pathologic states that impair function, such as hydrops of the gallbladder or a Courvoisier gallbladder secondary to carcinoma distal to the cystic duct. The sonographer should obtain a careful clinical history, including the last time the patient has eaten solid foods. The sonographer should carefully scan for pathologic conditions that could cause sludge to form.

Sludge typically appears as a mildly echogenic homogeneous material layering in the most dependent portion of the gallbladder. Unlike stones, sludge will slowly slide to the most dependent portion of the gallbladder with a change in the patient's position and then demonstrate a fluid-to-fluid interface (Fig. 2-27). Total biliary sludge may make initial identification of the gallbladder difficult, since the entire lumen is filled with a parenchymal-like pattern (Fig. 2-28). The use of anatomic landmarks and a higher frequency transducer will allow the proper identification of this condition.

Benign Diseases of the Gallbladder Wall

Benign diseases of the gallbladder wall, called hyperplastic cholecytoses, refer to noninflammatory conditions that include adenomyomatosis, cholesterosis, neuromatosis, fibromatosis, and lipomatosis. **Adenomyomatosis** is characterized by excessive proliferation of the surface epithelium and a thickening of the muscle layer of the gallbladder wall. As the disease progresses, it causes the formation of diverticula, or pouches, that project outside the gallbladder lumen. **Cholesterosis,** or "strawberry gallbladder," is characterized by abnormal cholesterol deposits in the gallbladder wall and may be associated with gallstones. The lesions may be diffuse or localized. The localized form may have a single lesion or multiple polypoid lesions, which may be pedunculated and may interfere with function. The diffuse form does not always impair gallbladder function and may not appear on an oral cholecystogram. **Neuromatosis** and **fibromatosis** are both rare disease processes that cause the proliferation of nerve and fibrous tissue, respectively. **Lipomatosis** is an excessive buildup of fat layers in the gallbladder wall. All three of these conditions may or may not interfere with normal gallbladder function and may not demonstrate any abnormal patterns on an oral cholecystogram.

These benign diseases are often asymptomatic. When symptoms occur, they often mimic those of cholelithiasis—right upper quadrant pain, nausea, and vomiting—but are often found without the presence of gallstones. Adenomyomatosis is more common in women than in men, and its incidence increases after the age of 40. With these benign tumors, the risk of malignancy is low. If the pain is intractable, surgery may be performed to alleviate the symptoms. If the condition interferes with function, the level of ALP may be elevated, as in cholelithiasis.

The sonographic appearance of these conditions varies and may not be evident on sonography. Identifying the exact classification of benign diseases may be difficult. In general, the sonographer inspects the gall-

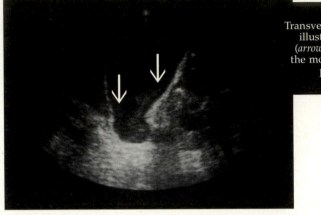

Fig. 2-27 Transverse sonogram illustrating sludge (*arrows*) layering in the most dependent portion of the gallbladder.

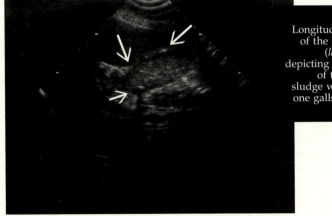

Fig. 2-28 Longitudinal image of the gallbladder (*large arrows*) depicting the pattern of total biliary sludge with at least one gallstone (*small arrow*).

bladder wall for irregular wall thickening, diverticula, and round or plaquelike solid projections in the lumen. Adenomyomatosis may present with flat, plaquelike lesions adherent to the wall, whereas cholesterosis tends to develop the more classic round, polypoid mass (Fig. 2-29). In some cases a comet tail artifact may be demonstrated in the layers of the wall (Fig. 2-30). This has been associated with the deposition of cholesterol crystals in the wall layers.[6] In either case the sonographer must prove that these masses are attached to the wall by changing the patient's position, noting that the mass moves with the wall and that it does not move to the most dependent portion of the gallbladder. Most polyps are hyperechoic, nonshadowing masses, but some may produce a small acoustic shadow. If a mass produces a shadow but does not move, the differential diagnosis should include the possiblility of an adherent gallstone. Besides a change in the patient's position, the sonographer may instruct the patient to cough. This action may dislodge a gallstone from the wall. The contractility of the gallbladder can be assessed by comparing the scans of the fasting patient with those obtained 30 minutes after the ingestion of a fatty meal.

The **porcelain gallbladder** refers to calcification of the gallbladder wall. The majority of patients are women, and gallstones are typically present. Researchers postulate a number of reasons for this condition. It may be the result of chronic inflammation of the gallbladder wall, which decreases the vascular supply. This vascular disruption leads, in turn, to progressive atrophy of the wall with the deposition of lime salts.[6] The calcification may involve a more localized portion of the wall or appear as a diffuse process. Since some types of porcelain gallbladder have an increased association with gallbladder cancer, surgery is usually indicated.

The typical sonographic pattern is marked acoustic shadowing that originates at the gallbladder wall interface, instead of stones in the lumen (Fig. 2-31). The sonographer should evaluate the gallbladder lumen, since the presence of stones or debris in the gallbladder may increase the risk of malignancy. If the sonographic examination does not allow the differentiation of gallbladder wall calcification from large stones, a plain-film radiograph of the abdomen will usually demonstrate the calcified gallbladder, as well as any gallstones in the lumen.

Carcinoma of the Gallbladder

Carcinoma of the gallbladder is the fifth most common carcinoma of the gastrointestinal tract and comprises 4% of all carcino-

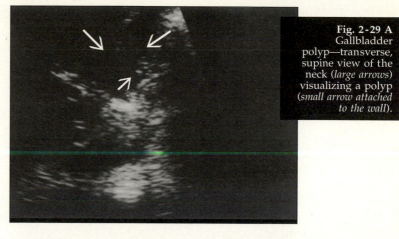

Fig. 2-29 A Gallbladder polyp—transverse, supine view of the neck (*large arrows*) visualizing a polyp (*small arrow attached to the wall*).

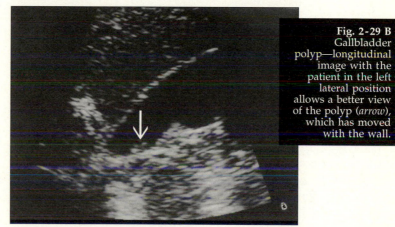

Fig. 2-29 B Gallbladder polyp—longitudinal image with the patient in the left lateral position allows a better view of the polyp (*arrow*), which has moved with the wall.

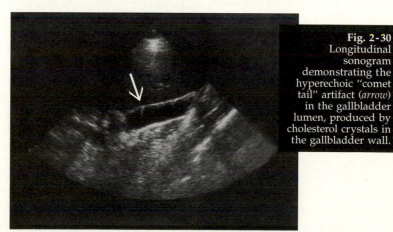

Fig. 2-30 Longitudinal sonogram demonstrating the hyperechoic "comet tail" artifact (*arrow*) in the gallbladder lumen, produced by cholesterol crystals in the gallbladder wall.

mas. It is found predominantly in women over 60 years of age; gallstones are also present in 90% of cases.[8] Approximately 80% of these tumors are adeno-carcinomas, with undifferenti-ated or squamous cell carcino-mas comprising the remainder. The metastatic spread is usually through the lymphatics to the duodenal, choledochal, or pan-creatic nodes, with a localized involvement of the venous sys-tem of the gallbladder. Direct extension into the liver can also occur. Typically the clinical diag-nosis occurs late in the disease process, and therefore the prog-nosis is often poor.

Usually the signs and symp-toms of gallbladder carcinoma are identical to those associated with cholelithiasis and cholecystitis. Ap-proximately 50% of the patients have jaundice, and 65% have a palpable right upper quadrant mass.[8] The laboratory findings do little to differentiate this condition from other benign pathologic con-ditions of the gallbladder. Typi-cally the ALP level is elevated, the SGOT/SGPT levels are mildly elevated, and the direct bilirubin level is increased in jaundiced patients. Fewer than 20% of these patients are diagnosed preopera-tively, and the carcinoma is often an incidental finding during rou-tine cholecystectomy.

Carcinoma of the gallbladder can assume a variety of sono-graphic patterns and may be in-distinguishable from gallstones. Suggestive findings include a large, inhomogeneous, and irregular mass in the gallbladder lumen that is attached to the wall and a "loss" of the gallbladder wall/liver interface.[10] In later stages sonography may demonstrate a solid mass protruding from the gallbladder into the liver or other surrounding structures and may reveal more distant liver metastases and lymphadenopathy (Fig.

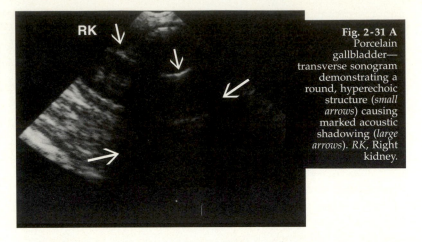

Fig. 2-31 A Porcelain gallbladder—transverse sonogram demonstrating a round, hyperechoic structure (*small arrows*) causing marked acoustic shadowing (*large arrows*). *RK,* Right kidney.

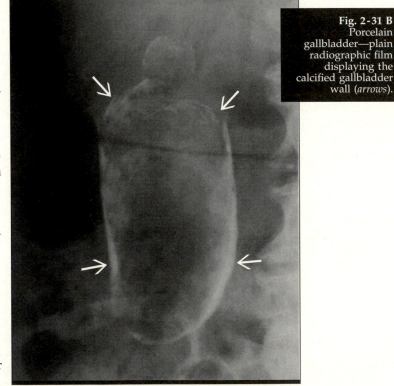

Fig. 2-31 B Porcelain gallbladder—plain radiographic film displaying the calcified gallbladder wall (*arrows*).

2-32). Because gallstones are present in most cases, the sonographer must look for and document any signs of distant metastases to narrow the differential diagnosis.

Cholangitis

Cholangitis, or infection of the biliary system, is most often associated with choledocholithiasis, or common duct stones. Other pathologic processes that may cause cholangitis include choledochal cysts and carcinoma of the bile duct. This inflammatory process may spread upward to include the intrahepatic biliary system, which can lead to hepatic abscesses.[9]

Usually this condition causes intermittent fever, upper abdominal pain, pruritus, and jaundice. Laboratory values are similar to those patients with common duct stones: elevated ALP levels, mildly elevated SGOT/SGPT levels, increased direct bilirubin (if the patient is clinically jaundiced), and an elevated white blood cell count.

There are several sonographic patterns associated with cholangitis. Dilated intrahepatic and/or extrahepatic ducts may be seen in cases of obstructive jaundice. Patients with AIDS may demonstrate thickened duct walls (Fig 2-33 A).[7] Occasionally, air in the biliary tree is seen as irregular, hyperechoic areas parallel to the portal vein branches that demonstrate the comet tail artifact or acoustic shadowing (Fig. 2-33 B).[4] To prove this pattern is air, the position of the patient should be changed; air

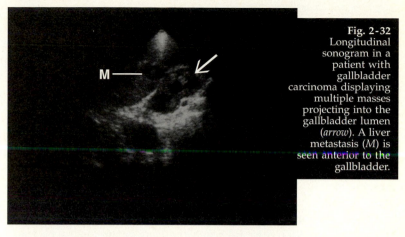

Fig. 2-32 Longitudinal sonogram in a patient with gallbladder carcinoma displaying multiple masses projecting into the gallbladder lumen (*arrow*). A liver metastasis (*M*) is seen anterior to the gallbladder.

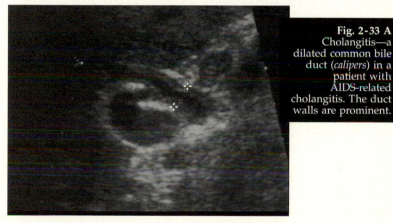

Fig. 2-33 A Cholangitis—a dilated common bile duct (*calipers*) in a patient with AIDS-related cholangitis. The duct walls are prominent.

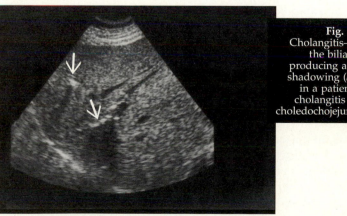

Fig. 2-33 B Cholangitis—air in the biliary tree producing acoustic shadowing (*arrows*) in a patient with cholangitis after a choledochojejunostomy.

will relayer in the most independent portion of the biliary system. Occasionally, a plain-film radiograph of the upper abdomen will verify the presence of air in the biliary tree. This pat tern may be indicative of an anaerobic cholangitis, although a choledochal jejunostomy or gallbladder fistula can also introduce air into the biliary system.

Cholangiocarcinoma

Cholangiocarcinoma, accounting for 3% of all cancer deaths in the United States, is equally divided among the sexes and usually occurs between the ages of 50 and 70.[16] The clinical advance of the disease is rapid, with death usually occurring within several months. Approximately one-third of the cases occur in the common bile duct, one-fifth at the junction of the cystic and common hepatic ducts, and one-fourth higher in the common hepatic duct. A cholangiocarcinoma that occurs at the junction of the left and right hepatic ducts with the common hepatic duct is referred to as the Klatskin tumor.

The main clinical symptoms of carcinoma of the bile ducts is marked jaundice. A palpable gallbladder is found when the level of the obstruction is distal to the cystic duct. Usually hepatomegaly is present, and ascites may occur if there is peritoneal metastasis. Laboratory tests reveal a moderate to severe elevation of the direct bilirubin (hyperbilirubinemia), elevated ALP, and normal to mildly elevated SGOT/SGPT levels.

Because these tumors start as intraluminal masses, obstruction usually occurs when the primary tumor mass is less than 1 cm in size. The sonographic signs of obstructive jaundice are evident and include a dilated extrahepatic biliary system proximal to the site of obstruction. Additional signs include a dilated intrahepatic biliary tree (Fig. 2-34) and an enlarged gallbladder, if the obstruction is distal to the cystic duct. With the use of a high-frequency transducer, the tumor may be demonstrated as an echogenic, intraluminal mass with dilatation proximal to this site and a normal or collapsed system distal to it (Fig. 2-35).

Choledocholithiasis

Choledocholithiasis, or common duct stones, are found in approximately 15% of cholecystectomy patients, but the incidence can be as high as 50% in elderly patients.[14] Usually these stones form in the gallbladder, pass through the cystic duct and proximal common bile duct, and lodge in the narrow pancreatic or ampullary portion of the distal duct. Small stones may pass through the ampulla and into the duodenum. In some instances the stones may spontaneously form in the ductal system. Common duct stones are the most common cause of obstructive jaundice.

A stone in the duct may cause muscular spasm and produce a sharp episode of pain. In the case of obstruction, the patient experiences intermittent, colicky right upper quadrant pain, often radiating to the right scapula. The obstruction can be

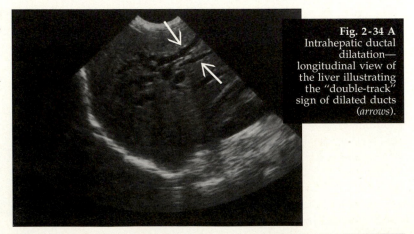

Fig. 2-34 A Intrahepatic ductal dilatation— longitudinal view of the liver illustrating the "double-track" sign of dilated ducts (*arrows*).

either complete or intermittent, especially if the stone is a "ball-in-valve" type. When obstruction is complete, jaundice progresses but is rarely severe, with only a moderately elevated direct bilirubin. The ALP is usually elevated, and the SGOT/SGPT levels may be mildly increased.

The sonographic patterns of choledocholithiasis include a hyperechoic intraluminal mass or masses that exhibit acoustic shadowing (Fig. 2-36) with a dilated duct proximal to the point of obstruction. However, small stones may not cause dilatation, which makes the demonstration of these stones a challenge.[2] The sonographer should scan the liver for evidence of intrahepatic dilatation. Usually gallstones are seen in the gallbladder, and occasionally stones may be demonstrated in the intrahepatic ducts. Because of the surrounding duodenum, finding a scanning window for the distal duct can be a challenge. Lateral and upright patient positions may allow adequate visualization.[5] Transverse scans demonstrating the stone in the duct lumen are crucial views (Fig. 2-37), since bowel contents may look like stones on longitudinal scans. When the cause of the obstruction cannot be documented with sonography, a percutaneous transhepatic cholangiogram may be necessary to document the level and cause of the obstruction.

Extrabiliary Causes of Obstructive Jaundice

After choledocholithiasis, the other causes of obstructive jaun-

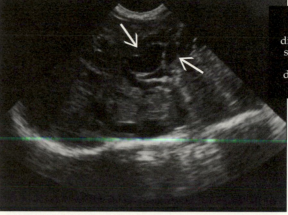

Fig. 2-34 B Intrahepatic ductal dilatation—tranverse scan depicting more severely dilated ducts (*arrows*) in the left lobe.

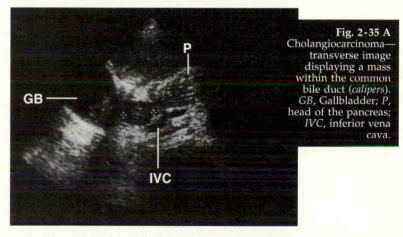

Fig. 2-35 A Cholangiocarcinoma—transverse image displaying a mass within the common bile duct (*calipers*). *GB*, Gallbladder; *P*, head of the pancreas; *IVC*, inferior vena cava.

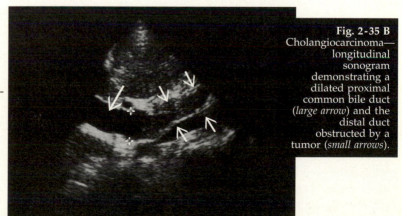

Fig. 2-35 B Cholangiocarcinoma—longitudinal sonogram demonstrating a dilated proximal common bile duct (*large arrow*) and the distal duct obstructed by a tumor (*small arrows*).

dice (in order of decreasing frequency) are carcinoma of the head of the pancreas and ampulla of Vater, carcinoma of the common bile duct, metastatic carcinoma (usually gastrointestinal), and direct extension of gallbladder carcinoma.[13] Liver metastases, especially in the area of the porta hepatis, can also cause obstructive jaundice.

The clinical symptoms of obstructive jaundice caused by extrabiliary masses are pruritus, progressive jaundice, and abdominal pain. Unexplained weight loss is associated with malignant entities. Prolonged obstruction can lead to hepatic cellular damage resulting in biliary cirrhosis. The direct bilirubin demonstrates a larger increase than that associated with common duct stones. The SGOT/SGPT levels are elevated in the presence of hepatocellular damage.

When the cause of the obstruction is proximal to the cystic duct, (e.g., in the area of the porta hepatis) the gallbladder and extrahepatic biliary tree distal to the obstruction are of normal or small size, and those biliary structures proximal to the obstruction are enlarged to varying degrees (Fig. 2-38). Malignancies in this region do not cause a Courvoisier gallbladder.

When the cause of obstruction is distal to the cystic duct, the biliary system proximal to the obstruction is dilated. In cases of neoplasm a Courvoisier gallbladder may be apparent. **Courvoisier's law** states that neoplasm is the most frequent cause of obstructive jaundice dis-

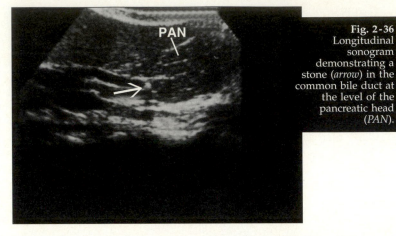

Fig. 2-36 Longitudinal sonogram demonstrating a stone (*arrow*) in the common bile duct at the level of the pancreatic head (*PAN*).

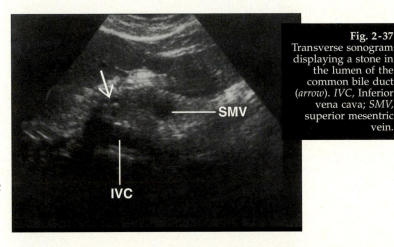

Fig. 2-37 Transverse sonogram displaying a stone in the lumen of the common bile duct (*arrow*). *IVC*, Inferior vena cava; *SMV*, superior mesentric vein.

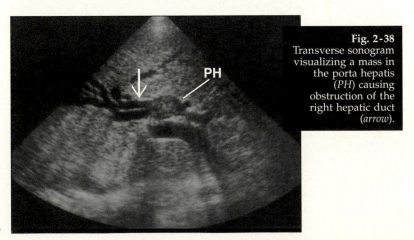

Fig. 2-38 Transverse sonogram visualizing a mass in the porta hepatis (*PH*) causing obstruction of the right hepatic duct (*arrow*).

tal to the cystic duct where the gall bladder is distended but has a normal wall (Fig. 2-39). The biliary system distal to the obstruction is normal or small in size. Examples of these types of neoplasms include (1) carcinoma of the head of the pancreas; (2) lymphoma in the periaortic, periduodenal, or peripancreatic area; (3) hyperplastic lymph nodes (benign) in the same areas; and (4) metastases or extension from gastric, duodenal, or colon carcinoma.

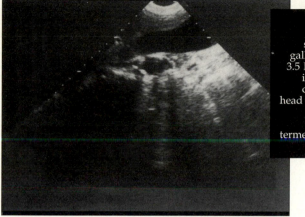

Fig. 2-39 Longitudinal sonogram of the gallbladder using a 3.5 MHz transducer in a patient with carcinoma of the head of the pancreas. This type of enlargement is termed a Courvoisier gallbladder.

TECHNICAL PITFALLS

Proper gain control is very important for adequately demonstrating the biliary system with a minimum of artifacts. For the intrahepatic biliary system, the gain controls are set with the same time gain compensation (TGC) curve that is used for hepatic imaging. For gallbladder imaging, the gain is initially set for hepatic imaging. The gallbladder should visualize as a cystic structure with an anechoic interior and distal acoustic enhancement. Depending on the scanning window used, the TGC and system gain may have to be decreased to display these characteristics. Finding an acoustic window where liver tissue is proximal to the gallbladder in the sound field will minimize reverberation artifacts and allow the operator to adjust the gain and focal zone controls more easily. Transducer selection plays a crucial role. Transducers should be selected to obtain the best resolution with adequate penetration. For superficial gallbladders, a 5.0 MHz and even a 7.5 MHz transducer may be necessary to adequately image the organ and to identify small stones, polyps, or sludge (Fig. 2-40).

Artifacts, such as reverberation and acoustic shadowing from the bowel, can lead to misdiagnoses. Several general rules can minimize this risk. The sonographer should always verify that the abnormality is consistently demonstrated in transverse and longitudinal planes, from several different scanning windows and in different patient positions. If the abnormality is not reproducible, the sonographer should mention this to the interpreting physician.

The sonographer should perform a preliminary sweep through the gallbladder, noting any questionable areas. The sonographer should verify the origin of any abnormality before recording images on hard copy. A common pitfall is mistaking a piece of a septa or fold for a polyp. The sonographer should always oblique the scanning plane while imaging this type of abnormality. Typically a polyp will continue to appear as a rounded mass, whereas a septa will lengthen and eventually connect to the rest of the septum. Initially a phrygian cap or fold in the gallbladder may visualize as a septum, but careful scanning will reveal the connection between the body and fundus.

Another source of the appearance of false sludge in the gallbladder is a side lobe artifact. Again, this artifact is related to the scanning angle and the normal curved shape of the gallbladder wall. At the critical angle, the interaction of the side lobes of the sound field with this reflector produces low-amplitude false echoes in the lumen of the gallbladder. However, if the sonographer changes the scanning window and thus the scanning angle to the gallbladder wall, the "sludge" disappears. This is why the sonographer must always ensure that sludge is reproducible from different scanning windows and with various patient positions.

Because many patients awaiting gallbladder sonography are initially in the emergency room, questions related to proper examination preparation are important. Many departments will

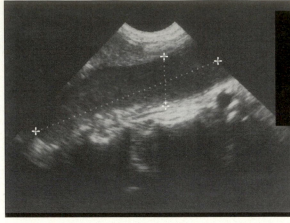

Fig. 2-40 Longitudinal sonogram of the same patient as in Fig. 2-39 performed with a 5.0 MHz transducer, which reveals total biliary sludge.

perform this examination regardless of patient preparation and regardless of how pathologic conditions may be interpreted. However, a partially contracted gallbladder may appear to have thick walls on sonography, and inadequate patient preparation may require a repeat examination to verify the cause of the wall thickening.

SUMMARY

This chapter has presented the most common types of biliary system pathology and some of the more rare diseases. Again, the clinical history and the results of the clinical laboratory tests play an integral role in the proper interpretation of the sonographic examination. Table 2-1 provides a brief summary of the clinical laboratory data related to the various disease processes. These values are for the "typical" presentation of the disease. Some patients will have superimposed conditions, such as biliary obstruction with coexisting cirrhosis of the liver. This and other combinations of different pathologies can make the interpretation of the laboratory tests ambiguous.

REFERENCES

1. Cohan RH, Mahony BS, et al: Striated intramural gallbladder lucencies on US studies: predictors of acute cholecystitis, *Radiology* 164:31, 1987.
2. Cronan JJ: US diagnosis of choledocholithiasis: a reappraisal, *Radiology* 161:133, 1986.
3. Darwees RMA, Dodd WJ, et al: Fatty-meal sonography for evaluating patients with suspected partial common duct obstruction, *AJR* 151:63, 1988.
4. Dolmatch BI, Laing FC, et al: AIDS-related cholangitis: radiographic findings in nine patients, *Radiology* 163:313, 1987.
5. Dong B, Chen M: Improved sonographic visualization of choledocholithiasis, *J Clin Ultrasound* 15:185, 1987.
6. Franquet T, Beslos JM, et al: Acoustic artifacts and reverberation shadows in gallbladder sonograms: their cause and clinical implications, *Gastrointest Radiol* 15:223, 1990.
7. Grumbach K, Coleman BG, et al: Hepatic and biliary tract abnormalities in patients with AIDS: sonographic-pathologic correlation *J Ultrasound Med* 8:247, 1989.
8. Harolds JA, Dennehy DC: Preoperative diagnosis of gallbladder CA by ultrasonography, *South Med J* 74:1024, 1981.
9. Ishida H, Yagisawa H, et al: Ultrasonography of acute obstructive suppurative cholangitis: serial observation by ultrasound, *J Clin Ultrasound* 15:51, 1987.

TABLE 2-1 CLINICAL LABORATORY TEST VALUES – BILIARY SYSTEM

	SGOT	SGPT	ALP	DIR BR	IND BR	Other Tests
CHOLELITHIASIS	Normal to Mild Increase	Normal to Mild Increase*	Increase	Normal to Mild Increase†		
CHOLECYSTITIS	Normal to Mild Increase	Normal to Mild Increase*	Increase	Normal to Mild Increase†		Increased WBC
BENIGN NEOPLASMS	Normal	Normal	Normal Increase	Normal		
GALLBLADDER CARCINOMA	Normal Increase	Normal Increase*	Increase	Normal Increase†	Normal Increase	
CHOLANGITIS	Normal Increase	Normal Increase*	Increase	Normal Increase†		Increased WBC
CHOLANGIO-CARCINOMA	Normal Increase	Normal Increase*	Increase	Moderate Increase	Normal Increase*	
CHOLEDOCHO-LITHIASIS	Normal Increase	Normal Increase*	Increase	Increase		
BILIARY CIRRHOSIS	Increase	Increase	Increase	Increase	Increase	

*Elevation of liver function test values depends on the presence of liver pathology and/or the severity and duration of the biliary system obstruction.

†The severity of the bilirubin elevation depends on the cause of the obstruction, whether it is partial or total, and the duration .

SGOT, Serum glutamic oxaloacetic transaminase; SGPT, serum glutamic pyruvic transaminase; ALP, alkaline phosphatase; DIR DR, direct bilirubin; IND BR, indirect bilirubin; WBC, white blood cell count.

10. Kumar A, Aggarwal S, et al: Ultrasonography of CA of the gallbladder: an analysis of 80 cases, *J Clin Ultrasound* 18:715, 1990.
11. Lover KL, Slasky BS, Skolnick ML: Sonography of cholesterol in the biliary system, *J Ultrasound Med* 4:647, 1985.
12. Malet PF, Baker J, et. al: Gallstone composition in relation to buoyancy at oral cholecystography, *Radiology* 177:167, 1990.
13. Malini S, Sabel J: Ultrasonography in obstructive jaundice, *Radiology* 123:429, 1977.
14. Parvelak SG, McNamara MP: Ultrasonography of choledocholithiasis, *J Ultrasound Med* 2:395, 1983.
15. Revter K, Raptopoulous VD, et al: The diagnosis of choledochal cyst by ultrasound, *Radiology* 136:437, 1980.
16. Schnur MJ, Hoffman JC, Koenigsberg M: Ultrasonic demonstration of intraductal biliary neoplasms, *J Clin Ultrasound* 10:246, 1982.
17. Shuman WP, Mack LA, et al: Evaluation of acute right upper quadrant pain: sonography and ^{99m}Tc-PIPIDA cholescintigraphy, *AJR* 139:61, 1982.
18. Wegener M, Borsch G, et al: Gallbladder wall thickening: a frequent finding in various non-biliary disorders—a prospective ultrasonographic study, *J Clin Ultrasound* 15:307, 1987.
19. Willi UV, Teele RI: Hepatic arteries and the parallel-channel sign, *J Clin Ultrasound* 7:125, 1979.

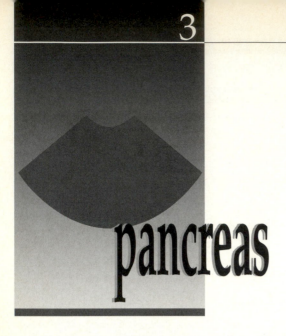

3

pancreas

INSTRUCTIONAL OBJECTIVES

At the completion of this chapter, the reader will be able to:

1. Describe the clinical problems that are typical reasons for sonography of the pancreas.
2. Identify on transverse and longitudinal illustrations and sonograms the major anatomic divisions of the pancreas, the pancreatic duct, the vascular landmarks, and the extrahepatic biliary system and the relationship of each to surrounding structures.
3. Describe the basic scanning protocol for sonography of the pancreas as defined by national professional organizations.
4. Describe the clinical laboratory tests used for evaluating pancreatic function, including serum amylase and serum lipase assays, as well as the specific disease processes they evaluate.
5. Describe the clinical symptoms and pathologic basis for the disease processes of the pancreas, including acute and chronic pancreatitis, abscess, pseudocyst, true cysts, benign islet cell tumors, and carcinoma of the pancreas.
6. Identify on sectional sonograms the above-mentioned disease processes of the pancreas, based on the sonographic pattern, the clinical history, and the results of other diagnostic procedures.
7. List several technical pitfalls associated with pancreatic sonography.

THE CLINICAL PROBLEM

The preliminary diagnosis for the patient who complains of epigastric pain usually includes diseases of the gastrointestinal tract such as peptic ulcer and pancreatic pathology such as pancreatitis and carcinoma. Because of its retroperitoneal location, the pancreas can pose a challenge for diagnostic evaluation. Another complicating factor is the typically late onset of symptoms for pancreatic carcinoma. Since patients may have jaundice accompanying the epigastric pain, the physician typically orders a sonographic examination of the biliary system and the pancreas. Pancreatic sonography presents a challenge for the sonographer because of the numerous vascular landmarks used for accurate identification of this rather small organ. Since the stomach and duodenum typically surround the pancreas, the sonographer must use different patient positions or give the patient water to drink to obtain a diagnostic examination.

NORMAL ANATOMY

The pancreas is a long, thin gland located in the anterior pararenal space of the retroperitoneal cavity. It is approximately 10 cm long, and the body and tail are approximately 2 cm in the posteroanterior dimension. The pancreas consists of the following subdivisions: head, uncinate process, neck, body, and tail (Fig. 3-1). The head of the pancreas is bordered superiorly, inferiorly, and laterally by the duodenum and posteriorly by the common bile duct and inferior vena cava. The uncinate process is an inferior extension of the head that courses toward the midline, posterior to the superior mesenteric vein and artery, and anterior to the aorta. The head constricts slightly, forming the neck and then widens to form the body. The body of the pancreas courses to the left, where it is anterior to the aorta, superior mesenteric artery, and splenic vein, and is posterior to the stomach. The tail of the pancreas lies in the lienorenal ligament and travels laterally and posteriorly, terminating in close proximity to the splenic hilum, posterior to the splenic flexure of the colon or stomach and anterior to the left kidney.

There are quite a few **arterial tributaries** that supply the pancreas. Three branches of the splenic artery—the dorsal pancreatic, pancreatica magna, and caudae pancreatis—supply the body and tail. The inferior pancreaticoduodenal artery, arising from the superior mesenteric artery, and the superior pancreaticoduodenal, arising from the gastroduodenal artery, supply the pancreatic head. The pancreatic veins are tributaries of the superior mesenteric and splenic veins.

The **pancreatic duct,** or the duct of Wirsung, traverses the length of the pancreas from left to right, slightly superior to the central axis of the gland. The duct transports the pancreatic

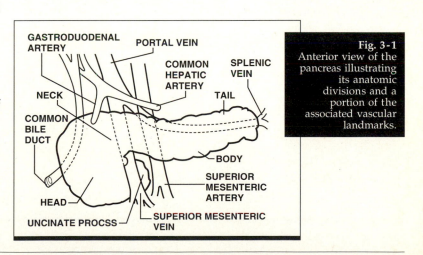

GASTRODUODENAL ARTERY
PORTAL VEIN
COMMON HEPATIC ARTERY
SPLENIC VEIN
NECK
TAIL
COMMON BILE DUCT
BODY
SUPERIOR MESENTERIC ARTERY
HEAD
UNCINATE PROCSS
SUPERIOR MESENTERIC VEIN

Fig. 3-1 Anterior view of the pancreas illustrating its anatomic divisions and a portion of the associated vascular landmarks.

enzymes to the duodenum where the enzymes aid digestion. Many small tributaries join the main duct before it courses through the pancreatic head. There the main duct joins the common bile duct before entering the duodenum. The **duct of Santorini,** or the accessory duct, may merge with the duct of Wirsung in the head or enter the duodenum directly through the minor ampulla (Fig. 3-2). Normal measurements for the pancreas and pancreatic duct are listed in Table 3.1.[4]

A number of vessels serve as landmarks for localizing the pancreas (Fig. 3-3). The **splenic vein** courses posterior and parallel to the body and tail of the pancreas and is usually the first structure seen on transverse scans. Posterior to the neck of the pancreas, the splenic vein merges with the **superior mesenteric vein (SMV)** at the portal-splenic confluence or junction. The SMV courses parallel to the inferior vena cava, and the uncinate process can be seen posterior to the SMV. Surrounded by the hyperechoic mesentery, the SMV lies anterior to

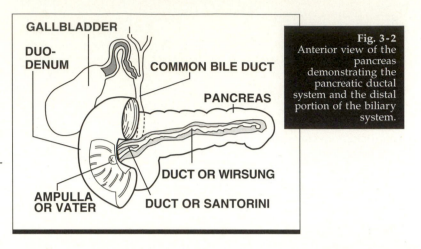

Fig. 3-2 Anterior view of the pancreas demonstrating the pancreatic ductal system and the distal portion of the biliary system.

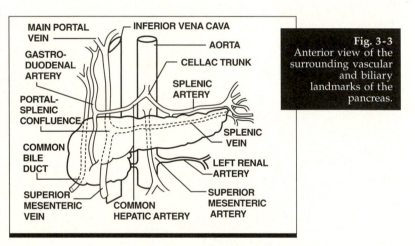

Fig. 3-3 Anterior view of the surrounding vascular and biliary landmarks of the pancreas.

TABLE 3-1 PANCREATIC MEASUREMENTS		
	ANTERIOR-POSTERIOR	*LENGTH*
HEAD	2.0 cm to 3.0 cm	2.4 cm to 4.8 cm
NECK	1.0 cm to 2.0 cm	
BODY	1.2 cm to 2.9 cm	2.4 cm to 3.6 cm
TAIL	2.0 cm to 2.8 cm	1.6 cm to 2.4 cm
DUCT	3.0 mm	

the aorta and posterior to the splenic vein. The renal arteries arise from the abdominal aorta in the region of the pancreas. The **left renal vein** courses posterior to the superior mesenteric artery and anterior to the aorta. The **gastroduodenal artery** arises from the common hepatic artery and courses inferiorly to the head of pancreas, where it travels along the anterolateral aspect (Fig. 3-4). The **common bile duct** travels along the posterolateral aspect of the pancreactic head, anterior to the inferior vena cava.

The pancreas lies in the **anterior pararenal space** of the retroperitoneal cavity. Since the pancreas does not have a true capsule, pancreatic pathology, such as an abscess, may spread into this space. The periaortic nodes are also located in the anterior pararenal space. The peritoneal cavity lies anterior to the pancreas. The **lesser sac** of the peritoneal cavity is located anterior to the pancreatic tail and posterior to the stomach. The lesser sac connects to the greater sac via the **foramen of Winslow,** which is situated at the level of the portal triad in the region of the lesser omentum. This connection allows pathologic conditions located in one of the potential spaces to spread to the other (Fig. 3-5).

CLINICAL LABORATORY TESTS

Amylase

Amylase is a digestive enzyme produced in the pancreas that aids in converting starches to sugars. This enzyme is also produced in the salivary glands, liver, and fallopian tubes. Amylase serum levels are increased in cases of inflammation of the pancreas.

In acute pancreatitis, the amylase levels are greatly increased starting 3 to 6 hours after the onset of clinical symptoms. The levels remain elevated for approximately 24 hours after the acute episode and then start to decrease. Elevated amylase levels also occur with chronic pancreatitis (acute attack), partial gastrectomy, obstruction of the pancreatic duct, perforated peptic ulcer, alcoholic poisoning, acute cholecystitis, and intestinal obstruction with strangulation.[17] Decreased amylase levels occur with hepatitis and cirrhosis of the liver. Because of the non-specificity of this test, some

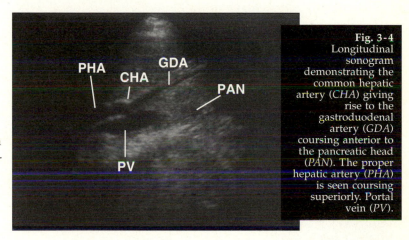

Fig. 3-4
Longitudinal sonogram demonstrating the common hepatic artery (*CHA*) giving rise to the gastroduodenal artery (*GDA*) coursing anterior to the pancreatic head (*PAN*). The proper hepatic artery (*PHA*) is seen coursing superiorly. Portal vein (*PV*).

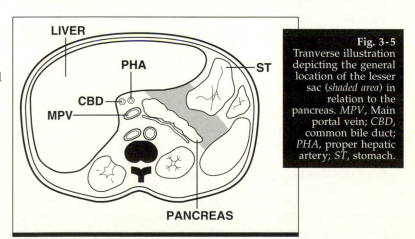

Fig. 3-5
Tranverse illustration depicting the general location of the lesser sac (*shaded area*) in relation to the pancreas. *MPV,* Main portal vein; *CBD,* common bile duct; *PHA,* proper hepatic artery; *ST,* stomach.

authorities believe that the diagnosis of acute pancreatitis should be based on the clinical symptoms. Sonographic evaluation may also allow a more specific diagnosis.

Lipase

Lipase is another enzyme produced primarily by the pancreas that changes fats to fatty acids and glycerol. As with amylase levels, serum lipase levels are increased after damage has occurred to the pancreas.

In acute pancreatitis, lipase levels may not be elevated until 24 to 36 hours after the onset of clinical symptoms. However, the lipase level remains elevated for a longer period of time (up to 14 days) than the amylase values. Therefore this test may be quite helpful, since some patients do not seek medical attention until several days after the attack. Increased lipase levels are also seen with obstruction of the pancreatic duct, pancreatic carcinoma, acute cholecystitis, cirrhosis, and severe renal disease.

Although the tests for bilirubin are not direct indications of pancreatic function, various pancreatic pathologic processes cause obstruction of the ampulla of Vater and/or the common bile duct. This obstruction is reflected in the bilirubin values. Increased conjugated or **direct bilirubin** levels are associated with carcinoma of the head of the pancreas and, occasionally, with acute pancreatitis.

RELATED IMAGING PROCEDURES

Plain-Film Radiograph and Upper Gastrointestinal Series

The plain abdominal radiograph may demonstrate pancreatic calcifications secondary to chronic pancreatitis, the renal halo sign of acute pancreatitis, water density mottling of acute pancreatitis, and a soft tissue mass effect from a pancreatic pseudocyst. The upper gastrointestinal series may demonstrate a widening of the duodenal loop caused by a mass in the head of the pancreas or displacement of the stomach caused by masses in the pancreatic body or tail.

Arteriography

Arteriography involves injection of an iodinated contrast material into the arterial system of the pancreas through a catheter inserted into the femoral artery. The catheter is then advanced into the origins of the pancreatic vessels. The primary function of arteriography is the differentiation of benign from malignant tumors of the pancreas. The importance of this technique has decreased with the widespread use of sonography, computed tomography (CT), and endoscopic retrograde cholangiopancre-atography. However, pancreatic arteriography may still be used for determining the resectability of malignant neoplasms. Arteriographic signs that a malignancy is not resectable include hepatic metastases, invasion or occlusion of the portal or superior mesenteric veins, and encasement by tumor of the celiac, superior mesenteric, hepatic, or gastric arteries. Arteriography is also useful for demonstrating small, highly vascular tumors that affect the endocrine function of the pancreas.[5]

ENDOSCOPIC RETROGRADE CHOLANGIOPANCREATOGRAPHY

Endoscopic retrograde cholangiopancreatography (ERCP) directly views the ampulla of Vater and portions of the pancreatic and common bile ducts by means of an endoscope that is passed through the esophagus and stomach and into the duodenum.

This is a highly specialized procedure usually performed by a gastroenterologist with the assistance of the radiology department. ERCP has an accuracy rate of approximately 95% for diagnosing carcinoma.[5] The course of the common bile duct and pancreatic duct is demonstrated after injecting iodinated contrast material and obtaining serial radiographs. Usually this procedure is contraindicated in the presence of acute pancreatitis. ERCP examinations do not obtain any information regarding metastatic involvement.

Nuclear Medicine Imaging

Currently no radionuclide can adequately visualize the pancreas with acceptable sensitivity and specificity. Hepatobiliary imaging can document obstructive jaundice and provide a differential diagnosis regarding its cause.

Computed Tomography

High resolution CT has a reported accuracy rate of nearly 100% in the detection of pancreatic carcinoma. Acute and chronic pancreatitis can be detected in approximately 95% of cases.[5] CT can also demonstrate dilated intrahepatic ducts and image the pancreas in the presence of bowel gas. Another advantage is that it allows recognition of metastases in the liver and retroperitoneal lymph nodes.

SCANNING PROTOCOLS AND TECHNIQUES

Most department protocols include transverse views of the pancreas as part of the biliary system examination. However, a complete sonographic examination of the pancreas requires both transverse and longitudinal images. The performance of transverse scans requires some initial survey scanning to determine the exact position of the gland. Usually the pancreas lies obliquely in the epigastric region with the head located more inferiorly than the body and tail (Fig. 3-6). Therefore the proper scanning plane is an oblique, transverse scan with the inferior portion of the angle located to the right of midline. Since the pancreas courses parallel to the splenic vein, the sonographer should first image the length of the splenic vein and then locate the pancreas anterior to it. Because the pancreas is almost completely surrounded by the bowel, the sonographer should always use the left lobe of the liver as an acoustic window. This approach may require moving superiorly and then applying a 10- to 15-degree caudal angulation. Usually it is easier to start with superior scans when localizing the pancreas. Identifying vascular landmarks are more easily seen by moving inferiorly, because the celiac trunk is the major landmark superior to the pancreatic area. Once this landmark is identified, the sonographer should move slightly infer-

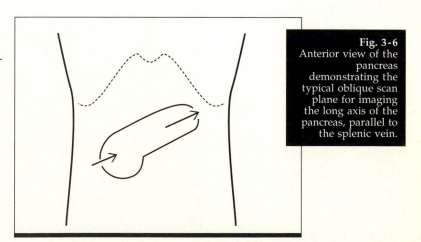

Fig. 3-6
Anterior view of the pancreas demonstrating the typical oblique scan plane for imaging the long axis of the pancreas, parallel to the splenic vein.

ior to the celiac trunk, looking for a portion of the splenic vein. Additional views of the pancreatic head, using a different scanning obliquity, may be necessary, particularly in the presence of pathologic conditions in this area. To prove that the pathologic disorder involves the pancreatic head, a scan must demonstrate that the head is attached to the pancreatic neck and body. This is also true for pathologic conditions in any area of the pancreas. A scan must demonstrate the pancreatic head and its relationship to surrounding pancreatic structures.

The pancreas can be very difficult to demonstrate in the presence of bowel gas. There are several procedures that may assist adequate visualization. Experimentation with patient position, including the right and left oblique, lateral, and upright positions, will often allow complete demonstration of the pancreas. If not contraindicated, the patient may drink 8 to 16 ounces of water. The sonographer should change the patient's position so that the water fills the portion of the gastrointestinal tract surrounding the area of the pancreas that is of interest. For example, filling the antrum of the stomach will allow visualization of the tail.

The box presented on this page is a suggested protocol for a complete examination of the pancreas.

This protocol would be an optimal study where complete visualization is possible. Figs.

BASIC SCANNING PROTOCOL

Transverse
- ✔ An oblique scan demonstrating the entire length of the pancreas (if possible)
- ✔ Distal pancreatic tail, anterior to the left kidney
- ✔ Body and proximal tail with splenic vein visualized posteriorly
- ✔ Neck of pancreas with portal-splenic confluence seen posteriorly
- ✔ Head of the pancreas, including common bile duct, with IVC seen posteriorly

Longitudinal
- ✔ Midline to right of midline
- ✔ SMV and portal-splenic confluence with pancreatic neck and uncinate process
- ✔ Pancreatic head with common bile duct

Left of Midline
- ✔ Body of pancreas with splenic vein, SMA, celiac axis, and aorta
- ✔ Tail of pancreas with splenic vein

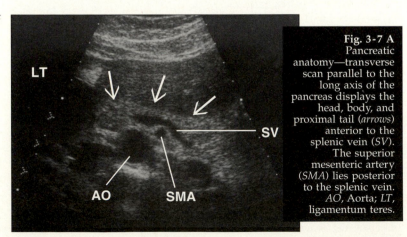

Fig. 3-7 A Pancreatic anatomy—transverse scan parallel to the long axis of the pancreas displays the head, body, and proximal tail (*arrows*) anterior to the splenic vein (*SV*). The superior mesenteric artery (*SMA*) lies posterior to the splenic vein. *AO,* Aorta; *LT,* ligamentum teres.

3-7 through 3-13 illustrate the scanning protocol. Longitudinal scans pose a problem for many beginning sonographers, since the surrounding vascular landmarks are harder to visualize, particularly for the tail. One technique for demonstrating the tail is to position the transducer to the right of midline and angle toward the patient's left. This achieves the "tunnel view" of the pancreatic tail with the splenic vein seen posteriorly (Fig. 3-14).

NORMAL SONOGRAPHIC PATTERNS

The sonographic pattern of the pancreas is classified according to its comparison with the normal liver parenchyma. In a younger patient the pancreas should be isoechoic to slightly hyperechoic to the liver. In elderly patients the pancreas may be more diffusely hyperechoic as a result of increased fat and fibrous tissue deposition as part of the normal aging process, but the gland still measures in the normal range.[10] As in all sonographic examinations, gain settings are important in establishing normal versus abnormal sonographic patterns. The system gain and time gain compensation (TGC) controls should be adjusted so that the interior of the prevertebral vessels contains at least a few sparse echoes. If the liver parenchyma is normal, the TGC may be set for adequate visualization of the liver, and only minor adjustments should be necessary for the pancreas. Proper transducer selection is crucial. A common error is the

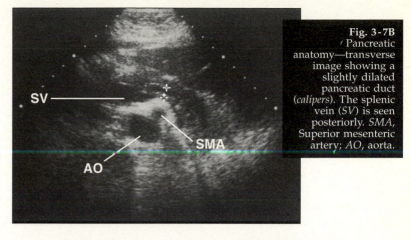

Fig. 3-7B Pancreatic anatomy—transverse image showing a slightly dilated pancreatic duct (*calipers*). The splenic vein (*SV*) is seen posteriorly. *SMA,* Superior mesenteric artery; *AO,* aorta.

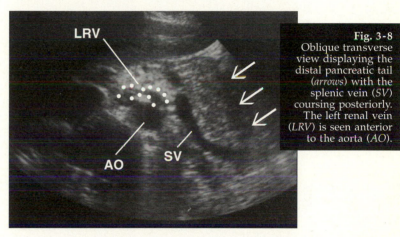

Fig. 3-8 Oblique transverse view displaying the distal pancreatic tail (*arrows*) with the splenic vein (*SV*) coursing posteriorly. The left renal vein (*LRV*) is seen anterior to the aorta (*AO*).

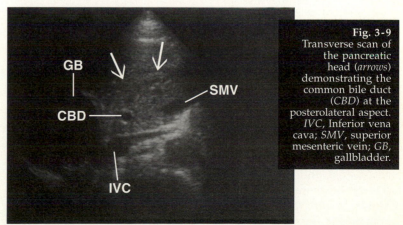

Fig. 3-9 Transverse scan of the pancreatic head (*arrows*) demonstrating the common bile duct (*CBD*) at the posterolateral aspect. *IVC,* Inferior vena cava; *SMV,* superior mesenteric vein; *GB,* gallbladder.

use of a lower frequency transducer for a superficial pancreas. In thin patients the pancreas may lie only a few centimeters from the anterior skin surface. A 5.0 or even 7.5 MHz transducer may be needed to demonstrate the pancreas.

CONGENITAL ANOMALIES

In general, congenital anomalies of the pancreas are rare. The condition termed **pancreas divisum** occurs when the duct of Wirsung and the duct of Santorini fail to join, and the duct of Wirsung is small and drains only the inferior portion of the pancreatic head. The duct of Santorini drains the majority of the gland. This anomaly may increase the patient's susceptibility to pancreatitis. Sonographically, pancreas divisum is demonstrable only with pancreatitis, which may allow the visualization of the ductal system.

Although still classified as rare, **annular pancreas** is the most common pancreatic anomaly and is characterized by a ring of pancreatic tissue encircling the second portion of the duodenum. The primary clinical symptom occurs with obstruction, which may be the source of dyspepsia. There is no specific sonographic pattern for annular pancreas, and often the only sign is a prominent pancreatic head. Other anomalies present in roughly 75% of cases include Down syndrome, tracheoesphageal fistula, and imperforate anus, each generally symptomatic early in life. Other very rare anomalies of the pancreas in-

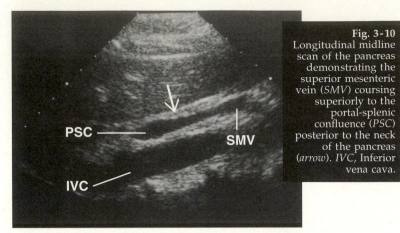

Fig. 3-10
Longitudinal midline scan of the pancreas demonstrating the superior mesenteric vein (*SMV*) coursing superiorly to the portal-splenic confluence (*PSC*) posterior to the neck of the pancreas (*arrow*). *IVC*, Inferior vena cava.

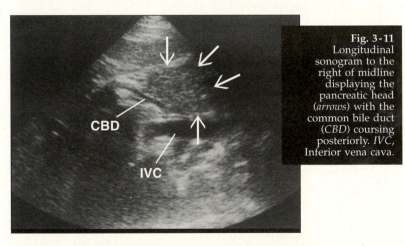

Fig. 3-11
Longitudinal sonogram to the right of midline displaying the pancreatic head (*arrows*) with the common bile duct (*CBD*) coursing posteriorly. *IVC*, Inferior vena cava.

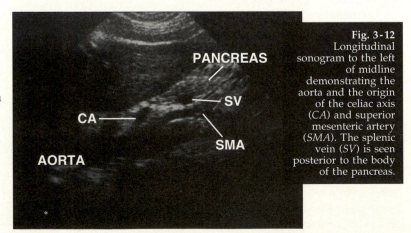

Fig. 3-12
Longitudinal sonogram to the left of midline demonstrating the aorta and the origin of the celiac axis (*CA*) and superior mesenteric artery (*SMA*). The splenic vein (*SV*) is seen posterior to the body of the pancreas.

clude pancreatic duct atresia, pancreatic hypoplasia, and partial or complete pancreatic agenesis.[13]

Cystic fibrosis is a multisystemic process that affects many of the mucus-secreting glands of the body. The major clinical symptoms are chronic infections of the lungs with obstruction and malabsorption syndromes caused by pancreatic dysfunction. On sonographic examination the pancreas appears diffusely hyperechoic as a result of microcyst formation. Occasionally, the cysts may attain a size that allows the display of the typical cystic pattern.

PATHOLOGIC PROCESSES OF THE PANCREAS

Acute Pancreatitis

Acute pancreatitis, or inflammation of the pancreas, causes the escape of pancreatic enzymes from the acinar cells into the surrounding tissues. The majority of the cases of acute pancreatitis stem from diseases of the biliary system and alcoholism. In the former case the presence of ductal stones does not have a high correlation with pancreatitis, although many patients have gallstones present in stool specimens. Alcoholics usually have a high protein concentration in the pancreatic juice, and often they have duodenal irritation. Other causes of acute pancreatitis include blunt abdominal trauma, viral infections, and excessive manipulation of the pancreas during surgery. Patients with pancreatic carcinoma may develop acute pancreatitis as the malignancy interferes with ductal secretion.

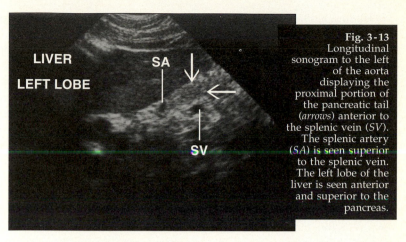

Fig. 3-13 Longitudinal sonogram to the left of the aorta displaying the proximal portion of the pancreatic tail (*arrows*) anterior to the splenic vein (*SV*). The splenic artery (*SA*) is seen superior to the splenic vein. The left lobe of the liver is seen anterior and superior to the pancreas.

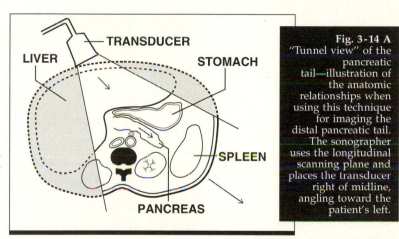

Fig. 3-14 A "Tunnel view" of the pancreatic tail—illustration of the anatomic relationships when using this technique for imaging the distal pancreatic tail. The sonographer uses the longitudinal scanning plane and places the transducer right of midline, angling toward the patient's left.

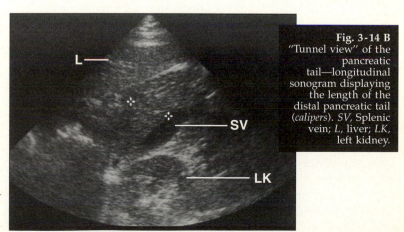

Fig. 3-14 B "Tunnel view" of the pancreatic tail—longitudinal sonogram displaying the length of the distal pancreatic tail (*calipers*). *SV,* Splenic vein; *L,* liver; *LK,* left kidney.

Hemorrhagic pancreatitis, the most severe form, consists of pancreatic tissue necrosis and hemorrhage caused by the leakage of the pancreatic enzymes out of the ductal system. These caustic enzymes cause the rupture of the pancreatic vessels, leading to acute hemorrhage. A heavy intake of alcohol over a rather short duration or the ingestion of a very large meal can lead to hemorrhagic pancreatitis.[8]

The clinical symptoms of acute pancreatitis include abrupt onset of epigastric pain, often radiating to the back, as well as nausea, vomiting, sweating, fever, and abdominal tenderness and distention.[6] The serum and urine amylase levels increase during the first 24 hours after the onset of symptoms and usually return to normal by the third day. Lipase levels rise more slowly and persist several days longer than the amylase levels. As previously mentioned, elevated amylase and lipase levels do not always indicate acute pancreatitis, and clinical symptoms should be given more weight for this diagnosis. Patients with acute hemorrhagic pancreatitis usually have an elevated white blood cell count and may have an elevated direct bilirubin level in the case of obstructive jaundice and an increased alkaline phosphatase level with the presence of common duct and/or gallstones. These patients have additional symptoms, including a decreased hematocrit and red blood cell count, a decreased serum calcium level hypotension, and may develop respiratory distress.[6]

The main sonographic finding in acute pancreatitis is an enlarged, edematous pancreas that is hypoechoic to the normal liver parenchyma (Fig. 3-15). This pattern is more readily apparent during the first hours after the acute attack, with a decrease in pancreatic size and a return to the normal pattern as the disease resolves. Usually the entire gland becomes enlarged, but occasionally only portions of it are affected (e.g., pancreatitis caused by trauma). If a patient has a history of repeated episodes of acute pancreatitis, the acute pattern may be superimposed on chronic changes. This pattern is more typical in alcoholics. The sonographer should check for an enlarged pancreatic duct, which should measure no greater than 2 to 3 mm.[12] Acute

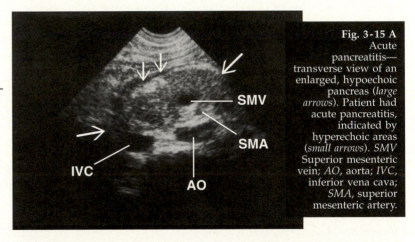

Fig. 3-15 A Acute pancreatitis—transverse view of an enlarged, hypoechoic pancreas (*large arrows*). Patient had acute pancreatitis, indicated by hyperechoic areas (*small arrows*). *SMV* Superior mesenteric vein; *AO*, aorta; *IVC*, inferior vena cava; *SMA*, superior mesenteric artery.

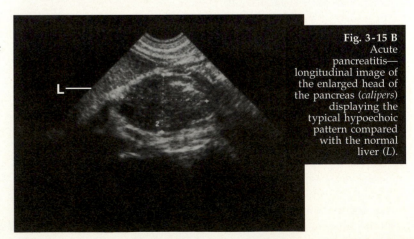

Fig. 3-15 B Acute pancreatitis—longitudinal image of the enlarged head of the pancreas (*calipers*) displaying the typical hypoechoic pattern compared with the normal liver (*L*).

pancreatitis can cause a paralytic ileus that may obscure the pancreatic area. If the clinical history does not reveal a cause for the attack, the sonographer should scan the liver for signs of cirrhosis and the biliary system for evidence of stones. In approximately 20% of cases the cause for the acute attack remains unknown. The sonographic pattern in acute hemorrhagic pancreatitis varies according to the clotting stage of the blood in the gland. In the acute stages of the attack the pancreas usually appears diffusely hypoechoic. The sonographer should check for adjacent collections of blood in the pancreatic bed. As the time from onset increases, the pattern may change to complex.[8] Complications from acute pancreatitis include the development of infection, or phlegmon, in the adjacent retroperitoneal and peritoneal spaces, pseudocyst, hemorrhage, and abscess. The physician may request a follow-up examination if clinical symptoms indicate the development of one of these complications.

Chronic Pancreatitis

Chronic pancreatitis, or chronic relapsing pancreatitis, results from a series of bouts with acute pancreatitis, which causes progressive fibrosis and destruction of the pancreatic cells. The majority of cases of chronic pancreatitis occurs in patients with a long history of alcohol abuse and repeated attacks of acute pancreatitis. Chronic pancreatitis caused by gallstones is rare, particularly after cholecystectomy. In the late stages of the disease the fibrosis of the pancreatic tissues causes alternating areas of strictures and dilatations in the ductal system and may lead to the development of retention cysts. In the very late stages calcifications occur in the ductal system but rarely in the parenchyma itself.[1]

The clinical symptoms of chronic pancreatitis include recurrent bouts of epigastric pain radiating to the back, as well as anorexia, nausea, vomiting, and constipation. In the later stages the pain changes from intermittent to continuous, with narcotic addiction common. In contrast, patients with gallstone-induced pancreatitis may have recurrent attacks, but they rarely cause the fibrotic changes associated with alcoholic pancreatitis.[1]

Elevation of the amylase and lipase values may occur during acute attacks. ERCP is very helpful in diagnosing chronic pancreatitis. The presence of pancreatic calcifications on radiographic examination also verifies the presence of this disease.

In the early stages of chronic pancreatitis the sonographic pattern mimics that of acute pancreatitis—an enlarged, hypoechoic gland. However, this pattern becomes difficult to diagnose when the liver has undergone cirrhotic changes. In the later stages of the disease the pancreas decreases in size, has irregular borders, and becomes hyperechoic in comparison with the normal liver parenchyma. The examination may also reveal the presence of ductal calcifications and dilated, tortuous pancreatic ducts (Fig. 3-16). Occasionally, the calcifications become so prominent that strong acoustic shadowing interferes with the identification of surrounding vascular landmarks and the gland itself. The sonographer should carefully check for the formation of pseudocysts and other complications of alcohol abuse such as splenomegaly and ascites.

Pseudocysts

Pancreatic pseudocysts account for three fourths of all cystic masses of the pancreas. Pseudocysts, unlike true cysts, have a fibrous lining that surrounds a collection of pancreatic juice and necrotic debris. Usually this structure results from a disruption of the ductal system of the pancreas. Most pseudocysts are unilocular, although some are multilocular. The most common location for pseudocyst development is in the lesser sac in close proximity to the tail. However, they may arise anywhere in the gland and occupy adjacent areas such as the transverse mesocolon and omentum, and even distant sites such as the mediastinum and pelvis. The location depends to a large extent on the site of disruption and the extent of injury.

The two primary causes of pseudocyst development are alcoholic pancreatitis and traumatic injury to the pancreas. There is a high incidence of pseudocyst with alcohol abuse. The typical patient is a man in his forties or fifties with a prior history of pancreatitis. The clinical symptoms include persistent pain, fever, and ileus, usually starting 2 to 3 weeks after an acute attack of pancreatitis or trauma to the pancreas. Nausea, vomiting, and anorexia are present in approximately 20% of the cases, and a palpable mass is present is 75%.[6] Usually patients with a pancreatitic pseudocyst have persistently elevated amylase levels.

The typical pseudocyst appears sonographically as a cystic mass in the area of the pancreas (Fig. 3-17). Typically the walls are thicker than in a true cyst and may contain calcifications and echogenic debris. The sonographer must ensure that a fluid-filled stomach or bowel loop is

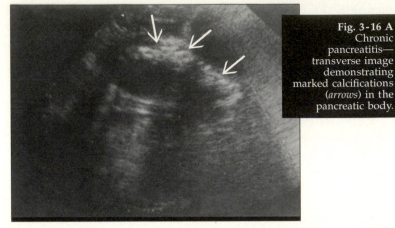

Fig. 3-16 A Chronic pancreatitis—transverse image demonstrating marked calcifications (*arrows*) in the pancreatic body.

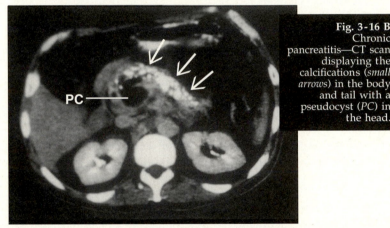

Fig. 3-16 B Chronic pancreatitis—CT scan displaying the calcifications (*small arrows*) in the body and tail with a pseudocyst (*PC*) in the head.

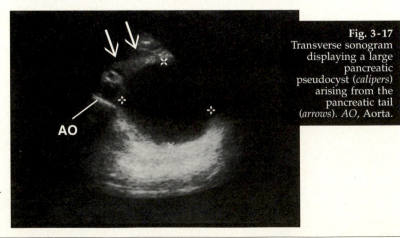

Fig. 3-17 Transverse sonogram displaying a large pancreatic pseudocyst (*calipers*) arising from the pancreatic tail (*arrows*). *AO,* Aorta.

not mistaken for a pseudocyst. If not contraindicated, the patient may drink water; the sonographer may then identify the microbubble production in the stomach. If the patient has a nasogastric tube, the stomach may be aspirated, or a repeat examination may be performed. The sonographer should check the surgical history for evidence of any surgical drainage procedures, such as a marsupilization. This history will affect the sonographic interpretation. Serial sonographic examinations may be necessary to monitor the maturation of the pseudocyst wall, which normally takes 4 to 6 weeks. At maturation, surgical drainage procedures can be performed, although a pseudocyst may undergo spontaneous regression and require no further treatment.

True Pancreatic Cysts

The walls of true pancreatic cysts contain an epithelial lining and are either congenital or acquired later in life. Although extremely rare, the congenital cysts can occur singly or in groups; the latter case includes polycystic disease. Dermoid cysts and fibrocystic disease fall into the congenital category. Acquired cysts encompass three types: retention, parasitic, and neoplastic cysts. A **retention cyst** is a dilatation of the pancreatic duct, almost exclusively a result of pancreatitis. **Parasitic cysts** are very rare in the United States. **Neoplastic cysts,** which are fairly uncommon, include the benign cystadenoma and the malignant cystadenocarcinoma. The cystadenoma occurs more frequently than the malignant variety.[7] All of these neoplastic cysts, including the cystadenocarcinoma, grow slowly, occur more frequently in women than in men, and are most common in patients over 60 years of age.

Because they are slow growing, these cysts may remain asymptomatic for years. When symptomatic, the patient often develops an abdominal mass. Other symptoms are dyspepsia and jaundice. Cystadenocarcinoma may present with additional symptoms such as unexplained weight loss, a Courvoisier gallbladder, and upper abdominal pain radiating to the back.

Usually these lesions display all the sonographic features of a cyst: smooth, regular wall, anechoic interior, and distal acoustic enhancement. In fact it may be difficult to distinguish between the benign and malignant varieties or to differentiate these true cysts from pseudocysts. The clinical history and pertinent clinical laboratory tests will help narrow the differential diagnosis. The sonographer should check for a history of adult polycystic disease and scan the kidneys for evidence of bilateral cystic involvement. Although rare, polycystic disease may involve the pancreas (Fig. 3-18). If the clinical history excludes other possibilities, single or multiple cysts in an elderly woman should make the sonographer suspicious of cystadenoma or cystadenocarcinoma.

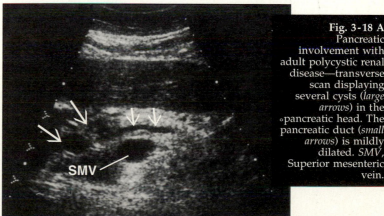

Fig. 3-18 A Pancreatic involvement with adult polycystic renal disease—transverse scan displaying several cysts (*large arrows*) in the pancreatic head. The pancreatic duct (*small arrows*) is mildly dilated. *SMV,* Superior mesenteric vein.

SMV

Carcinoma of the Pancreas

Carcinoma, the most common neoplasm of the pancreas, occurs in the head of the pancreas in approximately 75% of cases, with the remainder occurring in the body and tail. Adenocarcinoma is the most common type of pancreatic carcinoma. It arises from the ductal system in 90% of cases, with the remaining 10% arising from the acinar cells.[15] The primary malignancy is usually quite small and is surrounded by a region of pancreatitis, particularly when the lesion is located in the head. The duct of Wirsung may dilate and follow a tortuous course. The routes for metastatic spread include the stomach and duodenum, portal vein, inferior vena cava, lymph nodes, and liver.[13] Carcinoma of the pancreatic head, duodenum, and ampulla of Vater are often indistinguishable at surgery, particularly with the presence of pancreatitis.[16]

Unexplained weight loss is the primary symptom of pancreatic carcinoma. The patient may

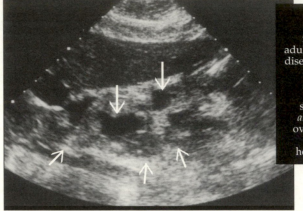

Fig. 3-18 B Pancreatic involvement with adult polycystic renal disease—longitudinal view of the pancreatic head demonstrating several cysts (*large arrows*), causing an overall enlargement of the pancreatic head (*small arrows*).

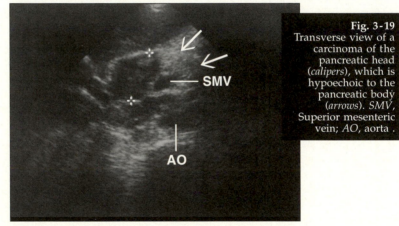

Fig. 3-19 Transverse view of a carcinoma of the pancreatic head (*calipers*), which is hypoechoic to the pancreatic body (*arrows*). *SMV*, Superior mesenteric vein; *AO*, aorta.

also complain of dull, aching pain in the midepigastric region, often radiating to the back. With carcinoma of the head of the pancreas, 75% of patients will experience progressive jaundice and may develop a Courvoisier gallbladder. Eighty percent of these patients already have liver metastases. The frequency of pancreatic carcinoma doubles in diabetic patients compared with nondiabetic patients.[13]

The most important clinical laboratory tests are those designed to evaluate obstructive jaundice and particularly those designed to demonstrate suspected masses in the pancreatic head. The direct bilirubin and alkaline phosphatase levels are elevated. Half of the patients will have abnormalities on radiographic examination, such as a widened duodenal loop or displaced antrum of the stomach.

Typically, carcinoma of the pancreas displays a hypoechoic, irregular mass in the head of the pancreas (Fig. 3-19), although it may be isoechoic, complex, or hyperechoic. Because clinical symptoms present late in this disease, the sonographer should evaluate the retroperitoneal lymph nodes and the liver for evidence of metastasis. With superimposed pancreatitis, the remainder of the gland may be large and edematous with a dilated pancreatic duct. All of these processes can distort the normal vascular landmarks, which can make identification of the pancreas difficult. When the mass is in the head of the pancreas, the sonographer must check for signs of obstructive jaundice—dilated common bile duct and intrahepatic ducts and a Courvoisier gallbladder. If the primary mass lies in the body or tail, the malignancy does not typically cause obstructive jaundice (Fig. 3-20). Scans must demonstrate the connection of the mass to the surrounding pancreatic tissue in order to specify the organ of origin. Giving the patient some water to drink may allow easier visualization of the mass and may allow proper identification of the organ of origin.

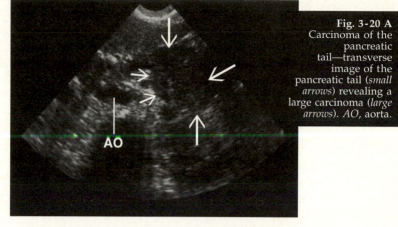

Fig. 3-20 A Carcinoma of the pancreatic tail—transverse image of the pancreatic tail (*small arrows*) revealing a large carcinoma (*large arrows*). *AO*, aorta.

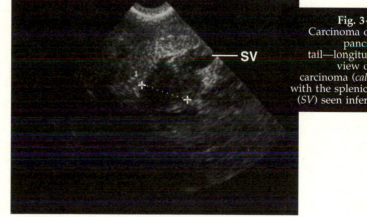

Fig. 3-20 B Carcinoma of the pancreatic tail—longitudinal view of the carcinoma (*calipers*) with the splenic vein (*SV*) seen inferiorly.

Benign Pancreatic Neoplasms

The most frequent benign tumor of the pancreas is the adenoma or islet cell tumor. These neoplasms develop in the beta cells of the pancreas and are often asymptomatic. Functional islet cell tumors secrete abnormal amounts of polypeptide hormone, and these tumors are subdivided according to the type of hormone that is oversecreted. The **insulinoma,** the most common type of islet tumor, oversecretes insulin, which causes hypoglycemia. In **Zollinger-Ellison syndrome,** the tumor causes an overproduction of gastrin. Glucagonoma syndrome is associated with hypersecretion of glucagon; somatostatinoma syndrome is associated with somatostatin. In Verner-Morrison syndrome, the neoplasm causes oversecretion of vasoactive intestinal polypeptide. Various bioassay tests will demonstrate the elevated hormone level. These functional tumors may be benign or malignant.[2]

Most patients with islet cell tumors are between the ages of 40 and 70, and the incidence is equally divided between men and women. Other symptoms vary depending on the specific overactive hormone. For example, the insulinoma causes hyperinsulinism, or large amounts of circulating insulin, which can produce severe hypoglycemia. If the blood glucose level falls rapidly, the main clinical symptoms are sweating, hunger, weakness, and tachycardia. If the blood glucose level drops slowly, the symptoms include headaches, mental confusion, visual disturbances, convulsions, and coma.[15]

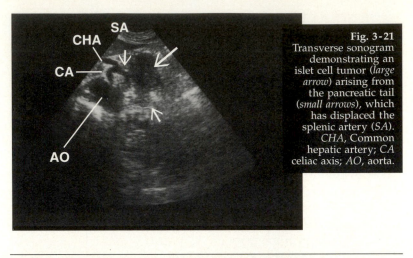

Fig. 3-21
Transverse sonogram demonstrating an islet cell tumor (*large arrow*) arising from the pancreatic tail (*small arrows*), which has displaced the splenic artery (*SA*). *CHA*, Common hepatic artery; *CA* celiac axis; *AO*, aorta.

When these tumors are small, sonographic examination typically demonstrates a round, homogeneous, discrete hypoechoic mass. The most common location is in the body and tail. Larger masses tend to demonstrate a more hyperechoic pattern[15] (Fig. 3-21). Insulinomas and gastrinomas are the most difficult masses to visualize on sonography. CT and magnetic resonance imaging may be more useful for detecting these tumors.

TECHNICAL PITFALLS

The most common problem in pancreatic sonography is nonvisualization of the gland. Using all the available techniques, such as water and various patient positions, the visualization rate for

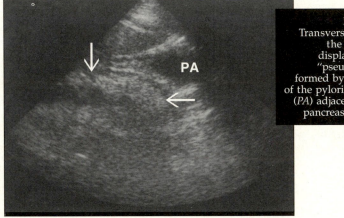

Fig. 3-22
Transverse scan of the pancreas displaying the "pseudo duct" formed by the wall of the pyloric antrum (*PA*) adjacent to the pancreas (*arrows*).

any ultrasound department should be in the 90% range.[3,9] On transverse scans the sonographer should initially search for a portion of the splenic vein, oblique the scanning path until the vein appears as a long tubular structure, and then look anteriorly for pancreatic tissue.

Another source of confusion is the duodenum, particularly when it is partially or totally distended. A common mistake is including the duodenum as part of the pancreatic head, which could lead to a false-positive diagnosis.[3] By using one of the alternative patient positions described previously, or by giving the patient water to drink, the sonographer can usually distinguish the duodenum from the pancreas. The duodenum, pylorus, and stomach can also cause errors in determining the size of the body and tail of the pancreas. The interface between the pancreas and duodenal or stomach wall can look like the pancreatic duct, which may lead the sonographer to include the structure in the pancreatic measurement[11] (Fig. 3-22). Before measuring, the sonographer should trace the course of the "duct." Typically it extends anterior to and more lateral than the pancreas. Evidence of peristalsis will also help the sonographer to avoid this pitfall. A portion of the splenic artery can also mimick the pancreatic duct.[14] The use of color-flow Doppler and tracing the course will alleviate this pitfall. In general, a longitudinal scan allows easier identification of the duct surrounded by pancreatic tissue and also demonstrates the surrounding vascular structures.

Another problem occurs in the thin patient. As mentioned previously, the pancreas is surprisingly superficial in these patients, and a higher frequency is essential in visualizing the pancreas. In addition, the pancreas in these individuals may lie quite inferiorly, even at the level of the umbilicus. A linear array may also improve the quality of the image. Looking for the pertinent vascular landmarks will allow the sonographer to localize the pancreas in this unique position. The "left-sided" pancreas poses another dilemma for the sonographer. The typical patient for this positional anomaly is a thin, elderly patient. Usually the superior mesenteric artery is located toward the left lateral border of the aorta; usually the body and tail are also more lateral, and the head of the pancreas is often anterior to the aorta instead of anterior to the inferior vena cava. The splenic vein and the body and tail of the pancreas may course in a more superior-to-inferior direction. Sorting out the vascular anatomy and obtaining the proper scan obliquity usually allow the proper identification of the pancreas.

TABLE 3-2   CLINICAL LABORATORY TEST VALUES – PANCREAS

	SGOT/SGPT	ALP	DIR BR	IND BR	AMYLASE	Other Tests
ACUTE PANCREATITIS	Normal	Normal Increase	Normal Increase†	Normal	Increase	Increased Lipase and WBC
CHRONIC PANCREATITIS	Normal Increase*	Normal Increase	Normal Increase†	Normal Increase*	Normal Increase	Normal Increased Lipase
PSEUDOCYST	Normal	Normal Increase	Normal Increase†	Normal	Increase	Increased Lipase
TRUE CYST	Normal	Normal	Normal	Normal	Normal Increase	
CARCINOMA, HEAD	Normal Increase*	Increase	Increase	Normal Increase*	Normal Increase	
CARCINOMA, BODY OR TAIL	Normal Increase*	Normal Increase	Normal Increase	Normal Increase*		
INSULINOMA	Normal	Normal	Normal	Normal	Normal	Increased Insulin
ZOLLINGER-ELLISON SYNDROME	Normal	Normal	Normal	Normal	Normal	Increased

*The liver function tests may be abnormal in the case of metastatic infiltration or cirrhosis.

†Elevation of the bilirubin depends on the site, cause, and duration of obstruction.

SGOT–serum glutamic oxaloacetic transaminase, SGPT–serum glutamic pyruvic transaminase, ALP–alkaline phosphatase, DIR DR–direct bilirubin, IND BR–indirect bilirubin, WBC–white blood cell count.

SUMMARY

The sonographer must again correlate the clinical symptoms and the results of the laboratory tests with the sonographic patterns demonstrated during the examination. As with any suspected malignant mass, scanning the liver and retroperitoneal lymph nodes for signs of metastases will often narrow the differential diagnosis. Any patient with a marked elevation of the direct bilirubin requires a careful evaluation of the pancreas for evidence of a malignancy. Table 3-2 summarizes the clinical laboratory test data with specific pathologic conditions of the pancreas.

REFERENCES

1. Alpern MB, Sandler MA, et al: Chronic pancreatitis: ultrasound features, *Radiology* 155:215, 1985.
2. Binkivitz LA, Johnson CD, Stephens DH: Islet cell tumors in von Hippel-Lindau disease: increased prevalence and relationship to the multiple endocrine neoplasias, *AJR* 155:501, 1990.
3. Crade M, Taylor KJW, Rosenfield AT: Water distension of the gut in the evaluation of the pancreas by ultrasound, *AJR* 131:348, 1978.
4. Craig M: *Pocket guide to ultrasound measurements,* Philadelphia, 1988, JB Lippincott.
5. Eisenberg R, Amberg J, editors: *Critical diagnostic pathways in radiology: an algorithmic approach,* Philadelphia, 1981, JB Lippincott.
6. Gonzalez AC, Bradley EL, Clements JL Jr: Pseudocyst formation in acute pancreatitis: ultrasonographic evaluation of 99 cases, *AJR* 127:315, 1976.
7. Hadidi A: Pancreatic duct diameter: sonographic measurement in normal subjects, *J Clin Ultrasound* 11:17, 1983.
8. Hashimoto BE, Laing FC, et al: Hemorrhagic pancreatic fluid collections examined by ultrasound, *Radiology* 150:803, 1984.
9. MacMahon H, Bowie JD, Beezhold C: Erect scanning of the pancreas using a gastric window, *AJR* 132:587, 1979.
10. Marks WM, Filly RA, Callen PW: Ultrasonic evaluation of normal pancreatic echogenicity and its relationship to fat deposition, *Radiology* 137:475, 1980.
11. McGahan JP: The posterior gastric wall: a possible source of confusion in the identification of the pancreatic duct, *J Clin Ultrasound* 12:366, 1984.
12. Parulekar SG: Ultrasonic evaluation of the pancreatic duct, *J Clin Ultrasound* 8:457, 1980.
13. Robbins SL, Cotran RS, editors: *The pancreas. In pathologic basis of disease,* Philadelphia, 1979, WB Saunders.
14. Sanders RC, Chang R: A variant position of the splenic artery mimicking the pancreatic duct, *J Clin Ultrasound* 10:391, 1982.
15. Shawker TH, Doppman JL, et al: Ultrasonic investigation of pancreatic islet cell tumors, *J Ultrasound Med* 1:193, 1982.
16. Shawker TH, Garra BS, Hill MC: The spectrum of sonographic findings in pancreatic carcinoma, *J Ultrasound Med* 5:169, 1986.
17. Wolfman NT, Ramquist NA, et al: Cystic neoplasms of the pancreas: CT and sonography, *AJR* 138:37, 1982.

4

urinary system

INSTRUCTIONAL OBJECTIVES

At the completion of this chapter, the reader will be able to:

1. Describe the clinical problems that are typical reasons for urinary system sonography.

2. Identify on transverse, longitudinal, and coronal illustrations and sonograms the major anatomic structures of the kidneys, including the medulla and renal pyramids, the cortex, calyces, renal pelvis, renal arteries and their veins and branches, the perinephric space, the quadratus lumborum and psoas major muscles, and the major structures and anatomic landmarks surrounding the kidneys.

3. Identify on transverse and longitudinal illustrations and sonograms the proximal and distal ureters, the urinary bladder and the major organs, and the anatomic landmarks used for the localization of each.

4. Describe the basic scanning protocol for sonography of the urinary system as defined by national professional organizations.

5. Describe the clinical laboratory tests used for evaluating the function of the urinary system, including the blood urea nitrogen, creatinine, urine pH, and urinary specific gravity, and tests for the presence of blood cells and casts in the urine.

6. Describe the clinical symptoms and pathologic basis for the disease processes of the urinary system, including renal anomalies, renal dysplasia, polycystic kidney diseases, simple cysts, obstructive uropathy, renal failure, benign and malignant renal tumors, renal abscess and hematoma, renal transplant complications, and anomalies, infections, and benign and malignant tumors of the ureters and bladder.

7. Identify on sectional sonograms the above-mentioned disease processes of the urinary system based on their sonographic appearance, the clinical history, and the results of other diagnostic procedures.

8. List several technical pitfalls associated with sonography of the urinary system.

THE CLINICAL PROBLEM

Renal function is crucial to life, and therefore it is imperative for the clinician to investigate any signs of renal dysfunction. Typically, clinical laboratory tests for the urinary system show abnormal values, which by themselves often do not differentiate the cause. Sonography plays an important role in differentiating medical renal diseases, such as renal failure, from obstructive uropathy caused by stones or tumors. Since the treatments are quite different for these two general disease processes, this differentiation on sonography provides very useful information to the clinician. The intravenous pyelogram (IVP) continues to serve as the radiographic standard for determining the status of renal function and as a screen for renal masses. If a mass is demonstrated on an IVP, a sonographic examination is usually requested to determine whether it is cystic or solid. To obtain a high-quality diagnostic examination, the sonographer must know and understand renal anatomy and physiology, pertinent clinical laboratory procedures, related diagnostic examinations, the technical aspects of an acceptable examination, clinical symptomology, and the sonographic characteristics of anomalous and pathologic disorders.

NORMAL ANATOMY

The kidneys are located in the retroperitoneal cavity, and each is approximately 11.25 cm long, 5.0 to 7.5 cm wide, and 2.5 cm thick. Table 4-1 contains the normal range of sonographic measurements.[4] Each lies in the paravertebral gutter adjacent to the vertebral column at an oblique angle, with the superior poles more medially located than the lower poles. Normally the presence of the liver causes the right kidney to lie more inferiorly than the left kidney. The right kidney is bordered by the liver and adrenal gland superiorly, by the abdominal wall posteriorly, by the hepatic flexure of the colon inferiorly and occasionally anteriorly, and by the duodenum medially. The left kidney is bordered by the abdominal wall and adrenal gland posteriorly, by the spleen and splenic flexure of the colon laterally, by the pancreas and duodenum medially, by the diaphragm superiorly, and by the intestines inferiorly (Fig. 4-1). Each kidney, encased in an outer fibrous capsule, is surrounded by perirenal fat, the thickness depending on the relative obesity of the individual. The perirenal space is defined by **Gerota's fascia** and extends superiorly to surround the adrenal glands and terminates inferior to the kidneys at the approximate level of the iliac crests. The **posterior pararenal space** lies posterior to the perirenal space and extends superiorly where it terminates adjacent to the diaphragm. The **quadratus lumborum** muscle is located posterior to each kidney. The **psoas major muscle** is located medial to each kidney. The **anterior pararenal space** is situated at the anterior aspect of the perirenal space. Chapter 7 contains illustrations of these potential spaces. Renal pathologic disorders may invade these potential retroperitoneal spaces.

The renal parenchyma consists of an outer layer, the **cortex,** and an inner layer, the **medulla.** In the medulla, a substructure termed the **renal pyramid** is often demon-

TABLE 4-1 RENAL MEASUREMENTS		
LENGTH	ANTERIOR-POSTERIOR	TRANSVERSE
9 cm to 12 cm	2.5 cm to 3.0 cm	4 cm to 5 cm

strated sonographically as a series of triangular structures with the bases pointing toward the cortex and the apexes pointing toward the renal hilum. The **renal hilum** is located at the medial aspect of each kidney, which provides the entrance and exit points for the renal vessels. The renal hilum or sinus contains a variable amount of adipose tissue, various vascular tributaries, lymphatics, and the calyces, which collect the urine produced by the kidneys. The renal pelvis is actually the expanded ureter as it courses superiorly through the hilum (Fig. 4-2).

The **right renal artery** arises from the abdominal aorta, travels transversely posterior to the inferior vena cava and the right renal vein, and enters the hilum of the right kidney, where it branches into numerous tributaries including the segmental, lobar, and arcuate arteries. The arcuate arteries course parallel to the bases of the renal pyramids. The **left renal artery** arises from the aorta and travels to the hilum of the left kidney, where it is posterior to the left renal vein and divides into the tributaries mentioned above (Fig. 4-3). Both **renal veins** exit their respective hilum and join the inferior vena cava, causing the right renal vein to be much shorter than the left. In the area of the renal hilum, the renal veins are anterior to the arteries (Fig. 4-4). The renal pelvis and ureter are located posterior to the renal arteries and adjacent to the hilum.

The ureters course inferiorly anterior to the psoas muscles.

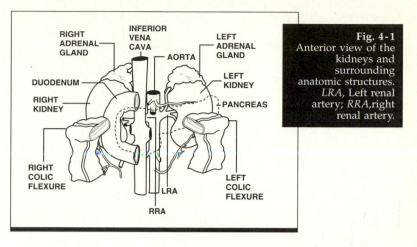

Fig. 4-1
Anterior view of the kidneys and surrounding anatomic structures. *LRA,* Left renal artery; *RRA,* right renal artery.

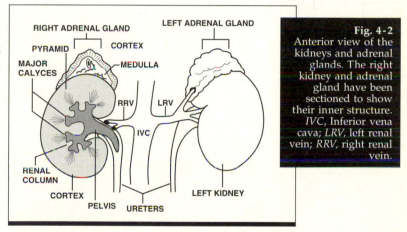

Fig. 4-2
Anterior view of the kidneys and adrenal glands. The right kidney and adrenal gland have been sectioned to show their inner structure. *IVC,* Inferior vena cava; *LRV,* left renal vein; *RRV,* right renal vein.

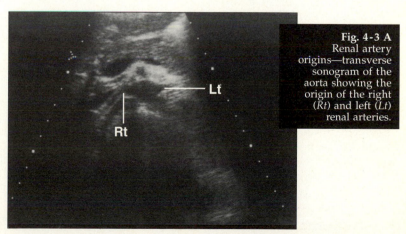

Fig. 4-3 A
Renal artery origins—transverse sonogram of the aorta showing the origin of the right (*Rt*) and left (*Lt*) renal arteries.

The **ureters** join the urinary bladder at the posterosuperior aspect of the bladder floor, or **trigone.** At the anterior apex of the trigone, the urethra leaves the bladder and courses through the prostate and penis in the male, whereas the female urethra has a much shorter course (Fig. 4-5).

CLINICAL LABORATORY TESTS

The main function of the kidneys is the production of urine. This function is very important to the maintenance of homeostasis, which is the balance between the intake and output of water and electrolytes, and the acid-base balance. Examples of some of the substances that cannot be maintained in normal blood concentrations in cases of renal dysfunction include sodium, potassium, chloride, and waste products (e.g., urea). The kidneys also play a role in the maintenance of normal blood pressure.

The functional unit of the kidney is the **nephron.** Each nephron consists of a series of ducts and other specialized subcomponents, such as the glomerulus, which filter reusable products that are transported to other organs for reprocessing. The nephron also removes waste products from the blood and transports the urine to the renal pelvis, where it travels through the ureters to the urinary bladder for elimination.

Blood Urea Nitrogen

Urea is the primary nonprotein waste product of protein catabolism. It is formed in the liver and

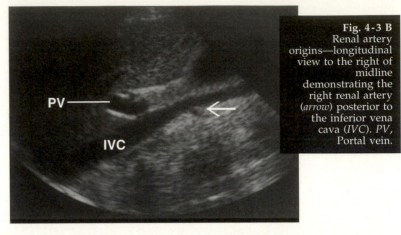

Fig. 4-3 B Renal artery origins—longitudinal view to the right of midline demonstrating the right renal artery (*arrow*) posterior to the inferior vena cava (*IVC*). *PV,* Portal vein.

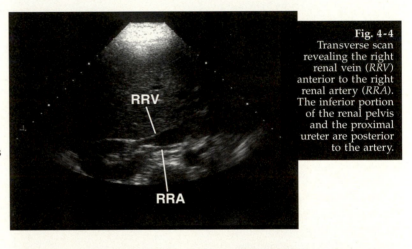

Fig. 4-4 Transverse scan revealing the right renal vein (*RRV*) anterior to the right renal artery (*RRA*). The inferior portion of the renal pelvis and the proximal ureter are posterior to the artery.

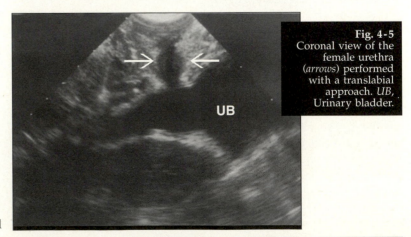

Fig. 4-5 Coronal view of the female urethra (*arrows*) performed with a translabial approach. *UB,* Urinary bladder.

transported via the blood to the kidneys, which excrete it into the urine. The blood urea nitrogen (BUN) assay, which measures the nitrogen portion of urea in the blood, is used as a gross index of glomerular filtration in the production and excretion of urea. Renal dysfunction and rapid protein catabolism produce an elevated BUN level. The amount of this increase depends on the amount of tissue damage, the extent of protein catabolism, and the renal excretion rate of urea nitrogen. The most common cause of an elevated BUN level is renal dysfunction caused by kidney disease or failure or urinary obstruction. Other causes include shock, dehydration, gastrointestinal hemorrhage, diabetes, and infection.

Creatinine

Creatinine is a by-product of muscle energy production that is specifically derived from the breakdown of muscle creatinine phosphate. The creatinine is removed from the muscle via the blood and is transported to the kidneys. The amount of creatinine produced is related to the person's muscle mass. The rate of this production is constant as long as the muscle mass remains constant. Renal dysfunction impairs creatinine excretion, which increases serum creatinine levels. The creatinine assay is used to monitor renal impairment and is more sensitive than the BUN assay. Causes of elevated serum creatinine include renal failure, chronic nephritis, and urinary tract obstruction.

Urinalysis

Hematuria is the presence of red blood cells or casts in the urine. This condition is one of the early manifestations of renal diseases such as acute failure or carcinoma. **Proteinuria** is the presence of protein in the urine. Any amount above a trace is abnormal. Usually proteinuria is the result of increased glomerular filtration of protein caused by renal diseases such as nephritis, polycystic disease, stones, and carcinoma. Other causes include ascites, fever, trauma, leukemia, and toxemia.

The presence of a large number of white blood cells in the urine usually indicates a urinary tract infection. White blood cell **casts** in the urine are associated with acute glomerular nephritis, pyelonephritis, and other renal inflammatory conditions.

Determination of the **urine pH level** is a screening test for renal and respiratory diseases and some metabolic disorders, and is also used to monitor diet and drug therapies. Urine pH is important in patients with renal calculi, because the calculous process partially depends on the pH of the urine. To adjust the pH to prevent stone formation, the patient is placed on a special diet to maintain a specific pH level. Alkaline urine (pH 7 or higher) is associated with urinary tract infections, chronic renal failure, and pyloric obstruction. Acidic urine (pH less than 7) is found in uncontrolled diabetes, pulmonary emphysema, and dehydration.

The test for **specific gravity** evaluates the kidney's ability to concentrate urine. This test compares the weight of urine with the weight of distilled water, which has a specific gravity of 1.00. The normal specific gravity of urine is 1.003 to 1.035. Examples of diseases with low urinary specific gravity (less concentration) include glomerular nephritis, pyelonephritis, renal failure, and diabetes insipidus. Examples of diseases with increased specific gravity (increased concentration) include diabetes mellitus, fever, hyperemesis, and diarrhea (excessive water loss). Specific gravity also depends on the hydration of the patient. For example, a large fluid intake by the patient will increase the urinary output, which may decrease the specific gravity.

RELATED IMAGING PROCEDURES

Plain Radiographic Film and Intravenous Pyelogram

The plain radiographic film, also known as the KUB (kidneys, ureters, bladder), provides information about the size, shape, and location of the kidneys. The information is limited by such factors as superimposing bowel gas, barium, overlying ribs, and motion artifacts. Renal and ureter stones containing calcium may be seen on this examination, but structural detail is limited without the use of contrast media.

The IVP, or excretory urography, examination gives more diagnostic information on both anatomic and physiologic abnormalities than the plain-film radiograph. The IVP consists of obtaining a series of timed radiographic films after the injection of an iodinated contrast material through a peripheral vein. The medium passes through the circulatory system and arrives at the kidneys. The nephrons process and excrete the material via the calcyces as part of the urine.

With normal renal function, the contrast material should adequately visualize the renal calyces, pelvis, and ureters. Usually this opacification occurs within several minutes after injection. Delayed excretion typically indicates impaired renal function. Enhancement of the collecting system with contrast material also assists in the demonstration of renal masses. This enhancement can also reveal a urinary tract obstruction by displaying dilated calyces, renal pelvis, and ureter. As the contrast medium collects in the urinary bladder, bladder masses and mass effects on the bladder contour can be seen.

The main disadvantages of the IVP include the following: (1) poor visualization in patients with acute and chronic renal failure, who have a moderate to marked increase in serum BUN and creatinine; (2) an inability to always distinguish solid from cystic tumors; and (3) obscured renal anatomy as a result of overlying bowel. Usually patients who are allergic to iodine cannot undergo this examination.

Another disadvantage is the nonspecificity of a mass effect between the calyces. This effect can be caused by a tumor or cyst, as well as by the presence of a column of Bertin, a benign congenital anomaly. In addition, fetal lobulation can distort the renal contour in a similar pattern produced by benign and malignant masses. Sonography can usually differentiate between these benign anomalies and neoplasms.

Although the IVP is the prime screening examination for renal pathology, it has some major limitations. Other modalities, including sonography, nuclear medicine, and computed tomography (CT), play important roles in the establishment of the final diagnosis.

Arteriography and Venography

Arteriography is performed by inserting a catheter into the femoral artery in the groin, advancing it to the origin of the renal artery, and injecting an iodinated contrast medium. Rapid, serial radiographs are taken. Malignant renal tumors often demonstrate a hypervascular pattern because of the presence of abnormal vessels in the mass. Usually, benign masses, such as a cyst, do not have an increased vascular supply and will typically displace the normal renal vessels. Arteriography has a high accuracy rate for the detection of renal malignancies, although some are missed because they are hypovascular. This procedure is invasive and therefore involves some morbidity and mortality risks.

Venography is performed by injecting iodinated contrast material through the femoral vein and opacifying the renal veins and inferior vena cava. This is the most direct method for determining the presence of tumor thrombus in the renal veins or inferior vena cava. The presence and extent of this type of renal carcinoma extension is very important for determining whether a tumor is resectable, as well as for defining the proper surgical approach.

Cystography

Cystography consists of the infusion of an iodinated contrast medium through a urethral cather inserted into the urinary bladder. Radiographs are then obtained. Cystography can demonstrate abnormalities in the shape or position of the bladder and reflux into the ureters. This technique can also demonstrate bladder diverticula, tumors, blood clots, and stones.

Percutaneous Nephrostomy

Percutaneous nephrostomy involves the placement of a catheter into an obstructed renal collecting system under fluoroscopic or sonographic guidance. Initially used for emergency drainage of an obstructed urinary tract, this procedure is now used for other reasons. The nephrostomy tube can alleviate a severe renal infection to determine the extent of renal function recovery. It can also serve as the first step in dissolving renal stones or establishing basket retrieval procedures.

Computed Tomography

CT has a high accuracy rate for the detection and characterization of renal masses. However, this procedure has several limitations. The differentiation between benign hemorrhagic cysts, necrotic tumors, and abscesses can be difficult. Postcontrast films taken after the venous injection of iodinated contrast material provide crucial information in establishing the diagnosis of a malignant neoplasm. Patients allergic to iodine cannot have this procedure. An advantage of CT is its ability to check for perirenal involvement from renal pathology and to localize distant metastatic sites. Other advantages include obtaining diagnostic information in obese patients and better delineation of tumors located in the medial aspect of the kidney and the peripelvic region. The ingestion of a contrast agent allows the differentiation of the bowel from soft tissue organs and masses.

Nuclear Medicine

Nuclear imaging with various ^{99m}Tc-labeled compounds provides an accurate method for determining the level of renal function and the severity of renal dysfunction. An advantage of the nuclear medicine scan over the IVP is its ability to evaluate renal function even with a moderate to severe increase in the values of serum BUN and creatinine. Flow studies can also be performed to rule out an arterial stenosis or to demonstrate the abnormal vascularity of a malignant tumor. However, the nuclear medicine scan is not as accurate as arteriography. Because nuclear imaging excels at monitoring renal function, this procedure is often performed on renal transplant patients to monitor for signs of rejection.

SCANNING PROTOCOLS AND TECHNIQUES

The routine scanning protocol for renal sonography consists of longitudinal, coronal, and transverse images. For the right kidney, the patient's position varies and includes supine, right posterior oblique, and right lateral positions. For a normal body habitus, supine and right posterior oblique positions using a subcostal approach on deep inspiration often allow good visualization of the kidney. When bowel gas interferes with this approach or when the patient is large, an intercostal approach may produce better images. A lateral patient position or the use of a lateral intercostal or subcostal approach will demonstrate the kidney in the coronal plane. This plane visualizes the calyces, renal pelvis, and proximal ureter and often provides the best documentation of renal obstruction. The left kidney provides the sonographer with a greater challenge, since soft tissue windows are limited in the left upper quadrant. The patient may stay in the supine position, but a lateral subcostal or intercostal scanning window will cause the right-handed sonographer to stretch across the patient. If this scanning position is awkward, it could cause muscle strain. The left posterior oblique or left lateral position alleviates this problem. Since the gastrointestinal tract occupies the more anterior recesses of the abdominal cavity, a midaxillary or posterolateral intercostal space provides greater access to the left kidney and allows the utilization of the spleen for imaging the upper- to mid-pole regions. If the intercostal spaces are small, or if the patient is heavy, a pillow placed under the lower rib cage and abdomen may allow easier access when the patient is in the lateral position. Another method is to simply have the patient place the arms above the head. For both kidneys, the sonographer should always include at least one image demonstrating the renal cortex with liver or spleen parenchyma to allow proper assessment of acute and chronic renal failure.

Longitudinal scans should course parallel to the long axis of each kidney. Experienced sonographers can simply rotate the transducer until an even amount of cortex appears in the upper and lower poles. For inexperienced sonographers or when a malrotation of the kidney appears, transverse scans can determine the long axis. After obtaining a transverse scan of the superior pole, the sonographer should place the transducer over the midpoint of the renal sinus, proceed to the midpole and inferior pole, and repeat the localization process. A straight line connecting the localization points should indicate the longitudinal scanning plane for the kidney (Fig. 4-6). In some cases placing the patient in the lateral position causes the kidney to rotate, so that the longitudinal plane of the kidney is parallel to the transverse body plane. Frequently, placing the patient supine allows a more normal scan plane orientation.

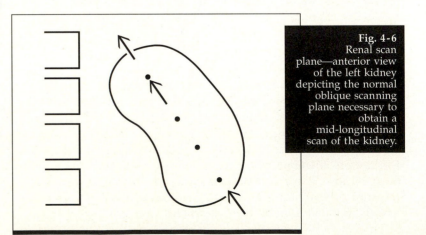

Fig. 4-6
Renal scan plane—anterior view of the left kidney depicting the normal oblique scanning plane necessary to obtain a mid-longitudinal scan of the kidney.

The basic scanning protocol for the kidneys is presented in the box on this page. All scans should be performed in sequence, and the exact number of images obtained varies with specific protocols and the type of pathology encountered. Figs. 4-7 through 4-10 illustrate the normal scanning protocol for renal sonography. Although not always documented on hard copy, the sonographer should scan medial, lateral, superior, and inferior to each kidney to ensure that no masses are present.

Usually a coronal view will allow visualization of the proximal ureter (Fig. 4-11). The midportion of the ureter courses posterior to the bowel, which often prevents its identification unless it is dilated. With a full urinary bladder, a dilated distal ureter may be seen posteriorly as it enters the trigone of the bladder (Fig. 4-11). Identification of the normal-sized ureter presents a challenge. However, the sonographer should watch for the "jet effect" of urine entering the bladder by either the use of color flow or the presence of hyperechoic microbubbles.

With a distended bladder, the course of the ureter may be traced as it ascends posterior to the bladder bilaterally. Because of its proximity to the iliac vessels, the sonographer should use color flow to verify that the structure is nonvascular.

When evaluating for bladder pathologic disorders, or to localize the cause of urinary tract obstruction, the patient's bladder should be full, but not overly distended. Longitudinal scans should include midline and right and left lateral views. Transverse scans should consist of inferior, midline, and superior views. Additional scans may be required depending on the type of pathologic conditions present.

BASIC SCANNING PROTOCOL

Longitudinal
- Medial aspect of the kidney (region of renal pelvis—a coronal scan may work better)
- Mid-long axis (for renal length measurement and demonstration of renal sinus and calyceal area)
- Lateral aspect

Transverse
- Superior pole (upper renal sinus)
- Midpole (demonstrating renal artery and vein—use for transverse and posteroanterior measurements)
- Inferior pole

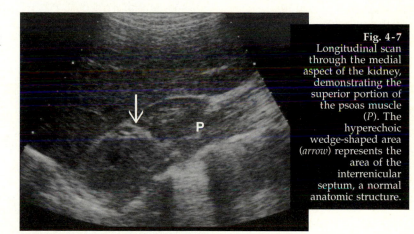

Fig. 4-7 Longitudinal scan through the medial aspect of the kidney, demonstrating the superior portion of the psoas muscle (*P*). The hyperechoic wedge-shaped area (*arrow*) represents the area of the interrenicular septum, a normal anatomic structure.

NORMAL SONOGRAPHIC PATTERNS

The normal sonographic pattern of the kidney demonstrates the hyperechoic renal sinus centrally and medially. The renal sinus contains the calyces, which distend with urine when obstructed. Normal physiologic function, which produces a small amount of urine in the calyces, should not be misidentified as hydronephrosis. If the patient drank 32 to 40 ounces of water to fill the bladder, the calyces may look very distended. The sonographer should always verify how much fluid the patient drank in order to interpret this pattern. A patient who has received nothing by mouth for a number of hours may become dehydrated to the point that a pathologic hydronephrosis may not visualize. The renal cortex should be hypoechoic to isoechoic when compared with the normal liver and spleen parenchyma. Usually an isoechoic pattern is normal if no renal dysfunction is present.[18] The renal pyramids may be isoechoic to slightly hypoechoic in the adult when compared with the normal renal cortical pattern. The pyramids are prominent and more hypoechoic in neonates and young children, and the sonographer must not mistake them for enlarged calyces. In adults with chronic renal failure, the pyramids may also appear more prominent because of the parenchymal changes in the cortex. In some patients the arcuate arteries may appear as one or a series of hyperechoic linear structures be-

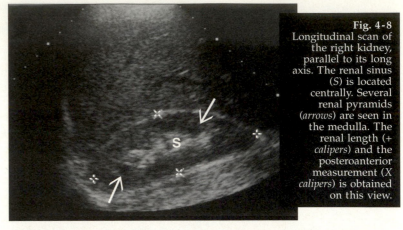

Fig. 4-8 Longitudinal scan of the right kidney, parallel to its long axis. The renal sinus (*S*) is located centrally. Several renal pyramids (*arrows*) are seen in the medulla. The renal length (+ *calipers*) and the posteroanterior measurement (*X calipers*) is obtained on this view.

Fig. 4-9 Transverse scan of the renal hilum depicting the renal vein and artery (*arrow*). The transverse length (+ *calipers*) is through the central portion of the kidney from the lateral to medial aspect of the cortex. The posteroanterior length (*X calipers*) forms a 90° angle with the transverse measurement.

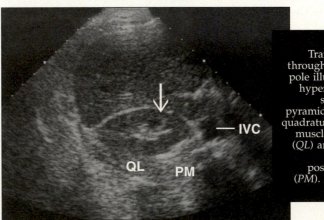

Fig. 4-10 Transverse scan through the inferior pole illustrating the hyperechoic renal sinus, a renal pyramid (*arrow*), the quadratus lumborum muscle posteriorly (*QL*) and the psoas muscle posteromedially (*PM*). *IVC*, Inferior vena cava.

tween the pyramids and the renal cortex. On transverse scans, the perinephric fat in obese individuals may appear as a moderately hyperechoic rim around the kidney. The psoas major muscle, located medial to the kidney, is best seen in transverse images. The quadratus lumborum muscle lies posterior to the kidney.

At the level of the renal hilum, the larger caliber renal vein courses anterior to the renal artery. The inferior portion of the renal pelvis and the proximal ureter lie posterior to the renal artery. The use of color flow and pulsed Doppler aid in the identification of these structures, particularly when evaluating for minimal hydronephrosis or for an extrarenal pelvis.

The normal ureter is a 1 to 2 mm tubular structure that is best seen proximally close to the renal pelvis and distally close to the urinary bladder. The distended urinary bladder should present as a thin-walled, anechoic structure. The sonographer should be aware of side lobe artifacts that can give the appearance of sludge in the bladder. Changing the scanning angle will usually eliminate this artifact.

CONGENITAL ANOMALIES

The sonographer will encounter a number of urinary system anomalies. A **column of Bertin,** a rather common anomaly, presents sonographically as a prominent invagination of cortical tissue in the medulla.[11] This disorder may cause a mass effect on IVP, but sonography reveals

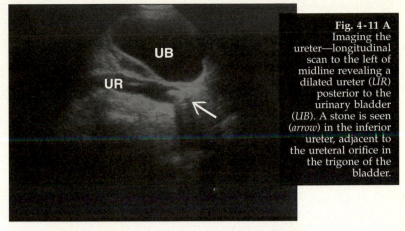

Fig. 4-11 A
Imaging the ureter—longitudinal scan to the left of midline revealing a dilated ureter (*UR*) posterior to the urinary bladder (*UB*). A stone is seen (*arrow*) in the inferior ureter, adjacent to the ureteral orifice in the trigone of the bladder.

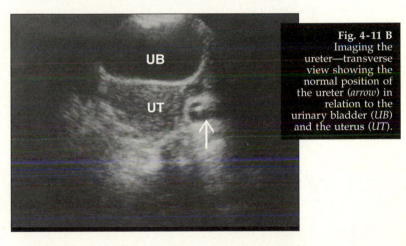

Fig. 4-11 B
Imaging the ureter—transverse view showing the normal position of the ureter (*arrow*) in relation to the urinary bladder (*UB*) and the uterus (*UT*).

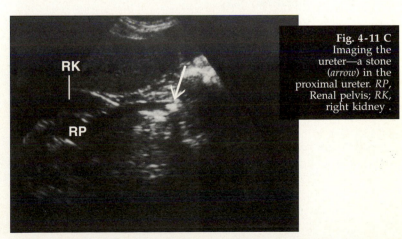

Fig. 4-11 C
Imaging the ureter—a stone (*arrow*) in the proximal ureter. *RP,* Renal pelvis; *RK,* right kidney .

that the mass is isoechoic to the surrounding cortex (Fig. 4-12). In **fetal lobulation** the normal embryologic lobulations persist and cause a scalloped outer renal margin.[16] This condition affects the left kidney more often than the right. On sonography this appears as one or several rounded "masses" distorting the renal capsule (Fig. 4-13), but the renal parenchyma has a normal pattern. On an IVP one lobulation is called a "dromedary hump," and a sonographic examination may be requested to verify that this is not a neoplasm.

Bilateral **renal agenesis** is a fatal condition. In unilateral renal agenesis the left kidney is usually absent, which causes physiologic hypertrophy of the right kidney. The sonographer must ensure that the kidney is not in an ectopic location. In utero the kidneys develop in the pelvis and later ascend to their normal position. A **pelvic kidney** occurs when one kidney fails to ascend to the normal position and remains in the pelvis. Patients with this type of anomaly may have a pelvic mass and associated pelvic pain. On sonographic examination, if a kidney does not visualize in the renal fossa, the sonographer should next scan the pelvis, preferably with a full urinary bladder. An ectopic kidney appears as a solid mass in the pelvis, but careful scanning reveals the reniform shape and normal patterns of the sinus and parenchyma (Fig. 4-14). Rarely, a kidney ascends into the thoracic cavity.

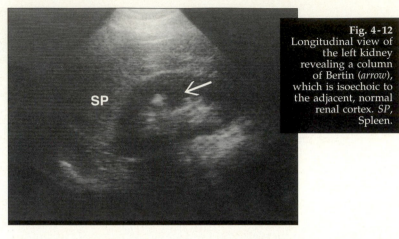

Fig. 4-12
Longitudinal view of the left kidney revealing a column of Bertin (*arrow*), which is isoechoic to the adjacent, normal renal cortex. *SP,* Spleen.

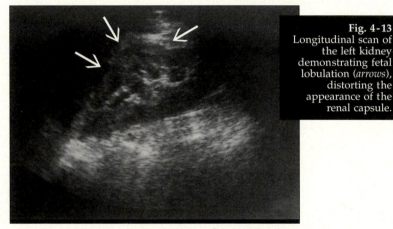

Fig. 4-13
Longitudinal scan of the left kidney demonstrating fetal lobulation (*arrows*), distorting the appearance of the renal capsule.

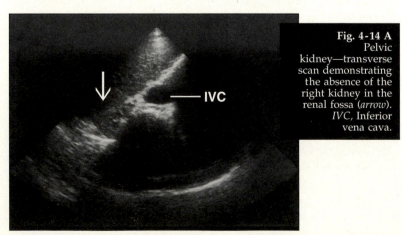

Fig. 4-14 A
Pelvic kidney—transverse scan demonstrating the absence of the right kidney in the renal fossa (*arrow*). *IVC,* Inferior vena cava.

Another example of this type of anomaly is the **horseshoe kidney**, which occurs when the kidneys remain joined by a band of fibrous or renal tissue. Usually this union occurs at the lower poles, and the root of the inferior mesenteric artery prevents the normal migration of the kidneys to the renal fossae. Other sites of union include the upper poles. Failure of the embryologic precursor tissue to divide into two kidneys produces one large renal mass of tissue, called a **unilateral fused kidney** or **crossed renal ectopia.** Usually both kidneys ascend into one renal fossa.

These anomalies are often incidental findings, as long as the ectopic location does not cause extrinsic pressure on the renal pelvis or ureter. In some patients a congenital malformation of the ureter may coexist with ectopia. This condition may lead to chronic renal infections or obstruction. The sonographer should note an elevation of the BUN and/or creatinine values or other clinical symptoms related to renal infection or failure.

Sonographically, the horseshoe kidney can prove challenging to image, since the connection may lie in the midabdomen obscured by the bowel. The sonographer should become suspicious of this condition when both kidneys appear lower than normal, the lower poles lie more medially, or the inferior portion of the kidney is ill-defined or abnormal in appearance (Fig. 4-15). The connecting band of tissue is classically located ante-

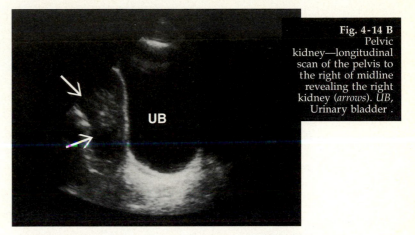

Fig. 4-14 B Pelvic kidney—longitudinal scan of the pelvis to the right of midline revealing the right kidney (*arrows*). *UB,* Urinary bladder .

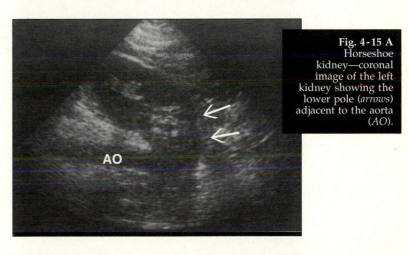

Fig. 4-15 A Horseshoe kidney—coronal image of the left kidney showing the lower pole (*arrows*) adjacent to the aorta (*AO*).

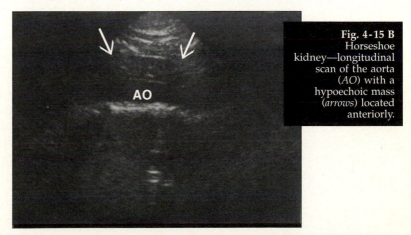

Fig. 4-15 B Horseshoe kidney—longitudinal scan of the aorta (*AO*) with a hypoechoic mass (*arrows*) located anteriorly.

rior to the aorta and may mimic the appearance of enlarged lymph nodes. The sonographic appearance of crossed fused ectopia varies according to the degree and site of the fusion. The sonographer may visualize two rather distinct kidneys in one renal fossa. However, a more typical pattern is a large, misshapen kidney. The documentation of a notch or indentation, usually seen in the posteroanterior dimension, is the most definitive sign of this anomaly.[13] The sonographer should also demonstrate that the parenchymal pattern is homogeneous and document the presence of each renal sinus area and two renal pelves. The verification that the opposite renal fossa does not contain a kidney should always be documented.

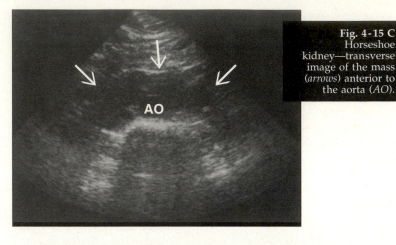

Fig. 4-15 C Horseshoe kidney—transverse image of the mass (*arrows*) anterior to the aorta (*AO*).

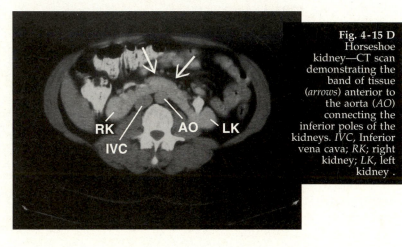

Fig. 4-15 D Horseshoe kidney—CT scan demonstrating the band of tissue (*arrows*) anterior to the aorta (*AO*) connecting the inferior poles of the kidneys. *IVC*, Inferior vena cava; *RK*; right kidney; *LK*, left kidney .

Another anomaly demonstrated by sonography is the **double collecting system.** With this condition there are two ureters draining the double collecting system of the kidney. In a normal kidney the typical sonographic pattern is two distinct, hyperechoic renal sinus areas on a longitudinal sonogram. If hydronephrosis is present, the affected system will usually show dilated calcyces and renal pelvis. The sonographer should follow the course of the ureter and determine the extent and site of obstruction.

PATHOLOGIC PROCESSES OF THE KIDNEY

Simple Renal Cyst

The simple renal cyst is one of the most common renal masses seen with sonography. Usually they occur in the renal cortex, although they can develop in the renal medulla and the peripelvic and parapelvic regions. They range in size from 1 to over 10 cm in diameter and can present as a solitary mass or in multiples. Typically they are asymptomatic, with normal BUN and creatinine values. Large cysts may cause pain or renal obstruction or exert pressure on surrounding structures. With obstruction the sonographer may find elevated BUN and creatinine values. Complications include infection and hemorrhage. An infected cyst may cause pain and fever, as well as the presence of white blood cells and casts in the urine. A substantial hemorrhage may produce a decreased hematocrit. Cysts are often incidental findings on sonography or may cause a mass effect on an IVP, which requires verification with sonography.

A simple renal cyst has smooth, thin walls that contain nonviscous fluid with no debris and exhibit acoustic enhancement (Fig. 4-16). Although most cysts are unilocular, some may contain septa. A complex pattern may indicate hemorrhage, infection, or necrotic malignancy. In these cases further investigation is indicated. If multiple cysts are seen in both kidneys, the possibility of polycystic disease must be investigated. Peripelvic cysts are located between the calyces and may be difficult to differentiate from hydronephrosis. However,

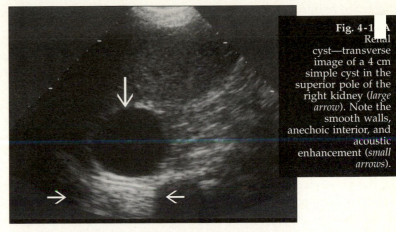

Fig. 4-16 A Renal cyst—transverse image of a 4 cm simple cyst in the superior pole of the right kidney (*large arrow*). Note the smooth walls, anechoic interior, and acoustic enhancement (*small arrows*).

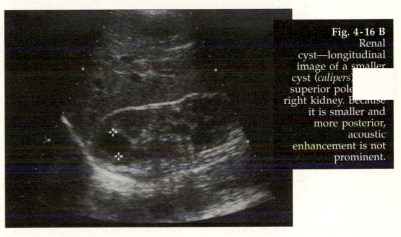

Fig. 4-16 B Renal cyst—longitudinal image of a smaller cyst (*calipers*), superior pole right kidney. Because it is smaller and more posterior, acoustic enhancement is not prominent.

unlike hydronephrosis, peripelvic cysts usually have thin walls and a circular appearance on both transverse and longitudinal views. The coronal plane may also prove useful in making this differentiation.

Polycystic Renal Diseases

Infantile polycystic disease is an inherited renal cystic disease and is characterized by dilated renal collecting tubules bilaterally and by liver involvement as a result of bile duct hyperplasia. This disorder is not related to adult polycystic disease. This disease is further divided into newborn and childhood types.

The newborn type of infantile polycystic disease develops in utero and results in nephromegaly and oligohydramnios. Usually the condition results in stillbirth or death several days after birth. Numerous complications, including renal failure, may develop in those patients who survive the neonatal period. The severity of the renal failure correlates with the abnormal elevation of BUN and creatinine values.

The childhood type of infantile polycystic disease usually occurs between the ages of 3 and 5. The clinical symptoms include hepatosplenomegaly, portal hypertension, and esophageal varices. This disease largely affects the liver with minimal renal involvement, although renal failure may occur.

Sonographically the newborn type presents as bilateral, hyperechoic kidneys as a result of microcysts. Occasionally, microcysts appear as cystic structures as they gain in size. The childhood type is characterized by multiple liver cysts. Associated fibrosis may cause hyperechoic areas within the liver parenchyma.[27]

Adult polycystic disease is an inherited trait that causes replacement of the renal parenchyma bilaterally with cysts of varying sizes. Cystic involvement of the liver occurs in approximately 33% of patients, and pancreatic involvement occurs in 10%. Involvement of other organs, such as the spleen and ovaries, is rare.

The formation of these renal cysts starts early in life but advances slowly; the clinical symptoms do not usually appear before 40 years of age. As the disease progresses, the renal function is impaired, and BUN and creatinine levels are elevated. The clinical symptoms include hematuria, hypertension, colicky pain, proteinuria, or a palpable mass. The disease is usually fatal without the use of hemodialysis and/or renal transplantation.

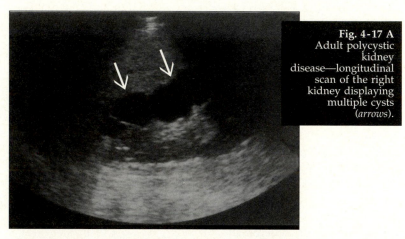

Fig. 4-17 A
Adult polycystic kidney disease—longitudinal scan of the right kidney displaying multiple cysts (*arrows*).

The typical sonographic pattern for adult polycystic disease is multiple cysts in both kidneys (Fig. 4-17). However, occasionally the disease is seen in one kidney; but when true polycystic disease involves only one kidney, it usually indicates that the disease has developed to a more advanced stage in that kidney.[12] The sonographer should scan the liver, pancreas, and spleen to rule out cystic involvement.

Renal dysplasia is a developmental anomaly that is not inherited. It is characterized by the formation of multiple renal cysts. Typically renal dysplasia occurs unilaterally and affects

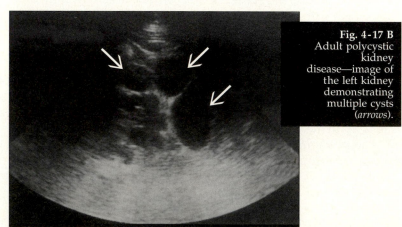

Fig. 4-17 B
Adult polycystic kidney disease—image of the left kidney demonstrating multiple cysts (*arrows*).

the entire kidney. However, it may occur in only one portion of the kidney, or it may affect both kidneys. Renal dysplasia is also referred to as unilateral polycystic disease, renal aplasia, and multicystic renal dysplasia.

Renal dysplasia is the most common form of renal cystic disease during the first month of life.[26] In neonates this benign condition usually presents first as a palpable abdominal mass. If not discovered during this period, renal dysplasia usually remains asymptomatic, although the patient may develop signs of infection or hematuria.

Typically, sonographic examination reveals multiple cysts in one kidney. The cyst walls may contain calcifications, and there is no cystic involvement of the liver or other organs.

Hydronephrosis

Obstruction of the renal collecting system has numerous causes and can occur anywhere between the minor calyces and the distal ureter. Some of the causes include renal, ureteral, and bladder stones or strictures; infections such as pyelonephritis; and benign or malignant tumors. Hydronephrosis is a dilatation of the renal calyces and pelvis resulting from an obstruction distal to these structures. An obstruction in the distal ureter or ureter-bladder junction may cause the proximal ureter to dilate. An obstruction at the level of the urethra may cause bilateral obstruction.

Generally when the obstruction is severe enough and of long duration, it will cause elevation of the BUN and creatinine levels. Obstruction caused by stones may cause flank pain, renal colic, nausea, and vomiting. The urine may contain red and white blood cells and protein. If an infection is present, there may be an elevated serum white blood cell count and bacteria in the urine. If a carcinoma is causing the obstruction, additional symptoms may include weight loss, gross hematuria, and evidence of metastasis.

Hydronephrosis appears sonographically as dilated cystic structures in the more medial aspect of the kidney (Fig. 4-18),

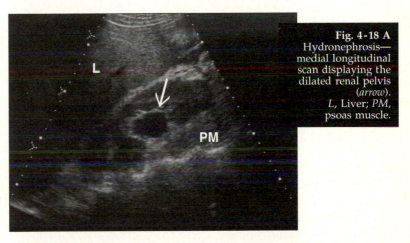

Fig. 4-18 A Hydronephrosis—medial longitudinal scan displaying the dilated renal pelvis (*arrow*). *L*, Liver; *PM*, psoas muscle.

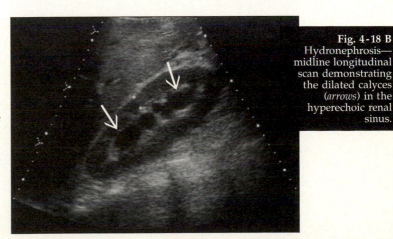

Fig. 4-18 B Hydronephrosis—midline longitudinal scan demonstrating the dilated calyces (*arrows*) in the hyperechoic renal sinus.

extending toward the midline anterior to the vertebra. Unlike peripelvic cysts, the dilated calyces have a thick, hyperechoic rim, since they are located in the renal sinus and appear circular on transverse scans and more ovoid on longitudinal views. A coronal scan can demonstrate the communication between the calyces and the renal pelvis and ureter, which allows the proper diagnosis (Fig. 4-19). Pulsed Doppler can provide additional information to assist the differentiation of obstructive from non-obstructive hydronephrosis.[3] A true obstruction appears to cause an increase in the vascular resistance at the level of the arcuate arteries. The normal mean resistive index (RI) is 0.63, whereas with obstructive uropathy the mean average is 0.77. However, the presence of various renal diseases can also increase the vascular resistance. An obstruction of longer duration can become infected and produce **pyonephrosis,** or a pus-filled collecting system, which typically appears as a sludgelike collection in the calyces.[9]

The current resolution capabilities of ultrasound equipment allow the sonographer to document small **renal calculi,** even in the absence of obstruction. The detection of renal stones is governed by the same rule as gallstone detection; it requires placing the area of interest in the focal zone of the transducer that has the best resolution possible with adequate penetration. Renal stones appear as hyperechoic structures located in the collect-

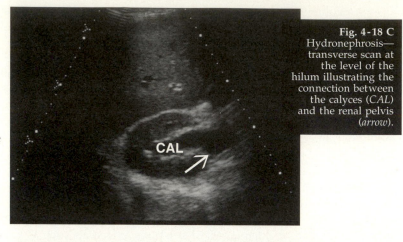

Fig. 4-18 C Hydronephrosis—transverse scan at the level of the hilum illustrating the connection between the calyces (*CAL*) and the renal pelvis (*arrow*).

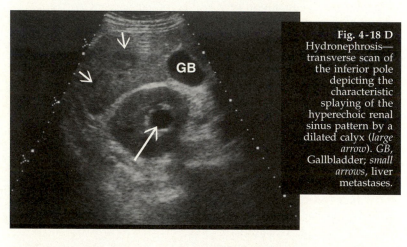

Fig. 4-18 D Hydronephrosis—transverse scan of the inferior pole depicting the characteristic splaying of the hyperechoic renal sinus pattern by a dilated calyx (*large arrow*). *GB,* Gallbladder; *small arrows,* liver metastases.

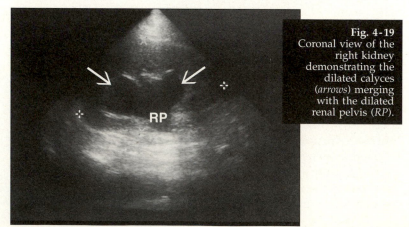

Fig. 4-19 Coronal view of the right kidney demonstrating the dilated calyces (*arrows*) merging with the dilated renal pelvis (*RP*).

ing system, which exhibits acoustic shadowing (Fig. 4-20). The use of various patient positions and scanning angles may be necessary to display these characteristics.

Benign Renal Tumors

Although not common in adults, there are several types of benign renal tumors. The **adenoma** is a type of alveolar papillary tumor that may be a precursor to malignancy. Typically adenomas are small and asymptomatic. Benign connective tissue tumors include fibromas, lipomas, myomas, angiomyolipomas, and hemangiomas. The most common symptom is painless hematuria. The angiomyolipoma contains a vascular supply that tends to bleed, producing flank pain.[1] Larger masses may interfere with renal function, indicated by elevated BUN and creatinine values.

Most solid benign renal tumors are difficult to differentiate from their malignant counterparts. Hemangioma, adenoma, and angiomyolipoma may present as rather discrete, hyperechoic masses[2] (Fig. 4-21). Often angiomyolipomas contain a high level of fatty tissue and usually occur as a solitary mass in the right kidney.[1] Fibromas or lipomas may appear as discrete, hypoechoic areas adjacent to or located in the renal sinus, or they may cause a diffuse process termed **renal sinus lipomatosis** (Fig. 4-22), which typically causes an inhomogeneous, prominent renal sinus pattern in the more obese individual. Any solid mass in the kidney requires

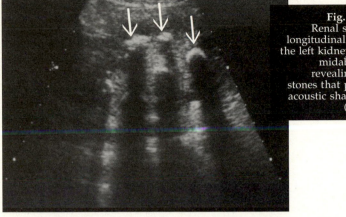

Fig. 4-20 A Renal stones—longitudinal scan of the left kidney in the midabdomen revealing large stones that produce acoustic shadowing (*arrows*).

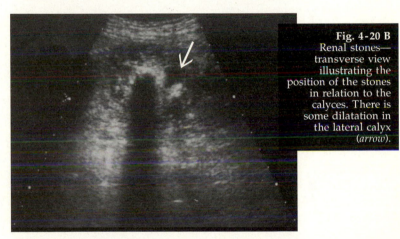

Fig. 4-20 B Renal stones—transverse view illustrating the position of the stones in relation to the calyces. There is some dilatation in the lateral calyx (*arrow*).

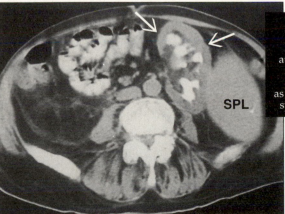

Fig. 4-20 C Renal stones—CT scan showing atypical inferior and medial positions of the kidney (*arrows*) as a result of massive splenomegaly (*SPL*).

further investigation because of the possiblity of malignancy. The use of pulsed Doppler may allow a more definitive diagnosis, since research has shown that benign renal tumors produce no Doppler signal.[22]

Renal Carcinoma

Renal cell carcinoma, or the hypernephroma, is the most common malignant renal tumor, accounting for three fourths of all renal malignancies. This neoplasm occurs more frequently in men than in women and metastasizes early to the lungs, liver, and long bones. Pathologists postulate that this malignancy arises from the renal tubule cells or develops from its benign counterpart, the renal adenoma. The renal cell carcinoma has a tendency to metastasize through the circulatory system, particularly the renal vein and inferior vena cava.

The clinical symptoms usually present after the tumor has metastasized. They include painless hematuria, fever, an enlarged palpable kidney, and evidence of metastasis. Usually clinical laboratory tests reveal red blood cells in the urine, and in cases of infection, these tests reveal bacteria and white blood cells in the urine. If the malignancy has caused a disruption of renal function, an elevation of the BUN and creatinine values occur. Tumor invasion and obstruction of the inferior vena cava causes engorged superficial veins and edema of the legs. The patient also suffers from anemia.

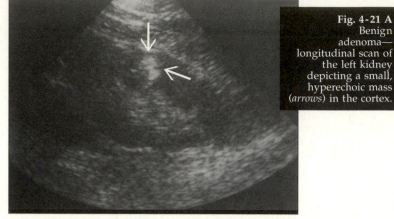

Fig. 4-21 A Benign adenoma—longitudinal scan of the left kidney depicting a small, hyperechoic mass (*arrows*) in the cortex.

Fig. 4-21 B Benign adenoma—transverse view of the left kidney depicting a small, hyperechoic mass (*arrow*) in the cortex.

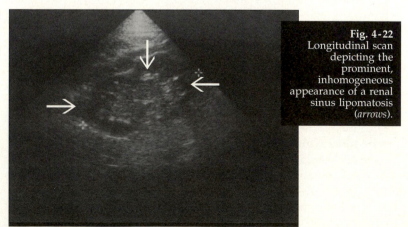

Fig. 4-22 Longitudinal scan depicting the prominent, inhomogeneous appearance of a renal sinus lipomatosis (*arrows*).

Because of the late onset of symptoms, often the primary tumor appears as a large mass that displaces and distorts the normal position of the kidney. The sonographic pattern ranges from hypoechoic, hyperechoic, to complex (Fig. 4-23). These tumors can contain areas of necrosis or cause renal obstruction.[21] Evaluation with pulsed Doppler in the presence of a vascular malignancy will typically demonstrate a frequency shift greater than 4.0 kHz, with either a large systolic-diastolic flow differential or a continuous signal.[22] Usually the flow pattern is in the periphery of the mass. Hypovascular carcinomas will not demonstrate these flow characteristics and may mimic a benign lesion. Whenever this condition is suspected, the sonographer should scan the area of the renal vein and the inferior vena cava. This malignancy has a marked tendency to invade the renal vein and extend into the inferior vena cava (Fig. 4-24). Because this tumor thrombus may be quite hypoechoic, the use of color Doppler may outline the position of the intraluminal mass. The retroperitoneal lymph nodes and the liver should be scanned for signs of metastasis.

The **transitional cell carcinoma** arises from the transitional epithelium that lines the renal pelvis, ureter, and bladder. It occurs more frequently in men than in women and seldom appears before the age of 50. The most common site for transitional cell carcinoma is the blad-

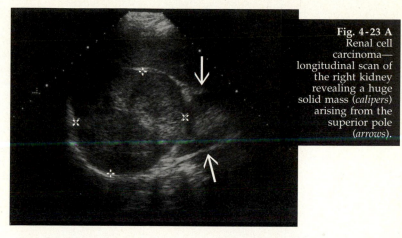

Fig. 4-23 A
Renal cell carcinoma—longitudinal scan of the right kidney revealing a huge solid mass (*calipers*) arising from the superior pole (*arrows*).

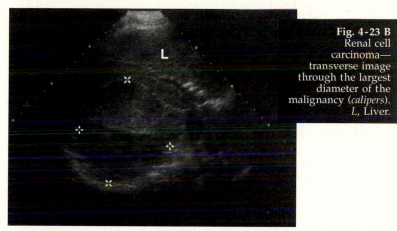

Fig. 4-23 B
Renal cell carcinoma—transverse image through the largest diameter of the malignancy (*calipers*). *L*, Liver.

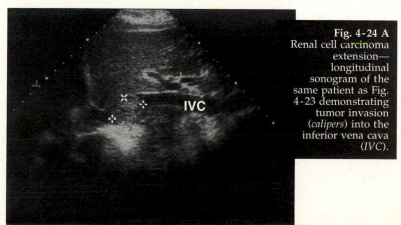

Fig. 4-24 A
Renal cell carcinoma extension—longitudinal sonogram of the same patient as Fig. 4-23 demonstrating tumor invasion (*calipers*) into the inferior vena cava (*IVC*).

der. The most common symptoms are gross hematuria and the passage of blood clots. The tumors tend to be multiple with metastasis to the ureter and bladder.

With sonography, these malignancies are difficult to differentiate from their benign counterparts. Their sonographic pattern ranges from hypoechoic to hyperechoic to the surrounding normal parenchyma and may present as a mass adjacent to the kidney, ureter, or bladder.[15] They

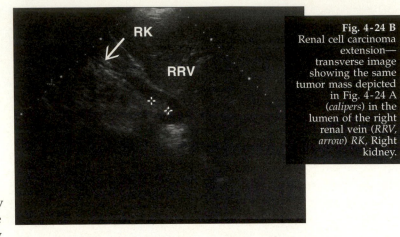

Fig. 4-24 B Renal cell carcinoma extension— transverse image showing the same tumor mass depicted in Fig. 4-24 A (*calipers*) in the lumen of the right renal vein (*RRV, arrow*) *RK*, Right kidney.

may appear as a solid mass in the renal pelvis. Transitional cell tumors are generally small and situated in or adjacent to the renal collecting system, appearing as filling defects on an IVP examination. These tumors may infiltrate to adjacent structures.

Renal lymphoma is a common metastatic pathway in patients with disseminated lymphomatous malignancies. The clinical symptoms include gross hematuria, fever, and weight loss. Usually the sonographic pattern consists of generalized renal enlargement with a diffuse hypoechoic pattern caused by cellular infiltration. However, a more localized invasion can occur.

Wilm's tumor, or nephroblastoma, characteristically occurs in children under the age of 8, with a peak incidence at 3 years. This is the most common solid renal tumor in children and accounts for 14% of renal malignancies. This malignant tumor metastasizes early to the liver, lung and brain. The most common clinical symptom is a large, asymptomatic flank mass. Other symptoms include weight loss, anorexia, hypertension, fever, and pain. Typically the sonographic pattern displays a well-defined, fairly homogeneous, large mass with the pattern ranging from hypoechoic to moderately hyperechoic.[23] These tumors can undergo necrosis, displaying central anechoic to cystic areas. The sonographer should scan the contralateral kidney and the liver for signs of metastases.

Hematoma

The kidneys are highly vascular organs and therefore are susceptible to hemorrhage secondary to trauma. Hemorrhage may also occur secondary to renal malignancies and may even occur spontaneously. The classification pattern for the extent of renal trauma consists of four general categories. The most common classification includes hematomas and/or lacerations that do not involve the collecting system. The second type includes hematomas and/or lacerations that involve the collecting system, allowing the extravasation of urine. The third type includes severely lacerated kidneys, which may disrupt the vascular supply. The fourth category, the most rare, includes laceration of the renal pelvis and/or the ureteropelvic junction.[19] For all categories, renal hematomas may occur and spread into the perinephric and paranephric spaces.

The symptoms correlate with the severity of the trauma. With minimal bleeding, the patient may complain of localized or flank pain. More massive trauma may produce severe pain, a decreased hematocrit, and signs of shock. The patient may show signs of acute renal failure, documented by increased BUN and creatinine levels. If the collecting system is involved in the injury, the patient may have gross hematuria.

The sonographic patterns for a renal hematoma vary with the clotting stages of blood. An actively bleeding hematoma may appear as a fairly homogeneous, hyperechoic area with acoustic enhancement. As the time from the initial injury increases, the pattern may range from solid to complex or cystic[19] (Fig. 4-25). Of great clinical significance is whether the calyces or the renal pelvis have been damaged, leading to the extravasation of urine. The sonographer should carefully examine the perinephric and paranephric spaces for urine collections (Fig. 4-26).

Renal Infections and Abscesses

Renal infections are a rather common clinical problem and include glomerulonephritis, acute tubular nephritis and necrosis, and pyelonephritis. The exact type depends on the type of bacteria involved and the portion of

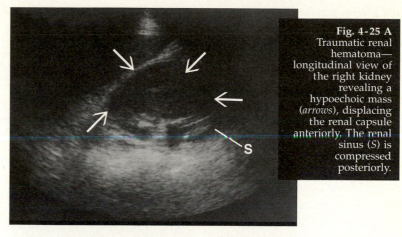

Fig. 4-25 A Traumatic renal hematoma— longitudinal view of the right kidney revealing a hypoechoic mass (*arrows*), displacing the renal capsule anteriorly. The renal sinus (*S*) is compressed posteriorly.

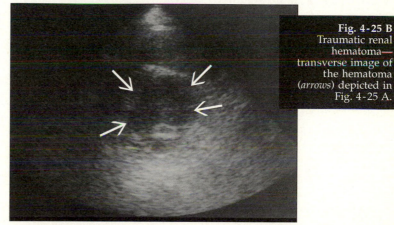

Fig. 4-25 B Traumatic renal hematoma— transverse image of the hematoma (*arrows*) depicted in Fig. 4-25 A.

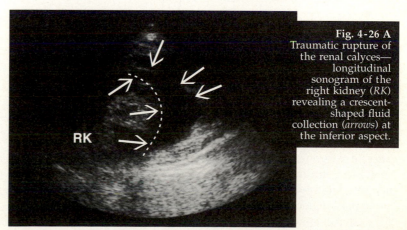

Fig. 4-26 A Traumatic rupture of the renal calyces— longitudinal sonogram of the right kidney (*RK*) revealing a crescent-shaped fluid collection (*arrows*) at the inferior aspect.

the kidney affected. **Acute pyelo-nephritis,** the most common type of renal infection, is usually caused by a bacteria that travels up the ureter from the bladder. This infection affects the lining of the calyces and pelvis and spreads into the renal parenchyma. In severe cases the infection leads to the production of a microabscess in the cortex. If untreated, further complications include the development of a renal carbuncle and a perinephric abscess.

Renal abscesses are classified according to their location. A **renal carbuncle** is an abscess that forms in the renal parenchyma. Usually a **perinephric abscess** is the result of a perforated renal abscess that leaks purulent material into the perinephric space contained by Gerota's fascia. The anterior and posterior para-nephric spaces can also become contaminated.

The presenting symptoms of renal infection generally include headache, malaise, anorexia, and a low-grade fever. These infections can cause acute renal failure, as indicated by elevated BUN and creatinine levels. The patient may also experience gross hematuria, and urine laboratory tests may reveal the presence of bacteria, protein, casts, and white blood cells. The clinical symptoms for a renal carbuncle vary from none to fever, leukocytosis, and flank pain. Classically a perinephric abscess causes a very high fever, flank pain, and boardlike rigidity of the abdominal wall.

Renal infections can be difficult to detect sonographically.

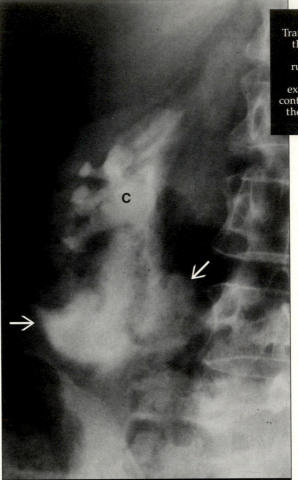

Fig. 4-26 B Traumatic rupture of the renal calyces—IVP depicting the ruptured collecting system (C) with extravasation of the contrast medium into the retroperitoneum (*arrows*).

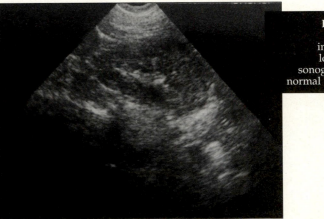

Fig. 4-27 A Renal inspection—longitudinal sonogram of the normal left kidney.

The most consistent sonographic sign is an enlarged kidney with either a hypoechoic or hyperechoic pattern compared with the normal parenchyma[17] (Fig. 4-27). The clinician often needs to know if the patient has hydronephrosis, since this can influence the patient's clinical management. Sonography plays a much larger role in evaluating for the presence of a renal carbuncle or perinephric abscess, both of which can be complications of a renal infection. A renal carbuncle appears as a discrete mass in the kidney, with the pattern ranging from cystic, to cystic with debris, to a more solid pattern (Fig. 4-28). Usually a perinephric and/or paranephric abscess visualizes as a fluid collection adjacent to the kidney (Fig. 4-29) or as a complex or even a solid mass adjacent to the kidney.

Chronic Renal Failure

Chronic renal failure, or renal insufficiency, may result from a variety of diseases that involve the renal parenchyma, or it may result from a systemic disorder that causes renal dysfunction. Examples include chronic glomerulonephritis and pyelonephritis, renal vascular disease, considerable exposure to substances toxic to the kidneys, chronic obstructive uropathy, and uncontrolled long-term hypertension and/or diabetes mellitus. Although the exact pathologic process varies with the causative factor, chronic renal failure is generally characterized by extensive scarring and fibrosis of the

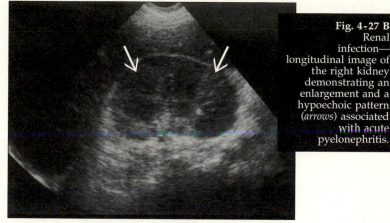

Fig. 4-27 B Renal infection—longitudinal image of the right kidney demonstrating an enlargement and a hypoechoic pattern (*arrows*) associated with acute pyelonephritis.

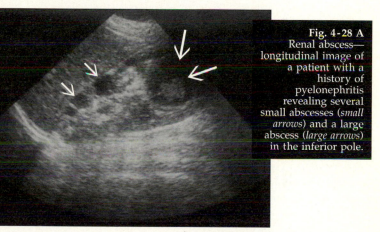

Fig. 4-28 A Renal abscess—longitudinal image of a patient with a history of pyelonephritis revealing several small abscesses (*small arrows*) and a large abscess (*large arrows*) in the inferior pole.

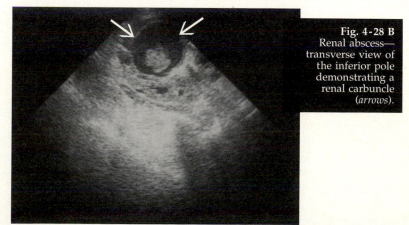

Fig. 4-28 B Renal abscess—transverse view of the inferior pole demonstrating a renal carbuncle (*arrows*).

renal parenchyma, which results in decreased renal size. Destruction of portions of the nephrons in conjunction with dilatation in other nephrons results in distorted renal architecture. Chronic long-term obstruction of the collecting system causes depression and destruction of the renal parenchyma, which may result in chronic renal failure. Patients with acquired immunodeficiency syndrome (AIDS) are also susceptible to the development of renal failure.[7]

The clinical symptoms of chronic renal failure include weakness and easy fatigability, headaches, nausea, vomiting, pruritus, polyuria, and nocturia. The patient may also develop hypertension and congestive heart failure. The clinical laboratory tests reveal anemia, elevated values of serum potassium, phosphate, BUN, and creatinine, and decreased levels of serum calcium and protein. The urinary specific gravity is low and fixed, and the patient may have proteinuria and red and white blood cells in the urine.

The typical sonographic pattern of chronic renal failure consists of bilaterally small kidneys with a hyperechoic pattern in the renal cortex (Fig. 4-30). Studies have classified the severity of renal failure into several categories with pathologic correlation. These studies are based on a comparison of the sonographic patterns of the liver or spleen, the renal sinus, and the renal cortex.[25] In the absence of renal dysfunction, the renal cortex is hypoechoic or isoechoic to the

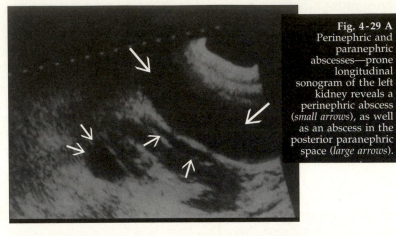

Fig. 4-29 A Perinephric and paranephric abscesses—prone longitudinal sonogram of the left kidney reveals a perinephric abscess (*small arrows*), as well as an abscess in the posterior paranephric space (*large arrows*).

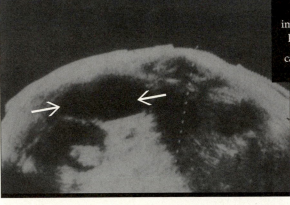

Fig. 4-29 B Prone transverse image depicts a large paranephric abscess (*arrows*). This was caused by a retained surgical sponge.

Fig. 4-30 A Chronic renal failure—longitudinal image of the right kidney (*arrows*) depicts a hyperechoic renal cortex in comparison with the liver (*L*). The renal sinus is actually hypoechoic in comparison with the renal medulla and cortex.

normal liver parenchyma. As the
disease progresses in severity,
the amount of fibrosis and atrophy in the cortex increases.
Grade 1 is assigned when the
renal cortex is isoechoic to the
liver parenchyma. Grade 2 is
used when the renal cortex is
hyperechoic to the liver but hypoechoic to the renal sinus.
Grade 3 occurs when the renal
cortex is isoechoic to the renal
sinus. The sonographer should
always obtain as complete a
clinical history as possible to cor-

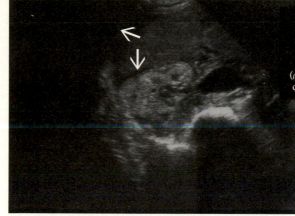

Fig. 4-30 B
Transverse scan of
the kidney that also
demonstrates
minimal ascites
(*arrows*) as a result of
chronic renal failure.

relate the history with the sonographic pattern. Subtle stages, as presented in Grade 1,
may require additional tests, such as a biopsy.

The kidneys decrease in size as the disease progresses. Consequently, the kidneys
become very difficult to demonstrate in severe cases. The use of the supine or left
posterior oblique position for the right kidney and the right lateral patient position for
the left kidney assist in the identification of the kidneys by using the liver and spleen
as acoustic windows. As mentioned previously, this technique also helps in staging the
disease by comparing the renal cortex with the normal hepatic and splenic parenchyma. Pulsed Doppler examination may reveal an increased resistive index, although
research has failed to demonstrate a correlation with specific parenchymal processes.[14]
Patients with renal failure and those undergoing dialysis may have renal cysts in
addition to the sonographic features of renal failure.

Renal Transplant

The transplanted kidney is usually placed in the right or left iliac fossa. This placement
is chosen because of the easy access to the external iliac vein and the internal iliac
artery (or hypogastric artery) for anastomosis of the allograft renal vein and artery.
This placement is also chosen because of its close proximity to the bladder, so that only
a short segment of ureter is necessary. The various sites of anastomosis dictate the
exact lie of the transplant. Hence the longitudinal axis of the transplant must be
determined for each patient (see Scanning Protocols and Techniques). The patient is
scanned in the supine position, and normally a higher frequency transducer can be
used because of the transplant's anterior location. The patient's bladder should be full,
especially when evaluating for fluid collections.

During the early postoperative period, anuria and oliguria are major clinical
problems. Causes for these complications include renal vein or artery thrombosis,
acute rejection of the kidney, urinary obstruction, and renal compression caused by
hematoma, seroma, lymphocele, or urinoma. During the later postoperative period,
the main clinical problem is rejection, although all of the early postoperative complications can occur months after transplantation. Acute rejection causes renal dysfunction, as indicated by elevated BUN and creatinine levels and decreased creatinine
clearance.

One of the most important roles of sonography in evaluating the renal transplant is the identification of extrarenal fluid collections. This is a very crucial role because the symptoms for acute rejection and these fluid collections are often indistinguishable. Usually these collections appear as cystic areas adjacent to the transplant. The sonographic differentiation between lymphocele, hematoma, or urocele is often difficult.

Sonography has also proved useful for evaluating the patency of the renal vessels with Doppler and color flow and for monitoring transplant rejection.[5] In cases of acute rejection, Doppler evaluation may demonstrate increased vascular resistance.[24,6] Documentation of flow reversal may provide more specific criteria.[10] Generally, acute rejection causes an increase in renal size and a hypoechoic parenchymal pattern. Chronic rejection, like chronic renal failure, can cause a decrease in renal size and a hyperechoic parenchymal pattern.

ABNORMALITIES OF THE URINARY BLADDER

Obstruction of the urinary bladder most often occurs in male patients and is usually caused by an enlarged prostate gland. Bladder tumors close to the urethra-bladder junction can also cause obstruction. The main clinical symptoms are decreased or no urination and, if prolonged, urinary tract infections and renal failure.

A diverticulum is an abnormal sac, or pouch, extending from a sacular or tubular structure, such as the urinary bladder. Diverticula are most commonly seen in the elderly, in whom the bladder musculature has weakened, or they are seen in the presence of urinary bladder tumors that have weakened the bladder wall. The primary clinical symptom is chronic urinary tract infections, as the urine becomes stagnant in the diverticula as a result of incomplete emptying.

Benign bladder tumors, such as the papilloma, are attached to the bladder wall by a stalk and generally do not deform the bladder wall. Usually malignant bladder tumors occur at the base of the bladder and often involve the ureteral orifice and the bladder neck. Men over the age of 50 are at the highest risk for bladder carcinoma. The transitional cell carcinoma is the most common form of malignancy. The main clinical symptom is hematuria, although the patient may also suffer from suprapubic pain and urinary tract infections.

Bladder obstruction usually appears sonographically as an overly distended, large bladder. Sometimes the cause of the obstruction is seen, such as an enlarged prostate or bladder tumor. If the obstruction has been prolonged, the patient may not feel the urge to urinate, since the innervation has been impaired. This condition is called **atonic bladder**, and in the elderly female patient the huge bladder must not be mistaken for a large cystic ovarian mass. The bladder may contain sludge in its most dependent portion, caused by sedimentation as a result of prolonged urine stagnation.

Bladder diverticula appear sonographically as abnormal, cystic pouches extending from the bladder wall (Fig. 4-31). The sonographer must differentiate diverticula from other types of cystic pathology, such as an ovarian cyst in the female patient. The oblique or lateral patient position is often necessary to display continuity of the diverticula with the normal bladder. Sludge may be demonstrated in the diverticula.

Carcinoma of the urinary bladder usually presents sonographically as an echogenic, irregular mass that disrupts the normally smooth bladder wall (Fig. 4-32), with extensions into the bladder lumen and invasion into surrounding structures in the advanced stages. Benign polyps and tumors typically have a more homogeneous, discrete sonographic appearance and do not distort the bladder wall. However, the pattern distinction is not totally specific, and any solid bladder mass requires further investigation.

TECHNICAL PITFALLS

Some of the technical pitfalls have already been described. Another example involves mistaking renal stones for gallstones.[8] If the sonographer uses a lateral scanning window for a gallbladder examination, a dilated renal pelvis containing stones can look similar to a gallbladder containing stones (Fig. 4-33). The sonographer must always demonstrate the relationship of the gallbladder to the main lobar fissure and right portal vein. The use of multiple scanning windows should also decrease the risk of making this mistake.

Proper gain settings are crucial for renal sonography. The cortical parenchymal pattern must be apparent on all images. Although renal cysts are a very common finding with sonography, the sonographer must always carefully assess the borders and interior of the lumen. The demonstration of acoustic enhancement is also important. Cysts under 2 cm may require a higher frequency transducer to properly display these characteristics. Because of the incidence of

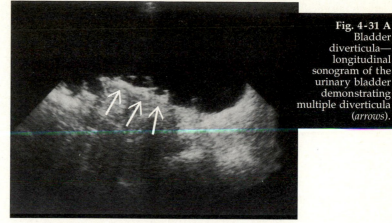

Fig. 4-31 A Bladder diverticula—longitudinal sonogram of the urinary bladder demonstrating multiple diverticula (*arrows*).

Fig. 4-31 B Transverse view depicts two bladder diverticula (*arrows*).

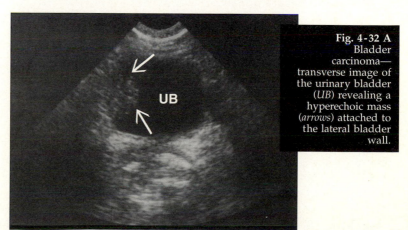

Fig. 4-32 A Bladder carcinoma—transverse image of the urinary bladder (*UB*) revealing a hyperechoic mass (*arrows*) attached to the lateral bladder wall.

cystic malignancies (such as the renal cell carcinoma), any cystic mass that does not fully meet all criteria for a cyst requires further investigation.[20]

As in all sonographic examinations, the sonographer must examine other anatomic areas, based on the abnormal findings in the kidneys. In the case of obstruction the sonographer should scan the ureters and urinary bladder to identify the level and cause of the obstruction. A solid or complex renal mass should be evaluated for signs of malignancy using pulsed Doppler. The renal vein and IVC should be evaluated for evidence of tumor invasion. A suspected hematoma or abscess requires the examination of the perinephric and paranephric spaces.

SUMMARY

The clinical history and the results of the various clinical laboratory tests again play an important role in the establishment of the differential diagnosis. The best clinical interpretation results from the evaluation of multiple renal function tests and urinalysis. The presence and severity of renal dysfunction always has an impact on the sonographic interpretation where the pattern changes are subtle or borderline. Table 4-2 contains a summary of typical clinical laboratory test findings with specific renal pathology.

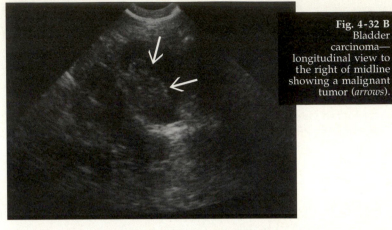

Fig. 4-32 B Bladder carcinoma—longitudinal view to the right of midline showing a malignant tumor (*arrows*).

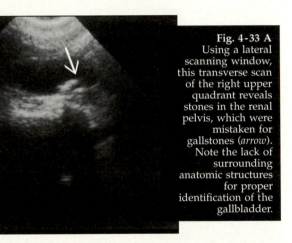

Fig. 4-33 A Using a lateral scanning window, this transverse scan of the right upper quadrant reveals stones in the renal pelvis, which were mistaken for gallstones (*arrow*). Note the lack of surrounding anatomic structures for proper identification of the gallbladder.

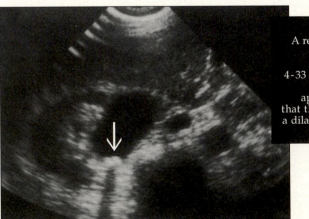

Fig. 4-33 B A repeat sonogram of the patient featured in Fig. 4-33 A. The use of a more anterior approach verifies that the stones are in a dilated renal pelvis (*arrow*).

TABLE 4-2   CLINICAL LABORATORY TEST VALUES – KIDNEY

	BUN	CREA	PROTEIN	HEMATURIA	BACTERIA	Other Tests
SIMPLE CYST	Normal	Normal	-	-	-	
POLYCYSTIC DISEASE	Increase	Increase	+	+	-/+	
HYDRONEPHROSIS	Increase	Increase	+		-/+	Increased WBC, if infected
BENIGN NEOPLASM	Normal	Normal	-/+	-/+		
RENAL CELL CARCINOMA	Increase	Increase	+	+	-/+	Increased WBC, if infected
TRANSITIONAL CELL CARCINOMA	Normal Increase*	Normal Increase	-/+	+		
LYMPHOMA	Normal Increase*	Normal Increase	-/+	+		
HEMATOMA	Normal Increase*	Normal Increase	-	+		Decreased Hematocrit
RENAL INFECTION	Normal Increase*	Normal Increase	+	-/+	-/+	Increased WBC
RENAL FAILURE	Increase	Increase	+	+	-/+	Decreased Serum Calcium and Serum Protein

*The presence and severity of renal dysfunction depends on the location and extent of pathology.

BUN, blood urea nitrogen; CREA, creatinine; BACTERIA, presence in the urine; WBC, white blood cell count in the serum.

REFERENCES

1. Bosniak MA, Megibow AJ, et al: CT diagnosis of renal angiomyolipoma: the importance of detecting small amounts of fat, *AJR* 151:497, 1988.
2. Bosniak MA: The small (≤3.0 cm) renal parenchymal tumor: detection, diagnosis, and controversies, *Radiology* 179:307, 1991.
3. Bude RO, Platt JF, et al: Dilated renal collecting systems: differentiating obstructive from nonobstructive dilation using duplex Doppler ultrasound, *Urology* 37:123, 1991.
4. Craig. *Pocket guide to ultrasound measurements*, Philadelphia, 1988, JB Lippincott.
5. Desberg AL, Paushter DM, et al: Renal artery stenosis: evaluation with color Doppler flow imaging, *Radiology* 177:749, 1990.
6. Grant EG, Perrella RR: Wishing won't make it so: duplex Doppler sonography in the evaluation of renal transplant dysfunction, *AJR* 155:538, 1990.
7. Hamper UM, Goldblum LE, et al: Renal involvement in AIDS: sonographic-pathologic correlation, *AJR* 150:1321, 1988.
8. Hewitt MJ, Older RA: Clyceal calculi simulating gallstones, *AJR* 134:507, 1980.
9. Jeffrey RB, Laing RC, et al: Sensitivity of sonography in pyonephrosis: a reevaluation, *AJR* 144:71, 1985.
10. Kaveggia LP, Perrella RR, et al: Duplex Doppler sonography in renal allografts: the significance of reversed flow in diastole, *AJR* 155:295, 1990.

11. Lafortune M, Constantin A, et al: Sonography of the hypertrophied column of Bertin, *AJR* 146:53, 1986.

12. Lawson TL, McClennan BL, Shirkhoda A: Adult polycystic kidney disease: ultrasonographic and computed tomographic appearance, *J Clin Ultrasound* 6:297, 1978.

13. McCarthy S, Rosenfield AT: Ultrasonography in crossed renal ectopia, *J Ultrasound Med* 3:107, 1984.

14. Mostbeck GH, Kain R, et al: Duplex Doppler sonography in renal parenchymal disease: histopathologic correlation, *J Ultrasound Med* 10:189, 1991.

15. Ostrovsky PD, Carr L, Goodman J: Ultrasound of transitional cell carcinoma, *J Clin Ultrasound* 13:35, 1985.

16. Patriquin H, Lefaivre JF, et al: Fetal lobulation: an anatomo-ultrasonographic correlation, *J Ultrasound Med* 9:191, 1990.

17. Piccirillo M, Rigsby CM, Rosenfield AT: Sonography of renal inflammatory disease, *Urol Radiol* 9:66, 1987.

18. Platt JF, Rubin JM, et al: The inability to detect kidney disease on the basis of echogenicity, *AJR* 151:317, 1988.

19. Pollack HM, Wein AJ: Imaging of renal trauma, *Radiology* 172:297, 1989.

20. Pollack HM, Banner MP, et al: The accuracy of gray-scale renal ultrasonography in differentiating cystic neoplasms from benign cysts, *Radiology* 143:741, 1982.

21. Press GA, McClennan BL, et al: Papillary renal cell carcinoma: CT and sonographic evaluation, *AJR* 143:1005, 1984.

22. Ramos IM, Taylor KJW, et al: Tumor vascular signals in renal masses: detection with Doppler US, *Radiology* 168:633, 1988.

23. Reiman TAH, Siegel MJ, Shackelford GD: Wilms tumor in children: abdominal CT and US evaluation, *Radiology* 160:501, 1986.

24. Rifkin MD, Needleman L, et al: Evaluation of renal transplant rejection by duplex Doppler examination: value of the resistive index, *AJR* 148:759, 1987.

25. Rosenfield AT, Siegel NJ: Renal parenchymal disease: histo-pathologic correlation, *AJR* 137:793, 1991.

26. Sanders RC, Nussbaum AR, Solex K: Renal dysplasia: sonographic findings, *Radiology* 167:623, 1988.

27. Wernecke K, Heckemann R, et al: Sonography of infantile polycystic disease, *Urol Radiol* 7:138, 1985.

5

adrenal glands

INSTRUCTIONAL OBJECTIVES

At the completion of this chapter, the reader will be able to:

1. Describe the clinical problems that are typical reasons for sonography of the adrenal glands.
2. Identify on transverse, coronal, and longitudinal illustrations and sonograms the major anatomic structures of the adrenal glands, including the cortex and medulla, the perinephric space, and the surrounding anatomic landmarks, such as the diaphragmatic crus and the aorta and inferior vena cava.
3. Describe the basic scanning protocol for sonography of the adrenal glands.
4. Describe the clinical laboratory tests used for evaluating the function of the adrenal glands, including plasma cortisol and plasma adrenocorticotropic hormone assays.
5. Describe the clinical symptoms and pathologic basis for the disease processes of the adrenal glands, including adrenal cysts, primary benign and malignant tumors, metastatic carcinoma, and the effects of Addison's disease and Cushing's syndrome.
6. Identify on sectional sonograms the above-mentioned disease processes of the adrenal glands, based on the sonographic appearance, the clinical history, and the results of other diagnostic procedures.
7. Discuss several technical pitfalls associated with sonography of the adrenal glands.

THE CLINICAL PROBLEM

Adrenal gland function is crucial to life. Consequently, signs of dysfunction always require clinical investigation. The clinical picture is clouded by the fact that the dysfunction of several different organs may produce similar symptoms. For example, pathology in the pituitary gland or in the adrenal gland may cause Cushing's syndrome. The differential diagnosis of a sudden onset of hypertension, particularly in a younger patient, must initially include the adrenal glands as the source of the problem. Several clinical laboratory tests may help narrow this wide differential diagnosis. The imaging modalities also play an important role in the initial clinical investigation. Although computed tomography (CT) generally allows better visualization of the normal adrenal glands, the current resolution capabilities of ultrasound equipment provide a higher sensitivity for the documentation of normal anatomy and may provide greater detail in the characterization of an adrenal mass.

NORMAL ANATOMY

The adrenals are paired glands that occupy the superomedial aspect of each kidney (Fig. 5-1). The right adrenal gland is bordered posteromedially by the diaphragm, anteriorly by the liver, anteromedially by the inferior vena cava, and inferolaterally by the right kidney. The left adrenal gland is bordered posteromedially by the diaphragm and aorta, anteriorly by the stomach, and inferolaterally by the left kidney. The diaphragmatic crus lies posteromedial to each adrenal gland and must not be misidentified as the adrenal. The tissue of each adrenal differentiates into the outer layer, called the cortex, and the inner layer, called the medulla. The adrenal glands are located in the retroperitoneal cavity in the perinephric space. Depending on the body habitus of the patient, a variable amount of adipose tissue surrounds each gland.

There are many arterial branches that supply the adrenal glands, arising from the abdominal aorta and from the renal and inferior phrenic arteries. The venous tributaries converge to form a single vein in each gland. The right adrenal vein directly enters the inferior vena cava, whereas the left adrenal vein enters the left renal vein, which then enters the inferior vena cava.

NORMAL PHYSIOLOGY

Each adrenal gland consists of an outer layer (the cortex) that surrounds the inner tissue (the medulla). These two layers function as separate endocrine glands, which secrete hormones directly into the circulatory system.

The cortex is divided into three layers, or zones. From the outer to the inner layer, they are called the zona glomerulosa, zona fasciculata, and zona reticularis. The zona glomerulosa secretes a group of steroids called

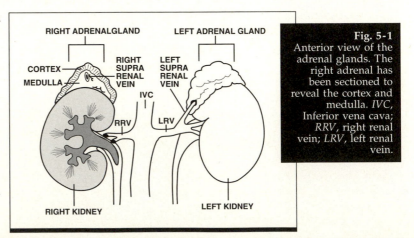

Fig. 5-1 Anterior view of the adrenal glands. The right adrenal has been sectioned to reveal the cortex and medulla. *IVC,* Inferior vena cava; *RRV,* right renal vein; *LRV,* left renal vein.

the **mineralocorticoids,** primarily aldosterone and deoxycorticosterone. Their primary function is the maintenance of sodium blood concentrations and electrolyte and fluid balance. The zona fasciculata secretes **glucocorticoids**, another group of steroids. The primary hormones are cortisol and corticosterone. These hormones promote normal protein, fat, and carbohydrate metabolism; and they assist in the immune system's response to stress and are essential to life. The innermost layer, the zona reticularis, secretes small amounts of glucocorticoids and sex hormones. These small secretions promote normal development of the bones and reproductive organs. If symptoms include precocious puberty, or if the patient develops secondary characteristics of the opposite sex, dysfunction of the adrenal cortex is included in the preliminary clinical diagnosis.

The adrenal medulla secretes **epinephrine** and **norepinephrine**. These hormones also assist in the body's response to stressful situations by controlling the "fight or flight" reaction characterized by tachycardia, vasoconstriction in the gastrointestinal tract, blushing, and "goose bumps." Although important, these hormones are not essential to life as are glucocorticoids.

CLINICAL LABORATORY TESTS

Serum Cortisol

Cortisol is a steroid secreted by the adrenal cortex that affects normal metabolism by stimulating liver gluconeogenesis and decreasing the cellular glucose utilization rate. It also inhibits the effect of insulin. Normally the cortisol secretion rate is higher in the early morning than in the evening. Decreased cortisol levels are associated with Addison's disease, hypothyroidism, and liver disease. Increased levels are seen in Cushing's syndrome, hyperthyroidism, stress, and some types of obesity.

Adrenocorticotropic Hormone Test

Adrenocorticotropic hormone (ACTH) is produced in the anterior pituitary gland and stimulates the adrenal gland to secrete cortisol and other glucocorticoids. The ACTH test helps differentiate between adrenal cortex pathology and hypopituitarism. Normally the administration of ACTH produces at least a 50% decrease in the eosinophil count 4 hours after injection. In the presence of adrenal cortex insufficiency, such as Addison's disease, the eosinophil count drops to less than 20%.

RELATED IMAGING PROCEDURES

Intravenous Pyelogram

The presence of a medial, superior mass that displaces the kidney may indicate the presence of an adrenal tumor. If the patient has severe hypertension or has an elevated blood urea nitrogen (BUN) level, an intravenous pyelogram (IVP) may be contraindicated. This procedure is not the method of choice for the evaluation of adrenal pathology.

Arteriography and Venography

Arteriography provides an accurate method for adrenal mass visualization and the characterization of its vascular supply. During the injection of the iodinated contrast medium, care must be taken to prevent adrenergic shock in patients with hypertension and those with excessive hormone production. A safer method for adrenal visualization is the venogram, which has a high accuracy rate for the diagnosis of adenoma.

Computed Tomography

Current CT examinations can reliably image the normal adrenal glands, as well as any masses. Biopsy procedures can be performed with CT guidance. This examination can also document extension of pathology into the surrounding retroperitoneal spaces, the perispinal areas, and the chest.

SCANNING PROTOCOLS AND TECHNIQUES

Although still a challenge, the sonographer can demonstrate the normal adrenal glands, particularly the right gland in a thin to average-size patient. Because each gland is a small "target area," knowledge of surrounding anatomy and landmarks plays a crucial role in adrenal sonography. The presence of a mass simplifies the scanning process, but identifying the correct organ of origin then becomes the challenge.

The standard scanning protocol consists of transverse, longitudinal, and/or coronal scans through the adrenal area. Because of the incidence of bilateral pathology, the routine protocol should include both glands. The position of the right adrenal in relation to the liver allows greater flexibility in patient positioning, since supine, left posterior oblique, or left lateral positions may allow adequate demonstration of the gland. The position of the left adrenal gland in relation to the stomach poses a greater challenge for adequate documentation, and the right posterior oblique patient position or the right lateral patient position is usually required. The coronal plane using the liver/spleen as an acoustic window often provides the best demonstration of the gland. Transverse survey scans of each adrenal area may allow easier identification, since more anatomic reference structures are demonstrated. For the right adrenal gland, the sonographer should localize the right kidney and move superiorly to the upper pole. The inferior vena cava (IVC) should be localized medial and anterior to the upper pole of the kidney. The sonographer should then concentrate on the lateral, posterior border of the IVC and look for a thin crescent-shaped structure anterior to the diaphragmatic crus. The right adrenal gland often appears as a Y-shaped or bilobular structure. Once localized, very small scanning movements will allow demonstration of the gland in the transverse plane. Coronal scans of the right gland are obtained by placing the transducer intercostally in the midaxillary plane or at a slightly posterior angle. To demonstrate the right adrenal, the sonographer should locate the IVC and upper pole of the kidney and angle slightly posterior from the IVC. For the left adrenal gland, the sonographer should localize the left kidney and move superiorly to the upper pole. Once the aorta is localized medial and anterior to the upper pole, the sonographer should search the area between the aorta, diaphragmatic

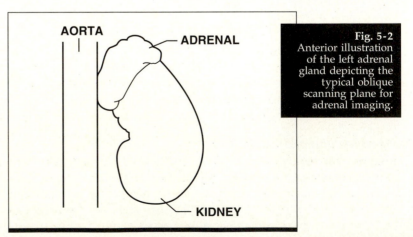

AORTA

ADRENAL

KIDNEY

Fig. 5-2 Anterior illustration of the left adrenal gland depicting the typical oblique scanning plane for adrenal imaging.

crus, and kidney for the left adrenal (Fig. 5-2). Typically the left gland lies medial to the upper pole of the kidney, lateral to the aorta, and posterior to the tail of the pancreas. Again, the sonographer should document the transverse dimensions of the gland and then rotate 90 degrees to obtain the longitudinal/coronal images. A rounded appearance, instead of a linear, crescent shape, suggests the presence of a small mass. The presence of moderate to large adrenal masses may allow adequate demonstration of the left adrenal with the patient in the supine position.

The scanning protocol for the adrenal glands is summarized in the box on this page.

NORMAL SONOGRAPHIC PATTERNS

The normal measurements for the adrenal glands range from 3 to 6 mm in thickness (posteroanteriorly) to 0.8 to 1 cm in length.[6] In the fetal and neonatal periods the adrenals are more prominent and approach a ratio of one third the size of the kidney. This size discrepancy occurs because of the prominence of the adrenal cortex during this period of development. The normal sonographic pattern during this period is of a prominent hypoechoic cortex surrounding the smaller hyperechoic medulla (Fig. 5-3). Although quite small, this same pattern exists in the normal adult adrenal gland (Fig. 5-4) with the cortex isoechoic to the normal liver/spleen parenchyma; the cortex may also be isoechoic to the perinephric fat.

BASIC SCANNING PROTOCOL

Transverse
- Images through the entire gland, including transverse and posteroanterior measurements

Longitudinal/Coronal
- Images through the entire gland, including a length measurement
- Any mass should be measured in all three dimensions

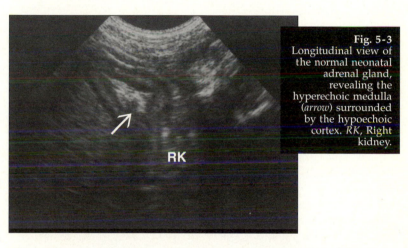

Fig. 5-3 Longitudinal view of the normal neonatal adrenal gland, revealing the hyperechoic medulla (*arrow*) surrounded by the hypoechoic cortex. *RK*, Right kidney.

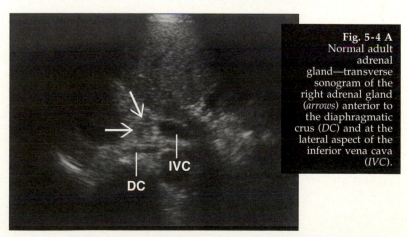

Fig. 5-4 A Normal adult adrenal gland—transverse sonogram of the right adrenal gland (*arrows*) anterior to the diaphragmatic crus (*DC*) and at the lateral aspect of the inferior vena cava (*IVC*).

With optimum resolution, the hyperechoic medulla can be differentiated. Since the diaphragmatic crus can mimic this sonographic pattern and is thin and long like the adrenal, the sonographer must document the adrenal in relation to the crus, which is posterior and medial to the glands.

PATHOLOGIC PROCESSES OF THE ADRENAL GLANDS

Adrenal Cysts

Adrenal cysts are usually unilateral, asymptomatic entities that may reach a rather large size. Occasionally a cyst may cause hypertension. These cysts may be congenital or acquired. The typical patient is a woman between 30 and 50 years of age. These cysts usually meet the sonographic criteria of a cyst: regular walls, anechoic interior, and distal acoustic enhancement (Fig. 5-5).

Calcifications in the walls may suggest a congenital formation. However, a pseudocyst or hemorrhagic cyst may have irregular borders and contain debris. Typically, pseudocysts are the result of hemorrhage. The sonographer must try to demonstrate the organ of origin by an accurate anatomic localization of the cyst. Since renal cysts are much more common, demonstrating an intact renal capsule adjacent to the cyst is crucial. Larger adrenal masses, including cysts, characteristically displace the kidney inferiorly and

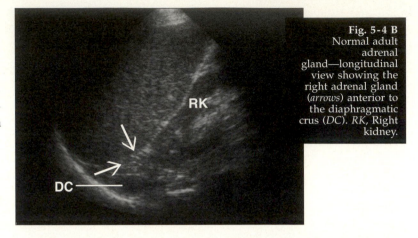

Fig. 5-4 B Normal adult adrenal gland—longitudinal view showing the right adrenal gland (*arrows*) anterior to the diaphragmatic crus (*DC*). *RK*, Right kidney.

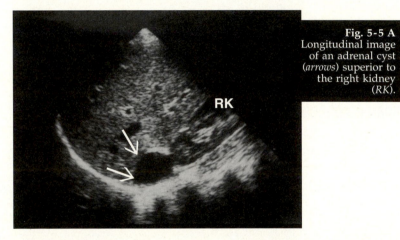

Fig. 5-5 A Longitudinal image of an adrenal cyst (*arrows*) superior to the right kidney (*RK*).

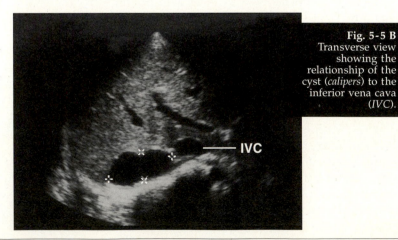

Fig. 5-5 B Transverse view showing the relationship of the cyst (*calipers*) to the inferior vena cava (*IVC*).

rotate the upper pole posterolaterally.

Adrenal Hemorrhage

During the early neonatal period, the adrenal cortex undergoes atrophy. Because of their large size and increased vascularity, the adrenals are susceptible to hemorrhage during this period. The hemorrhage most frequently occurs in the right adrenal. Factors that increase the risk of hemorrhage include fetal hypoxia and trauma during birth.[7]

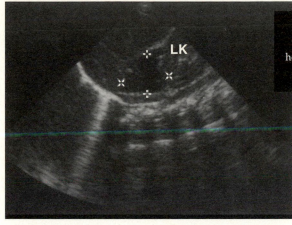

Fig. 5-6 Longitudinal image of an adrenal hemorrhage (*calipers*) superior to the left kidney (*LK*).

The clinical symptoms vary from asymptomatic to jaundice and a palpable right-sided mass. The hematocrit may be decreased with moderate to severe bleeding.

The classic sonographic pattern is a cystic mass contained in the adrenal component of the perinephric space (Fig. 5-6). As a result of the various clotting stages of blood, the pattern may appear complex. Although rare, the sonographer should evaluate the other adrenal gland for signs of hemorrhage. Adrenal hyperplasia may not be distinguishable from small or primarily solid hematomas.

Cushing's Syndrome

Cushing's syndrome is associated with excessive cortisol production in the adrenal cortex. This overproduction is typically a result of a benign hyperplasia, a benign tumor, or a malignant lesion in the adrenal cortex. It may also result from a primary tumor in the pituitary or hypothalamus.

Cushing's syndrome causes marked obesity in the trunk with a protuberant abdomen, a "moon face," and thin extremities. Other symptoms include menstrual irregularities in women, impotence in men, and weakness, headache, backache, hypertension, hirsutism, and easy bruising.

Plasma cortisol and urinary 17-hydroxycorticosteriods are increased. The patient is resistant to the actions of insulin, total eosinophil and lymphocyte counts are low, and the red and white blood cell counts are elevated.

Addison's Disease

Addison's disease occurs when the adrenal cortex does not produce adequate amounts of glucocorticoids and mineralocorticoids. The disease, once rare, is now more common because adrenal surgery is more prevalent, which causes hormonal insufficiency.

The clinical symptoms of Addison's disease include weakness, fatigue, anorexia, nausea, vomiting, and diarrhea. Other physical signs are increased axillary hair, increased skin pigmentation, and hypotension. Plasma cortisol levels are low to absent, serum sodium and chloride levels are low, and the plasma ACTH levels are elevated.

Primary Neoplasms of the Adrenal Cortex

Primary neoplasms of the adrenal cortex include hyperplasia, adenomas, and carcinomas. Hyperplasia, the most common cause of Cushing's syndrome, can be a result of increased ACTH production from a neoplasm of the pituitary or hypothalamus. Adenomas are usually benign tumors that can be quite small and still cause serious symptoms. Adrenocortical carcinoma occurs more often in the left adrenal gland than in the right.[8] Some neoplasms cause an increased production of sex hormones.

The primary clinical symptoms for cortical neoplasms are the same as those for Cushing's syndrome. Lesions that do not autonomously secrete adrenal steriods may cause no symptoms. Other symptoms may include hypertension and localized pain. Patients with a malignancy do not have as high an incidence of Cushing's syndrome as do patients with other types of neoplasms. The urinary 17-ketosteroids often help differentiate between the types of cortical tumors. These levels are low to normal in Cushing's syndrome when caused by adenoma, normal to high when caused by hyperplasia, and very high when caused by carcinoma.

Adrenal neoplasms range from hypoechoic and hyperechoic to complex on sonographic examination (Fig. 5-7). Laboratory and other diagnostic tests offer more specific information concerning the precise pathologic classification. The primary role of sonography is identifying the mass as adrenal in origin and ruling out bilateral involvement before treatment. Sonographic accuracy decreases in the identification of hyperplasia compared with discrete masses.

Tumors of the Adrenal Medulla

Primary tumors of the adrenal medulla include the pheochromocytoma, the ganglioneuroma, and the neuroblastoma.

The **pheochromocytoma** is a rare medullary tumor that arises in the pheochrome tissue in one or both adrenal glands or in the sympathetic nerve chain. Other sites include the retroperitoneum, the mediastinum, and the pelvis. Approximately 90% of these tumors occur in the adrenals, and a small percentage may be malignant.[3] The clinical symptoms of pheochromocytoma include attacks of headache, visual blurring, severe sweats, hypertension, and tachycardia. Laboratory tests reveal elevated levels of urinary catecholamines and their metabolites and high levels of blood and urinary epinephrine and norepinephrine during or following an attack. A pheochromocytoma appears sonographically as a homogeneous mass.[2]

The **ganglioneuroma** is a rare benign tumor consisting of mature ganglioneurons that are usually encapsulated and may contain areas of calcification. The most common location is in the thorax. The clinical symptoms range from asymptomatic to epi-

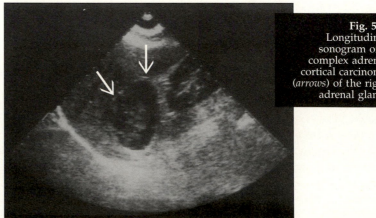

Fig. 5-7 Longitudinal sonogram of a complex adrenal cortical carcinoma (*arrows*) of the right adrenal gland.

sodes of hypertension. Most patients are under the age of 20. Typically, a ganglioneuroma displays as a discrete mass with at least a partial capsule and may contain calcifications.[5]

The **neuroblastoma** is a malignant tumor that typically occurs in children under 6 years of age. These tumors are more common in the left adrenal gland. They are highly malignant and metastasize early with a poor prognosis. The prognosis is better when the child is one year old or younger. Clinically these tumors can be confused with Wilm's tumor of the kidney. The clinical symptoms of neuroblastoma may include a palpable mass, hepatomegaly, weight loss, vomiting, hypertension, and abdominal pain. The clinical laboratory tests may indicate anemia, elevated urinary catacholamines, and the urinary metabolite homovanillic acid. These neoplasms are highly vascular and metastasize early to the bones, lymph nodes, liver, brain, and lungs. Neuroblastomas are usually large, solid masses that often

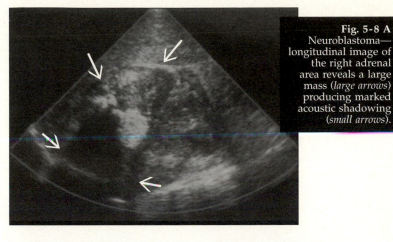

Fig. 5-8 A Neuroblastoma—longitudinal image of the right adrenal area reveals a large mass (*large arrows*) producing marked acoustic shadowing (*small arrows*).

Fig. 5-8 B Neuroblastoma—scan of the left upper quadrant displays a left adrenal mass (*arrows*).

have a complex pattern caused by both necrosis and calcification[1] (Fig. 5-8). Typically this pattern is much different from that of a Wilm's tumor, which tends to be more homogeneous. The sonographer should check for bilateral adrenal involvement, as well as lymphadenopathy and liver metastases, to narrow the differential diagnosis of neuroblastoma.

Metastatic Adrenal Disease

Metastases to the adrenal glands have been reported with carcinoma of the stomach, lungs and breasts, melanoma, and large cell primaries. Bronchogenic carcinoma has one of the highest incidences of adrenal metastasis (33%), followed by breast carcinoma. These tumors are frequently bilateral and can attain a large size.

The sonographic pattern ranges from hypoechoic to hyperechoic (Fig. 5-9). Large masses may contain central areas of necrosis.[4] Large metastatic deposits may make the identification of the organ of origin difficult. Bilateral masses in the upper abdomen increase the suggestion of an adrenal origin.

TECHNICAL PITFALLS

Because the normal adrenal glands are usually isoechoic to the liver/ spleen and perinephric fat, the acoustic power, overall gain, and time gain compensation (TGC) controls require settings similar to those used for liver and renal sonography. Setting the gain too high will mask the appearance of the adrenal. The sonographer should evaluate the pattern of the normal renal cortex. If this area presents as a hyperechoic pattern, the sonographer should decrease the gain settings. Transducer selection depends on patient size and position, which affects the scanning depth of the adrenal glands. The transducer selected should place the adrenal in the focal zone and employ the highest resolution with adequate penetration. Normally this would be a 3.5 MHz transducer.

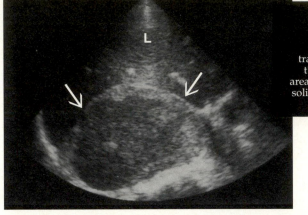

Fig. 5-9 A Metastasis from bronchogenic carcinoma— transverse scan of the right adrenal area reveals a large, solid mass (*arrows*). *L*, Liver.

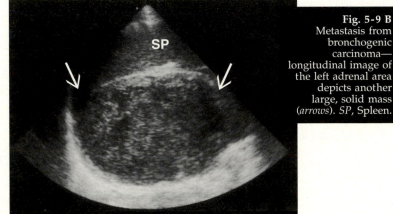

Fig. 5-9 B Metastasis from bronchogenic carcinoma— longitudinal image of the left adrenal area depicts another large, solid mass (*arrows*). *SP*, Spleen.

The major technical pitfall is nonidentification of the glands as a result of inadequate recognition of anatomic landmarks. Another pitfall is assigning a mass an adrenal origin when it actually relates to the kidney. The sonographer should remember that large adrenal masses usually displace the kidney inferiorly and rotate it posterolaterally. For any size of mass, the sonographer should demonstrate an intact renal capsule in relation to the lesion. Identification of an anterior displacement of the retroperitoneal fat plane by a mass can allow the differentiation of a retroperitoneal or a peritoneal origin.

SUMMARY

Although not a common sonographic examination, adrenal sonography requires detailed knowledge of surrounding anatomic structures to visualize normal-size glands. A more common situation that requires these skills is identification of the organ of origin of a mass located in the posterior and inferior aspect of the liver. The patient's clinical history, symptoms, and the results of pertinent clinical laboratory tests also assist both the sonographer and the interpreting physician in refining the differential diagnosis. Table 5-1 summarizes the findings of pertinent clinical laboratory tests related to adrenal pathology.

TABLE 5-1   CLINICAL LABORATORY TEST VALUES – ADRENAL GLANDS

	CORTISOL	*ACTH*	*17-HYD*	*Other Tests*
CUSHING'S SYNDROME	Increase	Increase	Increase	Resistant to Insulin
ADDISON'S DISEASE	Decrease		Decrease	Decreased Serum Sodium Chloride
ADRENAL CYST	Normal	Normal	Normal	
HEMORRHAGE	Normal	Normal	Normal	Decreased Hematocrit
CORTICAL ADENOMA	Increase	Increase	Normal	
CORTICAL HYPERPLASIA	Increase	Increase	Normal Increase	
CORTICAL CARCINOMA	Normal	Normal	High Increase	
PHEOCHROMOCYTOMA	Normal	Normal	Normal	Increased Epinephrine, Norepinephrine, Increased Urinary Catecholamines
NEUROBLASTOMA	Normal	Normal	Normal	Increased Urinary Catecholamines

17-HYD, 17-Hydroxycorticosteroids.

REFERENCES

1. Amundson GM, Trevenen CL, et al: Neuroblastoma: a specific sonographic tissue pattern, *AJR* 148:943, 1987.
2. Bowerman RA, Silver TM, et al: Sonography of adrenal pheochromocytomas, *AJR* 137:1227, 1981.
3. Dunnick NR: Adrenal imaging: current status, *AJR* 154:927, 1990.
4. Forsythe JR, Gosink BB, Leopold GR: Ultrasound in the evaluation of adrenal metastases, *J Clin Ultrasound* 5:31, 1977.
5. Jasinski RW, Samuels BI, Silver TM: Sonographic features of retroperitoneal ganglioneuroma, *J Ultrasound Med* 3:413, 1984.
6. Marchal G, Gelin J, et al: High-resolution real-time sonography of the adrenal glands: a routine examination? *J Ultrasound Med* 5:65, 1986.
7. Murphy BJ, Casillas J, Yrizarry JM: Traumatic adrenal hemorrhage: radiologic findings, *Radiology* 169:701, 1988.
8. Prando A, Wallace S, et al: Sonographic findings of adrenal cortical carcinoma, *Pediatr Radiol* 20:163, 1990.

general abdomen

INSTRUCTIONAL OBJECTIVES

At the completion of this chapter, the reader will be able to:

1. Describe the clinical problems that are typical reasons for the sonographic evaluation of the peritoneal cavity.

2. Identify on transverse and longitudinal illustrations and sonograms the major anatomic structures of the peritoneal cavity, including the anatomic divisions of the gastrointestinal tract, parietal peritoneum, and subdivisions of the visceral peritoneum.

3. Describe the basic scanning protocol for sonography of the gastrointestinal tract and peritoneal cavity.

4. Describe the clinical laboratory tests used for evaluating disease processes of the peritoneal cavity, including white blood cell count, red blood cell count, and hematocrit.

5. Describe the clinical symptoms and pathologic basis for the disease processes of the gastrointestinal tract and peritoneal cavity, including gastrointestinal carcinoma and obstruction, appendicitis and abscess formation, ascites, primary and secondary malignancies of the peritoneum, and abdominal abscesses and hematomas.

6. Identify on sectional sonograms the above-mentioned disease processes of the gastrointestinal tract and peritoneal cavity, based on their sonographic appearance, the clinical history, and the results of other diagnostic procedures.

7. Identify on transverse and longitudinal illustrations and sonograms the major anatomic structures of the anterior abdominal wall.

8. Describe the basic scanning protocol for the anterior abdominal wall.

9. Describe the clinical symptoms and pathologic basis for the disease processes of the anterior abdominal wall, including abscesses, hematomas, hernias, benign and malignant primary neoplasms, and metastatic processes.

10. Identify on sectional sonograms the above-mentioned disease processes of the anterior abdominal wall, based on their sonographic appearance, the clinical history, and the results of other diagnostic procedures.

11. List several technical pitfalls associated with sonography of the gastrointestinal tract, peritoneal cavity, and anterior abdominal wall.

THE CLINICAL PROBLEM

Although sonography does not play a primary role in diagnosing abnormalities of the gastrointestinal (GI) tract, the sonographer may document these diseases as incidental findings as part of a survey scan of the abdomen. Also, the discovery of liver metastasis requires a careful examination for the primary malignancy when the site is not known at the time of the examination. Unfortunately, many patients experience the first symptoms when distant metastasis has already occurred. The early symptoms for acute appendicitis often mimic other infections and diseases, so that the initial clinical differential is quite broad. Today sonography plays a greater role in the workup of a patient for appendicitis. The clinical diagnosis of a patient with minimal ascites can be difficult, particularly in a more obese individual. With sonography these minimal fluid collections can usually be demonstrated. The cause for the ascites, such as cirrhosis of the liver or ovarian carcinoma, may also be evident on sonography. The postoperative patient with an elevated white blood cell count or a decreased hematocrit always poses a clinical dilemma—where is the source of the infection or bleeding? The sonographer can evaluate the wound site and the surrounding organs, anterior abdominal wall, and peritoneal spaces. Although computed tomography (CT) can evaluate these areas very well, sonography still plays a prominent role in the evaluation of the peritoneal cavity.

NORMAL ANATOMY

Stomach

The stomach is divided into four major sections: the fundus, body, pyloric antrum, and pylorus (Fig. 6-1). The fundus is the most superior portion of the stomach. The gastroesophageal junction is the union between the esophagus and the fundus and usually lies anterior to and left of the aorta. The fundus merges with the body, which tapers as it progresses medially and inferiorly to form the pyloric antrum. The pyloric antrum then joins the pylorus, which travels slightly to the right of the median plane before uniting with the first portion of the duodenum.

The arteries that supply the stomach are the right gastric, right gastroepiploic, left gastric, left gastroepiploic, and the short gastric branches of the splenic artery (Fig. 6-1). The left gastric arises from the celiac trunk but does not routinely visualize on sonographic examination. The venous tributaries merge into the venous counterparts of the major arterial branches. These empty into either the splenic or superior mesenteric vein or directly into the portal vein.

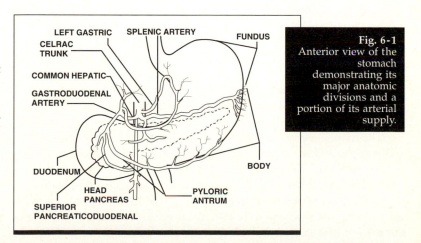

LEFT GASTRIC
CELRAC TRUNK
COMMON HEPATIC
GASTRODUODENAL ARTERY
DUODENUM
HEAD PANCREAS
SUPERIOR PANCREATICODUODENAL
SPLENIC ARTERY
FUNDUS
BODY
PYLORIC ANTRUM

Fig. 6-1 Anterior view of the stomach demonstrating its major anatomic divisions and a portion of its arterial supply.

Small Intestine

The small intestine is divided into three anatomic areas: the duodenum, jejunum, and ileum. The duodenum, the most proximal portion, follows an almost circular path. It consists of four segments: the superior (first), the descending (second), the horizontal (third), and the ascending (fourth) (Fig. 6-2.). The first segment is bordered medially by the pyloric valve of the stomach, laterally by the gallbladder, superiorly by the liver, posteriorly by

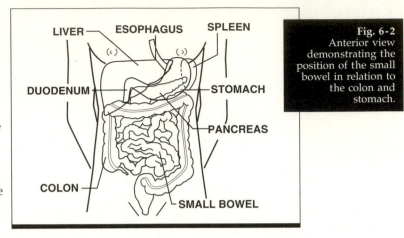

Fig. 6-2
Anterior view demonstrating the position of the small bowel in relation to the colon and stomach.

the gastroduodenal artery, common bile duct, and portal vein, and inferiorly by the head and neck of the pancreas. The second segment courses inferiorly along the right side of the vertebrae and is bordered medially by the head of the pancreas and common bile duct, anteriorly by the hepatic flexure of the colon, laterally by the gallbladder and right lobe of the liver, and posteriorly by the right kidney, psoas muscle, renal vessels, and inferior vena cava. The **ampulla of Vater** is located in the medial aspect of this segment, adjacent to the pancreatic head. The third segment courses medially from its junction with the second segment toward the left at a slightly superior angulation, coursing close to the head of the pancreas at its termination. The fourth segment ascends along the lateral aspect of the aorta and then courses anteriorly to merge with the jejunum. A large portion of the duodenum lies in the retroperitoneal cavity.

The remainder of the small intestine is composed of the jejunum and ileum. The division between these two segments is arbitrary because there is no distinct morphologic division. The ileum empties into the colon via the ileocecal valve.

The arteries supplying the duodenum are the right gastric, superior pancreaticoduodenal, and inferior pancreaticoduodenal. Various branches of the superior mesenteric and intestinal arteries supply the jejunum and ileum. The venous tributaries of the small intestine terminate in the splenic and superior mesenteric veins. Usually these smaller tributaries are not seen sonographically.

Large Intestine

The large intestine is divided into the cecum, appendix, colon, rectum, and anal canal. The cecum is a large, blind pouch that is inferior to the ileocecal valve and is situated in the right iliac fossa. The appendix is located inferior to the ileocecal valve and opens into the medial aspect of the cecum. The rectum is located inferior to the sigmoid colon and anterior to the sacrum. The inferior portion of the rectum leads into the anal canal, which terminates at the external anal sphincter.

The colon consists of the ascending, transverse, descending, and sigmoid segments (Fig. 6-3). The ascending colon originates at the cecum and ascends to the right lobe of the liver where it lies in the colic impression, which is a shallow, hepatic depression lateral to the gallbladder. At this level it turns medially to form the hepatic flexure. The transverse colon extends across the abdomen from the right hepatic flexure to the inferior border of the spleen where it turns inferiorly, forming the splenic flexure. The descending colon travels inferiorly from the splenic flexure along the lateral border of the left kidney and then courses medially into the pelvis. The sigmoid colon lies in the pelvis and is very movable. Generally it forms several loops in the pelvis before coursing inferiorly to join with the rectum.

The arterial system of the colon includes the ileocolic, right colic, middle colic, and inferior mesenteric and sigmoid arteries. The various venous tributaries of the colon merge to form several major branches that drain into the superior and inferior mesenteric veins. Many of these tributaries are not demonstrated sonographically because of the surrounding bowel.

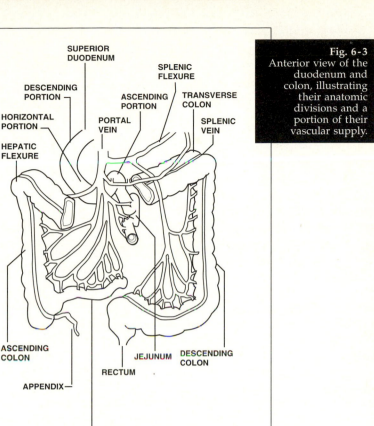

Fig. 6-3 Anterior view of the duodenum and colon, illustrating their anatomic divisions and a portion of their vascular supply.

Labels in figure: SUPERIOR DUODENUM, SPLENIC FLEXURE, DESCENDING PORTION, ASCENDING PORTION, TRANSVERSE COLON, HORIZONTAL PORTION, PORTAL VEIN, SPLENIC VEIN, HEPATIC FLEXURE, ASCENDING COLON, JEJUNUM, DESCENDING COLON, RECTUM, APPENDIX, TERMINAL ILIUM

Peritoneum and Potential Peritoneal Spaces

The peritoneum is a large, serous membrane that lines a large portion of the abdominopelvic cavity. The membrane that lines the anterior abdominal wall is called the **parietal peritoneum**. The posterior peritoneum divides the peritoneal from the retroperitoneal cavity. The **visceral peritoneum** consists of a series of serous membranes that surround the abdominal viscera, which include the liver, gallbladder, stomach, spleen, and small intestine, but which exclude most of the duodenum, colon, urinary bladder, and internal reproductive organs.

The folds of the peritoneum that suspend and enfold these organs are referred to with the prefix "meso." For example, the transverse mesocolon refers to the peritoneal fold that covers the transverse colon. The peritoneum also forms suspensory ligaments. Unlike the tough, fibrous ligaments found in skeletal joints, the peritoneal ligaments make up a layer of serous membrane and are portions of the peritoneum that extend between two organs. Examples of this type of ligament include the gastroduodenal and gastrosplenic ligaments. The hepatoduodenal ligament, also called the **lesser omentum**, courses between the lesser curvature of the stomach, the inferior aspect of the liver, and the first portion of the duodenum. The portal triad vessels course through the layers of the lesser omentum. The **greater omentum** attaches superiorly to the greater curvature of the stomach and spreads inferiorly like an apron to cover most of the abdominopelvic cavity. Located just posterior to the parietal peritoneum, the greater omentum contains a variable amount of adipose tissue and assists in maintaining internal temperature homeostasis.

The peritoneal folds and ligaments form several potential peritoneal spaces in the abdominopelvic cavity (Fig. 6-4). Although typically indistinguishable sonographically in a normal patient, pathologic processes such as ascitic fluid, tumors, abscesses, and hematomas may invade and occupy these spaces. These peritoneal spaces include the right and left subphrenic spaces, the right and left paracolic gutters, the colic spaces, the subhepatic space, and the pelvic spaces. All of the above-mentioned spaces are referred to as the **greater sac** of the peritoneal cavity. **Morrison's pouch** is the most dependent portion of the right subhepatic space, bordered inferiorly by the hepatic flexure of the colon and transverse mesocolon, medially by the duodenum and lesser omentum, and laterally by the abdominal wall. Minimal amounts of fluid in the upper abdomen in the supine patient will accumulate in Morrison's pouch (Fig. 6-5).

The **lesser sac,** or omental bursa, is a small extension of the peritoneal cavity that courses between the stomach and posterior abdominal wall (Fig. 6-6). More inferiorly, the lesser sac is

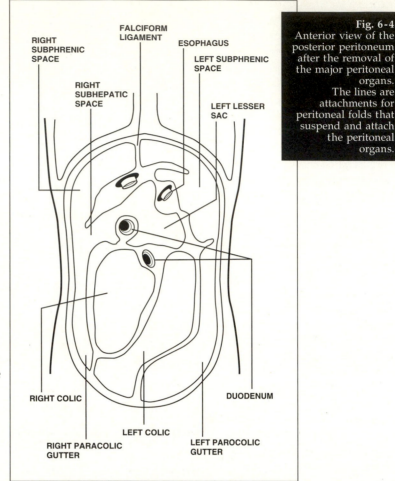

Fig. 6-4 Anterior view of the posterior peritoneum after the removal of the major peritoneal organs. The lines are attachments for peritoneal folds that suspend and attach the peritoneal organs.

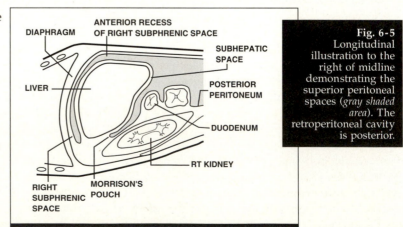

Fig. 6-5 Longitudinal illustration to the right of midline demonstrating the superior peritoneal spaces (*gray shaded area*). The retroperitoneal cavity is posterior.

bordered by the caudate lobe of the liver, the esophagus, the gastrophrenic ligament, the phrenicosplenic ligament containing the tail of the pancreas, the transverse mesocolon, and the first portion of the duodenum (Fig. 6-7). The lesser sac joins the greater sac via the **foramen of Winslow,** or epiploic foramen, which courses through the lesser omentum adjoining the portal triad vessels. Therefore pathology can extend through the epiploic foramen into the greater or lesser sac.[10]

In males the peritoneal cavity is a closed space without normal direct access from external sources. However, in females the fallopian tubes open directly into the peritoneal cavity. Consequently, bacteria and infections that enter through the vagina can gain direct access to the peritoneal cavity, which increases the risk of general peritonitis. The most dependent portion of the female pelvic peritoneum is the **pouch of Douglas,** or retrouterine space. The most dependent

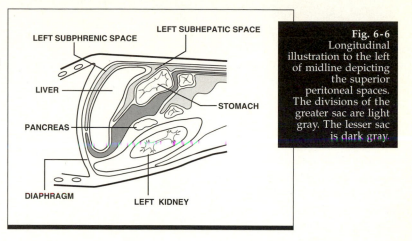

Fig. 6-6 Longitudinal illustration to the left of midline depicting the superior peritoneal spaces. The divisions of the greater sac are light gray. The lesser sac is dark gray.

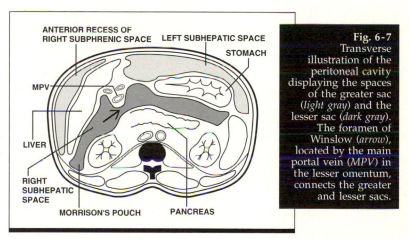

Fig. 6-7 Transverse illustration of the peritoneal cavity displaying the spaces of the greater sac (*light gray*) and the lesser sac (*dark gray*). The foramen of Winslow (*arrow*), located by the main portal vein (*MPV*) in the lesser omentum, connects the greater and lesser sacs.

portion of the male pelvis is the **retrovesicular space**. These pelvic spaces are discussed with greater detail in later chapters.

Anterior Abdominal Wall

The anterior abdominal wall consists of several layers of fat, fascia, and muscles. The skin forms the most superficial layer. Several layers of subcutaneous fat are posterior to the skin, the thickness depending on the relative obesity of the individual. The **linea alba** is a tendonlike band that is located at the midline of the abdomen, extending from the xiphoid process to the pubic symphysis. It is posterior to the subcutaneous fat layers (Fig. 6-8). The **rectus abdominus muscle** is located on either side of the linea alba and also extends the entire length of the anterior abdominal wall. Each rectus muscle is contained in the **rectus sheath,** which is joined at the midline. The lateral abdominal wall is composed bilaterally of the **external and internal oblique** and **transverse abdominus muscles.** The **peritoneum** forms the posteromedial boundary to these muscle groups.

CLINICAL LABORATORY TESTS

White Blood Cell Count

The main function of white blood cells, or leukocytes, is to control infection through phagocytosis of bacteria and other foreign organisms. Another important function is the production and distribution of antibodies specific to a particular microorganism. White blood cells are divided into two broad groups, based on whether the cells have granules in their cytoplasm. The first type, **granulocytes,** includes

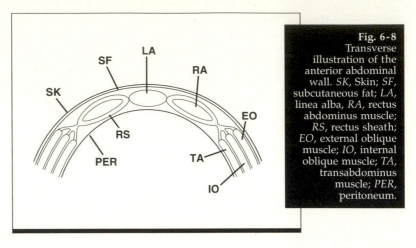

Fig. 6-8
Transverse illustration of the anterior abdominal wall. *SK*, Skin; *SF*, subcutaneous fat; *LA*, linea alba, *RA*, rectus abdominus muscle; *RS*, rectus sheath; *EO*, external oblique muscle; *IO*, internal oblique muscle; *TA*, transabdominus muscle; *PER*, peritoneum.

neutrophils, eosinophils, and basophils. The second group, **agranulocytes,** includes lymphocytes and monocytes. All white blood cells are formed in the bone marrow except lymphocytes. Lymhocytes are produced in the lymphatic tissue, such as the spleen, thymus, and tonsils.

A normal white blood cell (WBC) count is generally 5,000/mm^3 to 10,000/mm^3. A count above 10,000/mm^3 is called **leukocytosis.** Slight leukocytosis is usually an elevation to 20,000/mm^3. An increase to 30,000/mm^3 is moderate, and a count of 50,000/mm^3 above normal is a severe increase. Usually this elevation occurs with only one of the WBC types. Leukocytosis occurs with acute infections, hemorrhage, carcinoma, and acute leukemias.

Leukopenia is the term used when the WBC count is below 4,000/mm^3. This condition can occur with hypersplenisms, viral infections, leukemia, pernicious and aplastic anemias, and diabetes.

Red Blood Cell Count and Hematocrit

Red blood cells contain hemoglobin molecules that transport oxygen to the body cells. They also remove carbon dioxide from the cells and transport it to the lungs. The proper term for a mature red blood cell is an **erythrocyte.**

The red blood cell (RBC) count refers to the number of cells in 1 cc of blood. The normal values are 4.2 million/mm^3 to 5.4 million/mm^3 for men and 3.6 million/mm^3 to 5.0 million/mm^3 for women. A decreased RBC count can occur with Hodgkin's disease, leukemia, and hemolytic and pernicious anemias. A moderate to severe hemorrhage can also decrease the RBC count. An increased RBC count is seen in patients with polycythemia vera and severe diarrhea.

The **hematocrit** gives a more rapid determination of the RBC count by separating the cells from the plasma and formulating the total RBC mass. The procedure is performed in a capillary tube and is usually done on blood removed from the finger. The normal hematocrit values vary, but approximate values are 45 to 47 for men and 42 to 44 for women. Increased hematocrit levels are found in conjunction with shock, polycythemia vera, erthrocytosis, and severe dehydration. Decreased values are associated with anemias, leukemia, cirrhosis, and moderate to massive blood loss. The hematocrit is unreliable immediately after blood loss and transfusion.

RELATED IMAGING PROCEDURES

Radiography

The plain-film radiograph may demonstrate the presence of ascitic fluid, bowel obstruction, and air outside the digestive tract. It may also visualize abdominopelvic masses that displace normal organ shadows. Gastrointestinal radiographic procedures and the intravenous pyelogram (IVP) may also demonstrate pressure defects related to general abdominal pathology. Arteriography was once the method of choice for the localization of arterial hemorrhage sites, which can cause abdominal hematomas. However, nuclear medicine procedures are now the method of choice for localizing gastrointestinal bleeding.

Nuclear Medicine Imaging

Nuclear imaging procedures performed with gallium-67 citrate are very useful for detecting abdominopelvic abscesses and lymphadenopathy. This substance attaches onto white blood cells so that their migration and accumulation visualize. Both abscesses and lymphadenopathy appear as "hot spots" of radioactive concentration when compared with normal background levels. The main disadvantage of this procedure is the tendency of gallium to collect in the normal liver, spleen, and colon, which may mask an abscess.

Computed Tomography

In the study of general abdominal pathology, the main advantage of CT is its ability to identify normal bowel in relation to suspected abdominal pathology. The patient ingests a radiographic contrast medium to highlight the bowel. Another advantage is its clear, high-resolution images of the entire abdomen, resulting in anatomic relationships that are generally very discernible. A disadvantage of CT is that it cannot always differentiate between abscesses, hematomas, and necrotic tumors, because the density values for these processes can be similar. The use of an intravenous contrast medium can aid the differentiation.

SCANNING PROTOCOLS AND TECHNIQUES

The scanning protocol for sonography of the peritoneal cavity varies depending on the patient's clinical symptoms and the differential clinical diagnosis. For postoperative patients, where the referring physician wants to rule out abscess or hematoma formation, the protocol consists of transverse and longitudinal scans adjacent to the incision. The sonographer should use sterile techniques to prevent further wound complications. These precautions include placing the transducer in a sterile glove and using special sterile scanning gel packets. After the examination the patient's dressing should be changed, or the nursing staff should be notified that a clean dressing should be applied. The adjacent peritoneal spaces should also be checked for abscess or hematoma formation. When evaluating for ascites, the following potential spaces are evaluated in both transverse and longitudinal scanning planes:
- Splenic recesses and around the peripheral splenic borders
- Left subphrenic space
- Hepatic recesses and around the peripheral hepatic borders
- Right subphrenic space
- Subhepatic space (Morrison's pouch)

- Paracolic gutters
- Lesser omentum
- Lesser sac
- Transverse mesocolon
- Colic spaces—recesses around the intestinal loops
- Extrahepatic falciform ligament
- Pouch of Douglas or retrovesicular space
- Anterior to urinary bladder (space of Retzius)

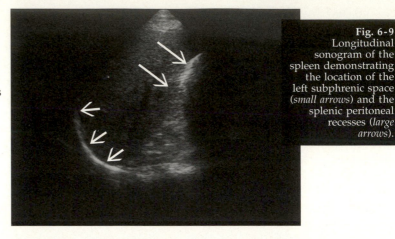

Fig. 6-9 Longitudinal sonogram of the spleen demonstrating the location of the left subphrenic space (*small arrows*) and the splenic peritoneal recesses (*large arrows*).

Figs. 6-9 through 6-14 illustrate this basic scanning protocol. Initially the patient is placed in the supine position, but oblique and decubitus positions may be necessary to display the potential spaces free of bowel gas imposition. If no pathologic condition is present, the sonographer should at least document the major spaces according to the department protocol. With pathology, more detailed scans are usually required and the cause of the abnormality should be investigated. For example, the sonographer should determine if the ascites is caused by cirrhosis of the liver or is the result of a malignancy. In the case of minimal fluid collections, the patient should be placed in the supine position for several minutes before scanning, so that gravity will cause the fluid to layer into the most dependent peritoneal spaces.

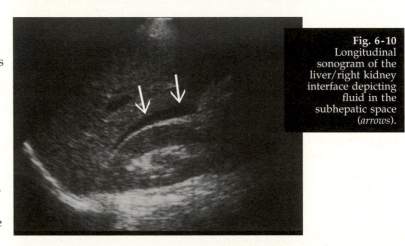

Fig. 6-10 Longitudinal sonogram of the liver/right kidney interface depicting fluid in the subhepatic space (*arrows*).

The acoustic power and gain controls for sonography of the general abdomen should be initially set using the liver to ensure that the time gain compensation (TGC) settings are balanced. In midabdominal scanning, the prevertebral vessels

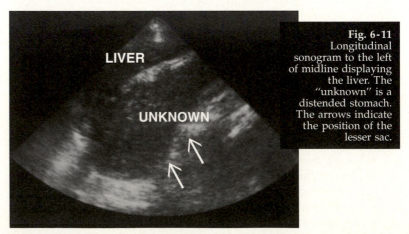

Fig. 6-11 Longitudinal sonogram to the left of midline displaying the liver. The "unknown" is a distended stomach. The arrows indicate the position of the lesser sac.

should barely demonstrate echoes in the lumens. Typically a 3.5 MHz transducer provides adequate penetration, although a 5.0 MHz transducer may provide adequate penetration for thin patients with optimum resolution. To evaluate the anterior abdominal wall and the wound in a postsurgical patient, a 5.0 MHz linear array provides a larger, superficial field of view and allows the necessary resolution for the anatomic divisions in the abdominal wall. Depending on the type of pathology and its locations, various patient positions and transducers may be required to place the area of interest in the focal zone of the transducer.

Sonography of the GI tract requires transverse and longitudinal images of the bowel segment of interest. The sonographer must recognize the various portions of the GI tract to accurately depict the surrounding soft tissue organs and to accurately identify the origin of pathology. To rule out appendicitis, sonographic examination has increased in frequency during the past several years. For this procedure the patient should have an empty urinary bladder to decrease the displacement and compression of the bowel in the iliac fossa. The scanning protocol includes transverse and longitudinal scans of the right iliac fossa, concentrating on the area adjacent to **McBurney's point**, which is the average surgical location of the appendix. McBurney's point is located by drawing a straight line between the

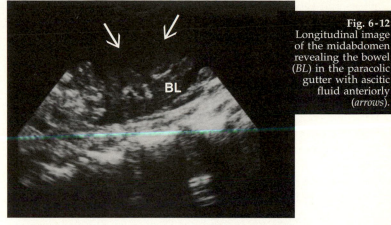

Fig. 6-12
Longitudinal image of the midabdomen revealing the bowel (*BL*) in the paracolic gutter with ascitic fluid anteriorly (*arrows*).

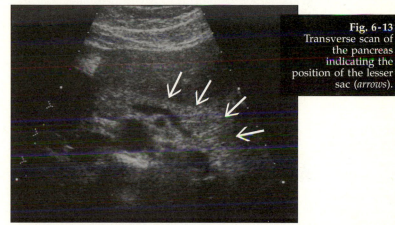

Fig. 6-13
Transverse scan of the pancreas indicating the position of the lesser sac (*arrows*).

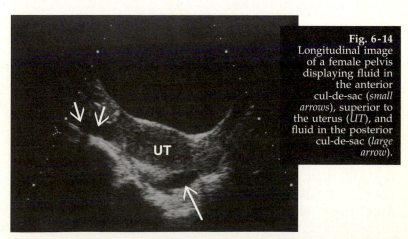

Fig. 6-14
Longitudinal image of a female pelvis displaying fluid in the anterior cul-de-sac (*small arrows*), superior to the uterus (*UT*), and fluid in the posterior cul-de-sac (*large arrow*).

umbilicus and the anterosuperior iliac spine and then moving approximately 2 inches along the line from the spine. Once this point is localized, the sonographer should apply pressure, at first lightly and then with increasing pressure. This procedure accomplishes two goals. First, it verifies if the patient is tender in the area of the appendix. Second, pressure during scanning will displace surrounding bowel loops and air so that the appendix may be localized.

For evaluating the anterior abdominal wall for suspected pathology, a linear array 5.0 MHz transducer offers a larger field of view and better resolution. The focal zone should be placed to correspond to the position of the abdominal wall layers. Transverse and longitudinal scans through the area of interest should be obtained. If the pathology is located on one side of the linea alba, scans of the unaffected side should be obtained for comparison. The use of a standoff pad may reduce reverberation artifacts and improve resolution.

NORMAL SONOGRAPHIC PATTERNS

In the normal patient the various potential peritoneal spaces are not routinely visualized. The sonographer documents only the area where the space is located. The normal GI tract has several characteristic patterns. The collapsed stomach or a bowel loop may display a small hyperechoic central area corresponding to the lumen and is referred to as the "bull's eye" or "target" sign (Fig. 6-15). A prominent or large hyperechoic area may be suggestive of a pathologic disorder such as carcinoma. The bowel may also appear complex as a result of the normal digestive process; it may contain air, which exhibits the "dirty shadow" sign; or it may display reverberation artifacts.

PATHOLOGIC PROCESSES OF THE PERITONEAL CAVITY

Ascites

Ascites is the accumulation of serous fluid in the peritoneal cavity. There are several causes of ascites, one of the more common is liver failure as a result of long-standing alcohol abuse. In liver failure, waste products, nutrients, and metabolites that are normally processed by the liver are instead channeled out of the tissue and into the peritoneal cavity. Ascites is a late manifestation of these diseases. Malignancy may be another cause of ascites. Chylous ascites results from a neoplasm obstructing the thoracic duct. The thoracic duct, the main primary duct of the lymphatic system, originates in the abdomen, ascends through the diaphragm, and drains into the left subclavian vein. An obstruction of this duct causes the release of a milky, fatty fluid into the pleural and peritoneal spaces. Other primary malignancies, particularly

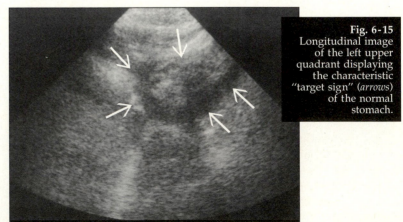

Fig. 6-15 Longitudinal image of the left upper quadrant displaying the characteristic "target sign" (*arrows*) of the normal stomach.

ovarian carcinoma, can cause malignant ascites. Whenever ascites is present without evidence of liver failure, an occult malignancy must be considered.

The primary clinical symptom associated with ascites is a distended abdomen with the presence of fluid waves when the abdomen is lightly palpated. However, this fluid wave may be difficult to see or differentiate in the case of minimal ascites or in the obese patient. If the ascites is secondary to liver failure, the liver enzymes are elevated. In the case of malignant ascites the patient may complain of weakness, unexplained weight loss in some areas, and a distended abdomen. Laboratory tests may reveal a decreased WBC count.

The typical sonographic characteristic of ascites is the presence of fluid in the most dependent portions of the abdomen and pelvis and in the intraperitoneal recesses surrounding the viscera (see Fig. 6-8 on page 124). In moderate to massive ascites, the bowel is matted and floating in the posterior, central area of the peritoneal cavity as a result of its attachment via the mesenteric root located adjacent to the posterior peritoneum. The ascitic fluid demonstrates two of the criteria of a cystic structure— through transmission and acoustic enhancement. The third characteristic, regular definite walls, is not present because the fluid conforms to any space available in the abdominopelvic cavity and relayers as a result of the effects of gravity. All the potential spaces identified in the preceding section should be checked. When malignant ascites is suspected, the sonographer should check the retroperitoneal lymph nodes and liver for evidence of further metastasis, the peritoneum for metastatic implants, and the location of the primary neoplasm.

Abdominal Abscesses and Hematomas

Approximately 85% of abdominopelvic abscesses appear after surgery or trauma. The hepatic recesses and perihepatic spaces are the most common sites for an abscess.[5] Another common site is in the pelvis. Free fluid collections below the transverse mesocolon often flow into the pouch of Douglas and perivesicular spaces. The right subhepatic space, another prime area, is accessible to free fluid that ascends the right paracolic gutter into Morrison's pouch, which is the most dependent portion of the right upper quadrant. When fluid fills Morrison's pouch, it spreads past the coronary ligament and travels into the right subphrenic space. Therefore the sonographer should always check the subhepatic space after the discovery of a right subphrenic collection.

Clinical symptoms of abdominal abscess include spiking temperature, weakness, malaise, and, occasionally, localized pain. Laboratory tests usually show an elevated WBC count and septicemia in severe cases. In postsurgical patients, open wounds draining purulent material that have positive bacterial cultures require further investigation for abscess formation.

Hematomas are typically the result of a surgical injury to the tissue or a blunt or sharp trauma to the abdomen. Symptoms of an abdominal hematoma include weakness and, occasionally, localized pain. The patient may show signs of shock if hemorrhage is moderate to severe. Laboratory tests may reveal a decreased hematocrit and RBC count, although this test may not be reliable if the hemorrhage is small or of recent development.

The sonographic pattern for an abdominal abscess often depends on the time elapsed between the formation of the abscess and the sonographic examination.[5]

Initially, abscesses appear as a
localized area of inflammation,
which produces edema. The
early sonographic pattern is typically hypoechoic compared with
the surrounding normal parenchyma. As a true abscess forms,
the typical pattern is cystic with
debris surrounded by irregular
walls. If located in a potential
space, the abscess will often con-
form to the shape of the surrounding organs and structures
(Fig. 6-16). Unlike free ascitic
fluid, an abscess contains thicker,
purulent material and is usually
walled off and therefore does not
readily relayer in the potential
space in response to gravity.

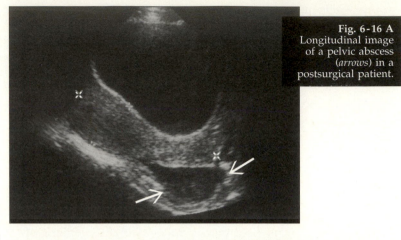

Fig. 6-16 A
Longitudinal image
of a pelvic abscess
(*arrows*) in a
postsurgical patient.

The sonographic appearance
of a hematoma also varies. An
actively bleeding or fresh hematoma may appear to have a
solid internal pattern with acoustic enhancement. As bleeding
stops and coagulation and liq-
uification occur, the pattern may
appear complex. An old hematoma reliquifies as part of the
body's natural healing process
and may possess a complex or a
totally cystic pattern.[11] If either

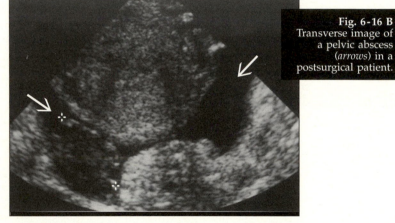

Fig. 6-16 B
Transverse image of
a pelvic abscess
(*arrows*) in a
postsurgical patient.

an abscess or a hematoma is discovered, the sonographer must scan all other potential
spaces for evidence of further contamination.

Peritoneal Malignancies

Primary peritoneal neoplasms are rare and include mesotheliomas. **Mesotheliomas**
arise from the epithelial cells of the peritoneum and pleura and classically grow as
thick sheets of tissue that extend from the anterior and posterior peritoneum and cover
the viscera. Malignant ascites may also be present.[6] Clinical symptoms include
weakness, unexplained weight loss, increased abdominal girth, and an decreased WBC
count. The prognosis is poor. Sonographically these tumors often present as a
placenta-like pattern emanating from the peritoneal layers, but they may also present
as localized, irregular solid masses (Fig. 6-17). Bowel loops may adhere to the tumor
mass. The sonographer should also check for lymphadenopathy and liver metastasis.

Metastatic deposits to the peritoneum are more common and are most often
associated with ovarian carcinoma and carcinoma of the stomach and colon. Symp-

toms include unexplained weight loss, fatigue, and specific symptoms depending on the location of the primary tumor. Their sonographic appearance includes sheetlike solid areas, as well as more localized, irregular projections attached to the anterior or posterior peritoneal lining (Fig. 6-18).

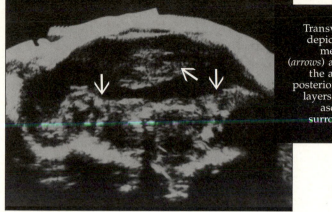

Fig. 6-17 Transverse image depicting a solid mesothelioma (*arrows*) arising from the anterior and posterior peritoneal layers. Malignant ascites is seen surrounding the masses.

PATHOLOGIC PROCESSES OF THE GASTROINTESTINAL TRACT

Bowel Neoplasms

Although sonography is not the primary diagnostic test for examining the GI tract, some bowel abnormalities can be diagnosed with sonography. Occasionally, primary tumors such as leiomyosarcoma and adenocarcinoma can be demonstrated sonographically, although care must be taken that normal stomach or bowel contents are not misinterpreted. The classic appearance of adenocarcinoma of the bowel is the "target sign," made up of a hyperechoic central area surrounded by a hypoechoic rim. Larger tumors may cause a bowel obstruction. Stomach car-

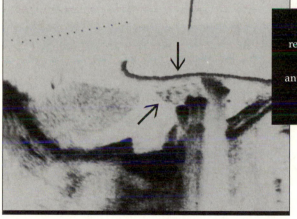

Fig. 6-18 Longitudinal scan revealing peritoneal implants (*arrows*) attached to the anterior peritoneum. The patient had a primary ovarian malignancy.

cinomas may also exhibit the "target sign" or present as a hypoechoic mass emanating from the gastric wall.[2] Endoscopic sonography is a newer technique that provides higher resolution of the mucous and muscular layers of the stomach and bowel. This allows earlier identification of neoplasms and a more accurate staging of the disease.[1] Usually any sonographic findings require further diagnostic testing, such as a barium radiographic study or endoscopy.

Bowel Obstruction

Adynamic or paralytic ileus results when nervous stimulation that causes peristalsis is interrupted, which may lead to a bowel obstruction. Some of the causes of adynamic ileus include direct intestinal tract irritation during surgery, peritoneal hemorrhage and peritonitis, pancreatitis, severe systemic infection, and severe traumatic injuries. Another category of bowel obstruction is mechanical in nature and includes fecal impaction, benign tumors or polyps, and adhesions from previous surgery or malignancies.

The clinical symptoms of bowel obstruction consist of abdominal pain, vomiting, severe constipation, and decreased to absent bowel sounds. Prolonged vomiting may cause an electrolyte imbalance. Serum amylase may be elevated. Decreased WBC and RBC counts may indicate malignancy.

The classic sonographic pattern for bowel obstruction is multiple, serpentine, dilated, fluid-filled loops of bowel. Occasionally the site and cause of the obstruction can be documented by noting the sudden collapse of the bowel loops distal to the site of obstruction.

Appendicitis

Acute appendicitis is the most common abdominal pathologic process that requires immediate surgery. This condition can occur at any age but is seen most frequently in patients between 20 and 40 years of age. The primary cause of acute appendicitis is obstruction of the appendix, usually in the form of a fecolith at its junction with the cecum. This causes the appendix to fill with its own mucinous secretions. Since the normal capacity of the appendix is less than 0.5 ml, rupture can occur relatively soon after obstruction.

The clinical symptoms of acute appendicitis consist of a slight fever and pain, usually located around McBurney's point. Laboratory tests reveal a moderately elevated WBC count. The symptoms for a ruptured appendix and consequent abscess formation include a tender, soft, palpable mass, spiking fever, and a markedly elevated WBC count. These symptoms, however, are not totally specific, and the differential clinical diagnosis must include pelvic inflammatory disease, ectopic pregnancy, and a twisted or ruptured ovarian cyst in the female patient, as well as gastroenteritis and mesenteric lymphadenitis.

Acute appendicitis is still not reliably seen with sonography, although the specificity and sensitivity have increased during the past few years. The primary diagnostic criteria on sonography is a noncompressible appendix.[12] Other signs include a wall greater than 2 mm thick and a diameter exceeding 6 to 7 mm in its greatest transverse dimension[3] (Fig. 6-19). The fecolith may visualize as a hyperechoic structure that may exhibit acoustic shadowing (Fig. 6-20). Color flow may reveal increased vascularity in the wall secondary to the infection. An appendiceal abscess may appear as a complex area adjacent to the ileocecal area in the right iliac fossa. It should be relatively noncompressible and exhibit no signs of peristalsis. These abscesses may wall off and remain localized, or they may spread into the other potential peritoneal spaces, such as the paracolic gutters and pelvic cul-de-sac. The sonographer should always scan all other potential spaces

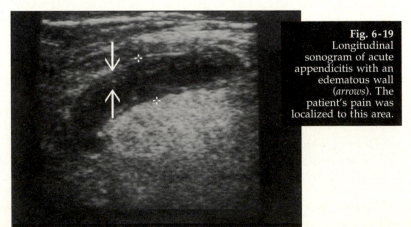

Fig. 6-19
Longitudinal sonogram of acute appendicitis with an edematous wall (*arrows*). The patient's pain was localized to this area.

when an appendiceal abscess visualizes sonographically. If the sonographer finds no evidence for appendicitis or abscess, other possible causes for the symptoms require investigation, such as a disorder of the female reproductive system.

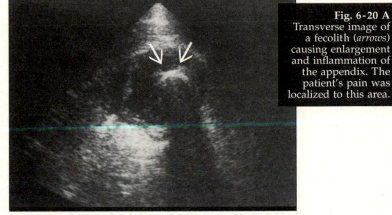

Fig. 6-20 A Transverse image of a fecolith (*arrows*) causing enlargement and inflammation of the appendix. The patient's pain was localized to this area.

PATHOLOGIC PROCESSES OF THE ANTERIOR ABDOMINAL WALL

Occasionally, palpable abdominal masses may be difficult to classify as intraabdominal in origin versus arising from within the anterior abdominal wall. Typically these masses are clinically suggestive of originating in the abdominal wall, but more detailed information is required regarding the exact pathologic entity. Sonography cannot always differentiate the exact etiology of a mass, but it can determine whether it is cystic, complex, or solid.

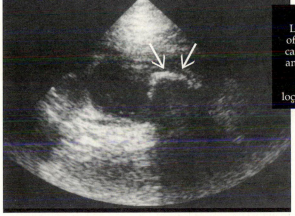

Fig. 6-20 B Longitudinal image of a fecolith (*arrows*) causing enlargement and inflammation of the appendix. The patient's pain was localized to this area.

Pathologic processes of the anterior abdominal wall can be classified into four categories. The first category consists of **normal anatomic variants.** Examples include prominent muscles in athletic individuals as well as incisional scars and keloid formations. The latter example typically causes acoustic shadowing. Another example is prominent vascular structures in the linea alba caused by severe portal hypertension.[9] These will appear as cystic tubular structures that will demonstrate flow with pulsed or color Doppler.

The second category consists of **abdominal wall hernias** that may allow loops of intestine to enter into the layers of the anterior abdominal wall. The main sonographic feature is a disruption in the hyperechoic, linear peritoneal interface just anterior to the normal bowel pattern. This disruption coupled with a mass in the abdominal wall is diagnostic of a hernia. The mass may contain only omentum and thus display as a solid mass. A herniated bowel may present as a complex mass or contain air with its related patterns.[13] The third group contains **neoplasms and metastatic processes** of the abdominal wall. This group includes benign lipomas, endometriomas, and fibromas. Sonographically, lipomas typically present as discrete, well-encapsulated solid masses in the abdominal wall (Fig. 6-21). Examples of malignant neoplasms include lymphoma, mesothelioma, melanoma, and bladder carcinomas. These malignancies tend to present a more inhomogeneous pattern than benign lesions, although correlation with the clinical history is always necessary to refine the differential diagnosis.

The fourth category consists of **inflammatory processes,** including abscesses, seromas, and hematomas. These masses may appear cystic, complex, or solid on sonographic examination. Rectus muscle hematomas usually appear as cystic masses with some solid components.[8] They are contained in the muscle or in the surrounding sheath. Typically they appear as a smoothly bulging mass on transverse views[7] (Fig. 6-22). Abdominal wall abscesses may appear cystic, complex, or solid[14] (Fig. 6-23). The sonographic pattern must be correlated with the patient's clinical history. The major sonographic sign that proves the mass is arising from the abdominal wall is the demonstration of an intact peritoneal layer posterior to the mass. If the peritoneum is disrupted, the mass may be arising from the abdominal cavity with extension into the abdominal wall.

TECHNICAL PITFALLS

The most common pitfall in abdominal sonography is the differentiation between normal bowel and pathologic processes. The sonographer should look for evidence of peristalsis and a

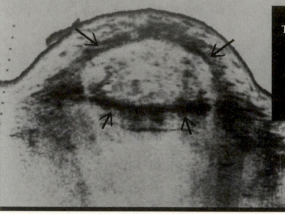

Fig. 6-21 A Transverse sonogram of a lipoma (*large arrows*) in the anterior abdominal wall. Note the intact peritoneum posteriorly (*small arrows*).

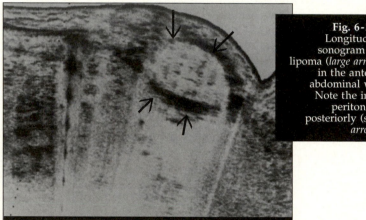

Fig. 6-21 B Longitudinal sonogram of a lipoma (*large arrows*) in the anterior abdominal wall. Note the intact peritoneum posteriorly (*small arrows*).

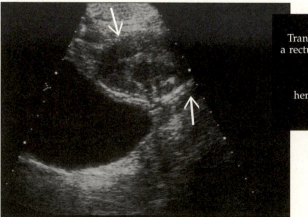

Fig. 6-22 A Transverse image of a rectus hematoma in a patient on anticoagulant therapy. The hematoma (*arrows*) was caused by sneezing.

change in the sonographic pattern. For the stomach and first portion of the duodenum, the sonographer can administer 16 to 32 ounces of water and check for the presence of microbubbles. Likewise a water enema may differentiate between normal rectum and sigmoid versus pathology in the posterior cul-de-sac. Changing the patient's position may allow differentiatiation of a free-fluid collection from an abscess or hematoma formation. The sonographer should always remember that ectopic organs, such as the kidneys, can initially appear as pathologic masses. Careful attention to gain controls will prevent the misidentification of solid versus cystic pathology.

The sonographer must always evaluate fluid collections in the upper abdomen in relation to the diaphragm.[4] Longitudinal scans allow the easiest identification. Fluid collections inferior to the diaphragm are in the peritoneal cavity. Fluid collections superior to the diaphragm are in the thoracic cavity (Fig. 6-24). This distinction is critical to the clinical management of the patient.

Another pitfall relates to misidentifying a large ovarian cyst for ascitic fluid. The sonographer should remember that the bowel loops float centrally in the abdomen with ascitic fluid, whereas cystic neoplasms displace the bowel. Using different scanning windows and angles will increase the possiblity of imaging the walls of the mass.

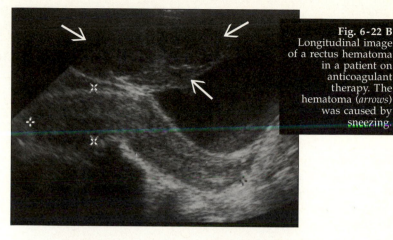

Fig. 6-22 B Longitudinal image of a rectus hematoma in a patient on anticoagulant therapy. The hematoma (*arrows*) was caused by sneezing.

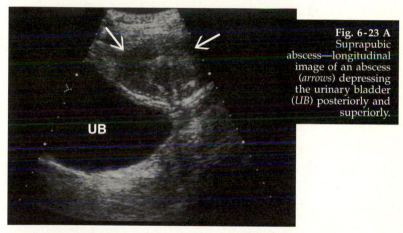

Fig. 6-23 A Suprapubic abscess—longitudinal image of an abscess (*arrows*) depressing the urinary bladder (*UB*) posteriorly and superiorly.

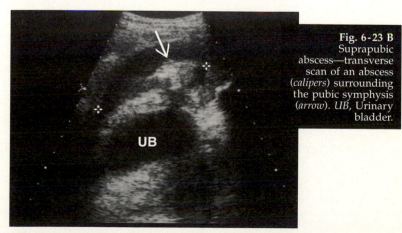

Fig. 6-23 B Suprapubic abscess—transverse scan of an abscess (*calipers*) surrounding the pubic symphysis (*arrow*). *UB*, Urinary bladder.

SUMMARY

Sonography offers a cost-effective and accurate method for the localization of free-fluid collections and masses in the peritoneal cavity. The sonographic evaluation of the bowel is still not considered a routine screening method for this type of pathology. However, the use of endoscopic sonography and the advent of new contrast agents, which will enhance the ultrasonic evaluation of these areas, may result in making this procedure more routine in the future. Table 6-1 summarizes the clinical laboratory test values with pertinent pathology as discussed in this chapter.

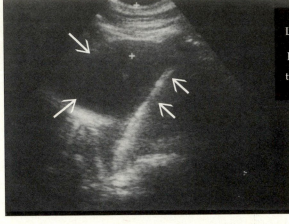

Fig. 6-24
Longitudinal view of the chest revealing pulmonic fluid (*large arrows*) superior to the diaphragm (*small arrows*).

TABLE 6-1   CLINICAL LABORATORY TEST VALUES – GENERAL ABDOMEN

	WBC	*RBC/HEMATOCRIT*	*Other Tests*
ASCITES	Normal Decrease	Normal	Increased Liver Function Tests in Cirrhosis + Malignant Cells*
ABSCESS	Increase	Normal	
HEMATOMA	Normal Increase	Decrease	
MESOTHELIOMA	Normal Decrease	Normal	+ Malignant Cells*
PERITONEAL METASTASES	Normal Decrease		+ Malignant Cells*
APPENDICITIS	Moderate Increase		

*Pathologic study of fluid sample.

WBC, White blood cell count; **RBC**, red blood cell count.

REFERENCES

1. Botet JF, Lightdale CJ, et al: Preoperative staging of gastric cancer: comparison of endoscopic US and dynamic CT, *Radiology* 181:426, 1991.
2. Fakhry JR, Berk RN: The "target" pattern: characteristic sonographic features of stomach and bowel abnormalities, *AJR* 137:969, 1981.
3. Jeffrey RB, Laing FC, Townsend RR: Acute appendicitis: sonographic criteria based on 250 cases, *Radiology* 167:327, 1988.
4. Landay M, Harless W: Ultrasonic differentiation of right pleural effusion from subphrenic fluid on longitudinal scans of the right upper quadrant: importance of recognizing the diaphragm, *Radiology* 123:155, 1977.

5. Lundstedt C, Hederstrom E, et al: Radiological diagnosis in proven intraabdominal abscess formation: a comparison between plain films of the abdomen, ultrasonography, and computerized tomography, *Gastrointest Radiol* 8:261, 1983.
6. O'Neil JD, Ross PR, et al: Cystic mesothelioma of the peritoneum, *Radiology* 170:333, 1989.
7. Rankin RN, Hutton L, Grace DM: Postoperative abdominal wall hematomas have a distinct appearance on ultrasonography, *Can J Surg* 28:84, 1985.
8. Spitz HB, Wyatt GM: Rectus sheath hematoma, *J Clin Ultrasound* 5:413, 1977.
9. Subramanyam BR, Balthazar EJ, et al: Sonography of portosystemic venous collateral in portal hypertension, *Radiology* 146:161, 1983.
10. Vincent LM, Mauro MA, Mittelstaedt CA: The lesser sac and gastrohepatic recess: sonographic appearance and differentiation, *Radiology* 150:515, 1984.
11. Wicks JD, Silver TM, Bree RL: Gray scale features of hematomas: an ultrasonic spectrum, *AJR* 131:977, 1978.
12. Worrell JA, Drolshagen LF, et al: Graded compression ultrasound in the diagnosis of appendicitis: a comparison of diagnostic criteria, *J Ultrasound Med* 9:145, 1990.
13. Yeh HC, Lehr-Janus C, et al: Ultrasonography and CT of abdominal and inguinal hernias, *J Clin Ultrasound* 12:479, 1984.
14. Yeh, HC, Rabinowitz JG: Ultrasonography and computed tomography of inflammatory abdominal wall lesions, *Radiology* 144:859, 1982.

retroperitoneal cavity

INSTRUCTIONAL OBJECTIVES

At the completion of this chapter, the reader will be able to:

1. Describe the clinical problems that are typical reasons for the sonographic evaluation of the retroperitoneal cavity.
2. Identify on transverse and longitudinal illustrations and sonograms the major anatomic divisions and structures of the retroperitoneal cavity, including the potential spaces, the prevertebral vessels, and the major retroperitoneal organs.
3. Describe the basic scanning protocol for sonography of the aorta and retroperitoneum.
4. Describe the clinical laboratory tests used for evaluating the disease processes of the retroperitoneal cavity, including the white and red blood cell counts.
5. Describe the clinical symptoms and pathologic basis for the disease processes of the retroperitoneal cavity, including aortic aneurysm, lymphadenopathy, primary and secondary neoplasms of the retroperitoneum, and abscess and hematoma formations.
6. Identify on sectional sonograms the above-mentioned disease processes of the retroperitoneum based on their sonographic appearance, clinical history, and the results of other diagnostic procedures.
7. List several technical pitfalls associated with sonography of the retroperitoneal cavity.

THE CLINICAL PROBLEM

Because of the posterior location of the retroperitoneal cavity, and because it is surrounded by the ribs, the clinical evaluation for pathology poses a challenge to the physician. A patient who has a fever of unknown origin will have a broad initial differential diagnosis. The various imaging modalities play a crucial role in narrowing this diagnosis by identifying the area of infection or by ruling out various anatomic areas in the search for the origin of the fever. A palpable midabdominal mass also poses a problem, since both peritoneal and retroperitoneal masses may be palpable. The pulsatile midabdominal mass always brings the possibility of an aortic aneurysm to the clinician's mind. However, a normal aorta in a thin patient can also present as a pulsatile mass. Sonography plays a significant role in the clinical workup of these types of patients. However, the presence of bowel gas can limit the diagnostic capabilities of the examination. The sonographer must understand the value of various patient positions and the pertinent anatomy to obtain the highest quality examination possible.

NORMAL ANATOMY

Prevertebral Vessels

The **abdominal aorta** originates at the diaphragm and travels inferiorly along the left side of the vertebrae until it bifurcates into the common iliac arteries at the level of the fourth lumbar vertebra. From superior to inferior, the main visceral branches of the aorta are:

- Celiac trunk
- Superior mesenteric artery
- Middle adrenal arteries
- Renal arteries
- Testicular and ovarian arteries
- Inferior mesenteric artery
- Common iliac arteries

Some of these branches are not essential landmarks used in abdominal sonography. There are normal variations associated with vessel origins. For example, the gastroduodenal artery may arise from the left or right hepatic artery instead of the common hepatic artery. For the celiac trunk there may be accessory or supernumerary branches. Therefore these vessels must be scanned sequentially so that each can be confidently identified. The major aortic branches and their tributaries pertinent to abdominal sonography are discussed below and are illustrated in Fig. 7-1.

The **celiac trunk** arises from the aorta, just inferior to the diaphragm. After a short course it divides into three branches: the left gastric, common hepatic, and splenic arteries. Usually the first to branch off the celiac, the left gastric artery courses anteriorly, superiorly, and toward the left through the lesser omentum to the cardiac portion of the stomach. This branch is not routinely visualized on sonography. The common hepatic artery (CHA) arises from the celiac trunk and travels transversely toward the right, posterior to the duodenum. At this point the gastroduodenal artery arises from the CHA. The CHA now changes direction and travels superiorly through the lesser omentum and gives rise to the cystic and right gastric arteries. The CHA continues to course superiorly as the proper hepatic artery. At the point it reaches the porta hepatis of the liver, it divides into the right, middle, and left hepatic arteries. As the largest branch of the celiac, the tortuous splenic artery travels transversely to the left along the superior border of the pancreas, sending tributaries to the pancreas and stomach. The splenic artery then courses anterior to the upper pole of the left kidney and enters the splenic hilum.

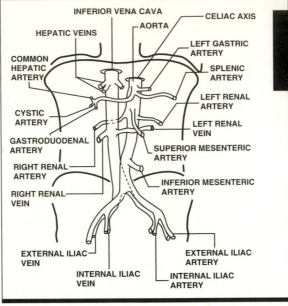

Fig. 7-1
Anterior illustration of the aorta and inferior vena cava with their major tributaires.

The **superior mesenteric artery** (SMA) arises from the anterior surface of the aorta at a variable distance inferior to the celiac trunk. It provides the vascular supply for the entire length of the small bowel except for the superior portion of the duodenum. The SMA is posterior to the splenic vein, and the splenic vein is posterior to the body and tail of the pancreas. This long vessel then travels inferiorly, anterior to the uncinate process of the pancreas and to the inferior portion of the duodenum, where it further descends into the mesentery and divides into numerous branches.

The **renal arteries** arise from either side of the aorta, just inferior to the origin of the superior mesenteric artery. The right renal artery, which is longer than the left, passes transversely anterior to the diaphragmatic crus and posterior to the inferior vena cava, the right renal vein, the head of the pancreas, and the inferior portion of the duodenum. The left renal artery travels transversely posterior to the left renal vein, the splenic vein, and the body of the pancreas. Each vessel branches into several tributaries to the adrenal glands before reaching the renal hilum, where each subdivides further.

The **right and left common iliac arteries** arise from the aorta at the approximate level of the fourth lumbar vertebra. They travel inferiorly at a diverging angle, and each then splits into the internal and external iliac arteries at the approximate level of the fifth lumbar and first sacral vertebrae. The internal iliac arteries supply the pelvic structures and organs, whereas the external iliac arteries supply the lower extremities.

The **inferior vena cava** (IVC) originates at the junction of the **common iliac veins** at the approximate level of the fifth lumbar vertebra and ascends along the right side of the vertebral column, in a more anterior plane than the spine. Along its course the IVC is posterior to the inferior portion of the duodenum, pancreas, common bile duct, portal vein, and posterior surface of the liver. In some instances the superior portion of the IVC is partially embedded in the liver parenchyma. In the upper abdomen the right kidney and ureter form the right lateral border of the IVC, and the caudate lobe of the liver and the aorta form the left border. From inferior to superior, the tributaries of the IVC are:

- Lumbar veins
- Testicular and ovarian veins

- Renal veins
- Adrenal veins
- Inferior phrenic veins
- Hepatic veins

Once again, not all of these tributaries are important sonographically. The vessels of primary interest are the renal and hepatic veins. The **right renal vein** has a shorter course than the left vein. It travels anterior to the right renal artery and enters the lateral aspect of the IVC. The **left renal vein** courses from the hilum of the left kidney, anterior to the left renal artery, crosses the aorta anteriorly, and passes posterior to the superior mesenteric artery. It enters the IVC at a slightly higher transverse plane than the right renal vein. The **hepatic veins** are the most superior tributaries of the IVC. The right, middle, and left hepatic veins converge at the posterior surface of the liver, adjacent to the diaphragm, and empty into the IVC, located in its fossa on the posterosuperior surface of the liver.

Retroperitoneal Cavity

The retroperitoneal cavity is bordered anteriorly by the posterior peritoneum, posteriorly by the spine, the psoas muscles, and the other back muscles, superiorly by the attachments for the diaphragm, and inferiorly by the pelvic brim. The retroperitoneal cavity contains the kidneys, adrenal glands, pancreas, aorta, IVC, lymph nodes, a major portion of the duodenum, and the ascending and transverse colon. The major potential spaces in the retroperitoneal cavity consist of the perinephric, the anterior paranephric, and the posterior paranephric spaces.[4] The **perinephric space** contains the kidneys, ureters, and adrenal glands. Its borders include **gerota's fascia** anteriorly and posteriorly, the diaphragm superiorly, the psoas muscle and lateral aspect of the prevertebral vessels medially, the iliac crest inferiorly, and the abdominal wall musculature laterally (Fig. 7-2). The prevertebral vessels are associated with the perirenal space, although the connective tissue surrounding these vessels usually prevents their involvement in the presence of general perirenal pathology. This space contains a variable amount of perirenal fat that is typically thickest at the inferior posterolateral aspect of the kidney.

The **anterior pararenal space** contains the pancreas, the majority of the duodenum, and the ascending and transverse colon. This space is bordered anteriorly by the posterior peritoneum, posteriorly by the anterior layer of Gerota's fascia, laterally by the fused anterior and posterior leaves of Gerota's fascia, inferiorly by the pelvic brim, and superiorly by the bare area of the liver (Fig. 7-3). This latter communication allows the possible spread of peritoneal pathology into the retroperitoneum, or vice

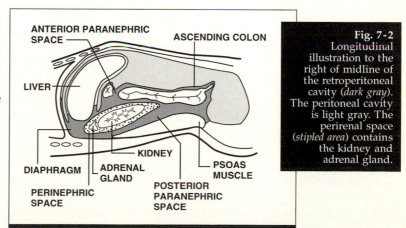

ANTERIOR PARANEPHRIC SPACE

ASCENDING COLON

LIVER

KIDNEY

DIAPHRAGM

ADRENAL GLAND

POSTERIOR PARANEPHRIC SPACE

PSOAS MUSCLE

PERINEPHRIC SPACE

Fig. 7-2 Longitudinal illustration to the right of midline of the retroperitoneal cavity (*dark gray*). The peritoneal cavity is light gray. The perirenal space (*stipled area*) contains the kidney and adrenal gland.

versa. Since the stomach and first portion of the duodenum lie in the peritoneal cavity, the second portion of the duodenum enters the retroperitoneal cavity through the posterior peritoneum and later reenters the peritoneal cavity, since the rest of the small bowel lies in this cavity. This space has no true anatomic barriers; consequently, pathologic processes such as infections can extend bilaterally. The **posterior pararenal space** contains no major organs; it contains only layers of fat, nerves, lymph nodes, and blood vessels. This space is bordered medially by the psoas muscle, superiorly by the diaphragm, and anteriorly by the posterior layer of Gerota's fascia, and it merges inferiorly with the anterior pararenal space (Fig. 7-4).

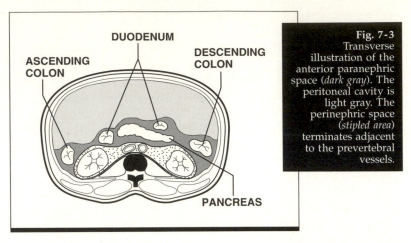

Fig. 7-3 Transverse illustration of the anterior paranephric space (*dark gray*). The peritoneal cavity is light gray. The perinephric space (*stipled area*) terminates adjacent to the prevertebral vessels.

Abdominal Lymph Nodes

The abdominal lymph nodes consist of the parietal and visceral nodes. The **parietal nodes** lie posterior to the peritoneum in the retroperitoneal cavity in close proximity to the aorta and IVC. The parietal nodes are subdivided further according to their location. These divisions include the epigastric, lumbar, common iliac, external iliac, internal iliac, iliac circumflex, and sacral groups. The lumbar group subdivides further into the lateral aortic, preaortic, and retroaortic subgroups, which literally surround the aorta. Generally the **visceral node** groups course with the blood vessels to supply the major organs, and they are divided into groups such as the liver, gallbladder, pancreas, stomach, small bowel, and large intestine. Most of these visceral nodes lie in the peritoneal cavity.

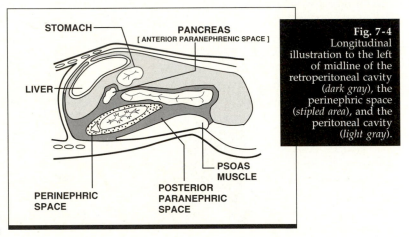

Fig. 7-4 Longitudinal illustration to the left of midline of the retroperitoneal cavity (*dark gray*), the perinephric space (*stipled area*), and the peritoneal cavity (*light gray*).

CLINICAL LABORATORY TESTS

The primary clinical laboratory tests that assist in the diagnosis of retroperitoneal pathology have been discussed in detail in the previous chapters. The **white blood cell (WBC) count** is elevated in cases of infection, with malignancies of the gastrointestinal tract and liver, with metastasis, and with leukemia. The WBC count is often decreased or totally absent with Hodgkin's and non-Hodgkin's lymphoma. The **red blood cell**

(RBC) count and **hematocrit** are decreased with moderate to severe hemorrhage and hematoma formation. Patients taking anticoagulant therapy and patients with hemophilia will have a lower hematocrit and an increased **prothrombin time.** These tests are periodically performed to monitor for signs of internal bleeding.

RELATED IMAGING PROCEDURES

Plain Abdominal Radiography

The plain abdominal radiographic examination may show calcifications in the aortic wall. These deposits are best demonstrated in a lateral view, because the aorta is projected free of the vertebral column. Because of unavoidable magnification, estimating the size of the aorta is not always accurate. Usually this examination does not visualize general retroperitoneal pathology, although the loss of the discrete borders of the ileopsoas muscles is an indication of pathologic involvement.

Computed Tomography

Computed tomography (CT) with contrast is often the method of choice for examining the retroperitoneal cavity. This area is delineated from the surrounding bowel and adjacent peritoneal spaces and organs. This examination can usually demonstrate parietal and visceral lymphadenopathy, the aorta and related wall calcifications, the origin of the renal arteries, and the fascial planes of the potential retroperitoneal spaces and adjacent muscles. An estimate of the size of aortic aneurysms can be performed, but the examination is usually ordered when a leaking aneurysm or other complications are clinically suggested.

Arteriography

Retrograde injection of the aorta with an iodinated contrast medium may be useful for the delineation of aneurysms and related complications such as dissection and leakages. The patency of aortic grafts may also be evaluated. This examination can also visualize the origins of the renal arteries and their position relative to the aneurysm. Arteriography is not always successful in the detection of mural thrombus formation. Only the true lumen may be demonstrated, which may result in underestimating the size of the aneurysm. Sonography excels at the visualization of the thrombus and at obtaining accurate measurements of the size of the aneurysm. Arteriography may also evaluate

---

BASIC SCANNING PROTOCOL

Transverse
- Proximal, from the level of the liver and diaphragm
- Mid, from the level of the pancreas, including the renal artery origins
- Distal, superior to bifurcation
- Bifurcation
- Right and left iliac arteries

Longitudinal
- Proximal, from the level of the diaphragm
- Mid, including the level of the pancreas
- Distal, from the level of bifurcation
- Bifurcation, including the courses of the right and left iliac arteries

the vascular supply of retroperitoneal neoplasms and aid in differentiating benign from malignant masses.

SCANNING PROTOCOLS AND TECHNIQUES

Aorta

The standard protocol for imaging the abdominal aorta consists of longitudinal and transverse images from the level of the diaphragm to the bifurcation into the common iliac arteries. An example of a scanning protocol for the aorta is provided in the box on the previous page.

Figs. 7-5 through 7-10 illustrate the standard protocol for the abdominal aorta. Usually the patient assumes the supine position, but coronal scans with the patient in the right or left oblique positions can display the aorta free of bowel gas superimposition. For most patients a 3.5 MHz transducer with the focal zone positioned in the far field provides adequate penetration with optimum resolution. A 5.0 MHz transducer may prove adequate for thin patients, particularly if the distal aorta is superficial. With a normal aorta, slight pressure while scanning may also improve the quality of the image. If possible, longitudinal/coronal scans should course parallel to the length of the aorta. A linear array transducer allows a larger field of view and therefore can image the length of the aorta in fewer images. If the course of the aorta is tortuous, the sonographer may need to perform several longitudinal scans at varying degrees of obliquity to image

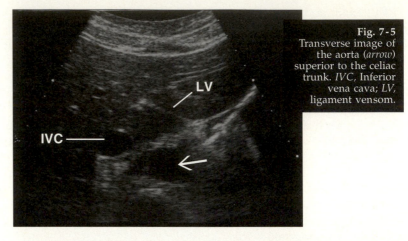

Fig. 7-5
Transverse image of the aorta (*arrow*) superior to the celiac trunk. *IVC,* Inferior vena cava; *LV,* ligament vensom.

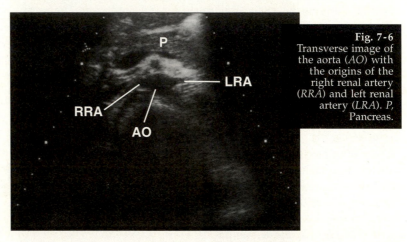

Fig. 7-6
Transverse image of the aorta (*AO*) with the origins of the right renal artery (*RRA*) and left renal artery (*LRA*). *P,* Pancreas.

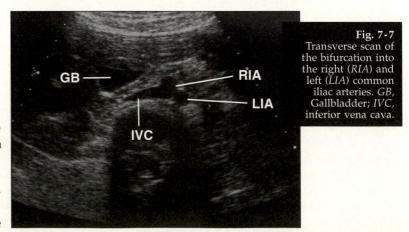

Fig. 7-7
Transverse scan of the bifurcation into the right (*RIA*) and left (*LIA*) common iliac arteries. *GB,* Gallbladder; *IVC,* inferior vena cava.

the entire aorta. Following the course of the aorta in the transverse plane will assist the sonographer in obtaining the proper longitudinal scanning planes. Since the iliac arteries diverge laterally from the bifurcation, transverse localization of their course can assist the sonographer in obtaining the proper obliquity for the longitudinal views. The coronal scanning plane can demonstrate both iliac arteries on one image. For an aneurysm, the largest postero-anterior and transverse dimensions of the aneurysm, as well as the true lumen, should be obtained on a transverse scan. The length of the aneurysm should be documented and measured on a longitudinal scan.

General Retroperitoneum

The scanning protocol for the retroperitoneal cavity will vary depending on the patient's symptoms and the clinical area of interest. Longitudinal/coronal and transverse images are always obtained for each area of interest. A 3.5 MHz transducer provides adequate penetration for the average patient. A 2.25 MHz transducer may be necessary for the obese patient, whereas a 5.0 MHz may be appropriate for thin patients. The patient is placed in the supine position for imaging the anterior pararenal space. The initial survey for the perinephric and posterior pararenal spaces is also performed with the patient in the supine position. Placing the patient in the lateral positions will allow better delineation of these spaces, since the sonogra-

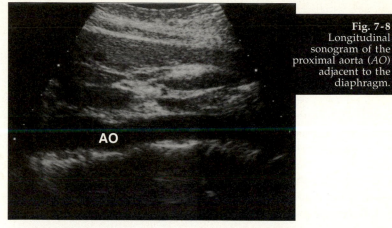

Fig. 7-8 Longitudinal sonogram of the proximal aorta (*AO*) adjacent to the diaphragm.

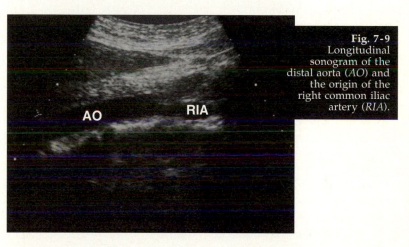

Fig. 7-9 Longitudinal sonogram of the distal aorta (*AO*) and the origin of the right common iliac artery (*RIA*).

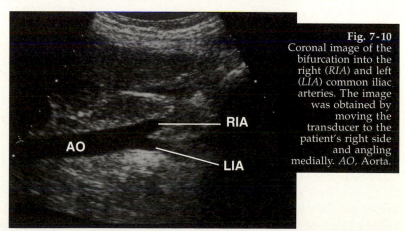

Fig. 7-10 Coronal image of the bifurcation into the right (*RIA*) and left (*LIA*) common iliac arteries. The image was obtained by moving the transducer to the patient's right side and angling medially. *AO*, Aorta.

pher can usually image these areas free of bowel gas. A full urinary bladder will assist the examination of the inferior recesses of the retroperitoneum, as well as the examination of the inferior peritoneal spaces.

Lymph Nodes

Since the retroperitoneal nodes lie adjacent to the aorta and IVC, the scanning protocol for these nodes is the same protocol that is used for the abdominal aorta. The coronal view allows excellent visualization of the medial nodes between the aorta and IVC. Again a 3.5 MHz transducer is the choice for most patients. With a normal aorta, slight pressure while scanning may displace the surrounding bowel gas and provide better delineation of the area. Although the patient normally lies supine, placing the patient in an oblique or lateral position may enhance the quality of the images. If the sonographer sees retroperitoneal lymphadenopathy, the surrounding visceral nodes should be scanned.

NORMAL SONOGRAPHIC PATTERNS

The **abdominal aorta** normally measures between 1 cm and 3 cm with a gradual tapering as it travels distally. The wall consists of three layers: the tunica adventitia, the tunica media, and the tunica intima. The tunica adventitia, the outer layer, is composed of white fibrous tissue. The tunica media, the middle layer, contains smooth muscle and white fibrous tissue. This muscle layer is quite prominent as a result of the relative high pressure in the aorta and the degree of vasoconstriction and vasodilatation. This layer is quite pronounced and accounts for the hyperechoic pattern of the wall on sonography. The inner lining, the tunica intima, is composed of epithelial tissue and undergoes changes in the presence of arteriosclerotic disease. At the proper gain settings the normal lumen should appear anechoic with a trace of echoes in it.

The **retroperitoneal spaces** are not routinely visualized sonographically. The sonographer must know the anatomic location of these spaces and document the normal surrounding landmarks. Since normal **lymph nodes** measure between 1 mm and 2 mm, they are not routinely visualized.

PATHOLOGIC PROCESSES OF THE RETROPERITONEAL CAVITY

Aorta

An **aneurysm** is an abnormal dilatation of a blood vessel that is usually caused by a weakened wall. There are several types of aneurysms (Fig. 7-11). The most common is the **fusiform** aneurysm where the entire diameter of the vessel enlarges, giving it a balloonlike appearance. A **saccular** aneurysm is a more localized weakness that causes a saclike bulge in a portion of the wall

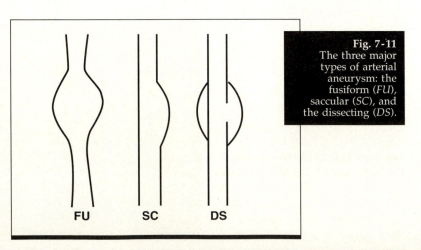

Fig. 7-11 The three major types of arterial aneurysm: the fusiform (*FU*), saccular (*SC*), and the dissecting (*DS*).

FU   SC   DS

diameter. A **dissecting** aneurysm occurs when the blood seeps between the wall layers, usually through an intimal tear. This can give the appearance of an extra lumen in addition to the normal lumen. A ruptured aortic aneurysm occurs when the outer arterial wall tears, allowing blood to escape into the retroperitoneal cavity.

Eighty percent of aortic aneurysms occur in the distal aorta, and the majority do not involve the renal artery origins. Aneurysms of the proximal abdominal aorta are rare. Most distal aortic aneurysms are of the fusiform variety and are a result of arteriosclerosis. Aneurysms that measure less than 5 cm may not be resected but should be followed with sonography on a periodic basis for evidence of enlargement. An aneurysm measuring less then 5 cm is sometimes referred to as an ectatic aorta. The sonographer will periodically see aortic grafts. The usual surgical technique is used to dissect the aortic wall, insert a Teflon or Dacron graft, and sew the original aortic wall around the graft to enhance its stability.

Many aortic aneurysms are asymptomatic and are found only through incidental radiographic or sonographic examinations. When symptoms are present, they may consist of a palpable, pulsatile midabdominal mass and mild to moderate midabdominal and lumbar pain. A ruptured aortic aneurysm is a true surgical emergency, since death can occur rapidly after rupture. The symptoms of a leaking or ruptured aneurysm are severe abdominal, back, and groin pain that increases when the patient is sitting or standing. The hematocrit and RBC count may be decreased if the rupture is large enough to cause moderate to severe hemorrhage. More than half of these patients can be saved if surgery is performed in time.

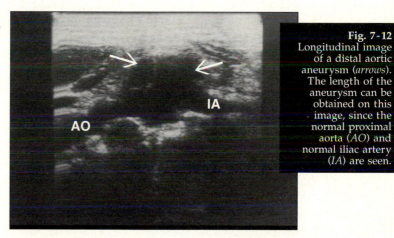

Fig. 7-12
Longitudinal image of a distal aortic aneurysm (*arrows*). The length of the aneurysm can be obtained on this image, since the normal proximal aorta (*AO*) and normal iliac artery (*IA*) are seen.

The typical sonographic appearance of an aortic aneurysm is an increased diameter greater than 3 cm in a segment of the aorta (Fig. 7-12). However, a smaller dilatation in the distal aorta may be considered abnormal. Many will contain mural thrombi, which are collections of cholesterol deposits projecting from the intimal lining (Fig. 7-13). The thickness of a mural thrombus, which governs the diameter of the true lumen, is very important to the surgeon because it affects the type and

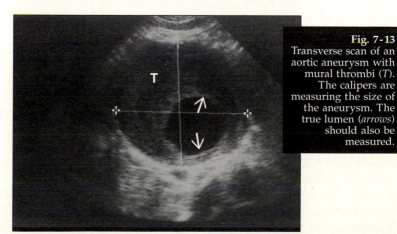

Fig. 7-13
Transverse scan of an aortic aneurysm with mural thrombi (*T*). The calipers are measuring the size of the aneurysm. The true lumen (*arrows*) should also be measured.

course of the aortic resection. A dissecting aneurysm appears sonographically as a fluid collection between the layers of the aortic wall or as an extra lumen (Fig. 7-14). Color flow will assist the sonographer in documenting whether blood flow is present in the true lumen, as well as in the area of dissection. If the renal arteries are involved in the aneurysm, surgery may be contraindicated. The use of color flow allows easier identification of the renal artery origins, particularly

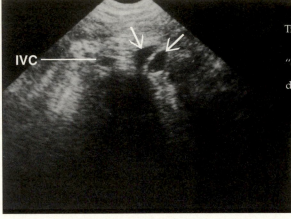

Fig. 7-14
Transverse sonogram of the distal aorta demonstrating the "double lumen" sign (*arrows*) of a dissecting aneurysm. *IVC*, Inferior vena cava.

the left renal artery. The typical appearance of a leaking or ruptured aortic aneurysm is a lack of continuity in the aortic wall that may be surrounded by a hematoma. Since the aortic wall is a specular reflector, the sonographer must change the scanning angle to ensure that the entire diameter is scanned at a 90-degree angle. Grafts placed in the aorta may also leak and cause hematoma formation. A normal graft appears as a hyperechoic inner wall surrounded by the remnants of mural thrombi and the original aortic wall.

Retroperitoneal Neoplasms

Primary retroperitoneal malignancies are rare, but metastatic disease is more common. These primary tumors arise from the tissues that comprise the retroperitoneal potential spaces, such as connective tissue, fat, fascia, muscle, vessels, nerves, and lymph nodes. Benign tumors include lipoma, fibroma, cystic teratoma or dermoid, neurofibroma, and hemangioma.[3] Retroperitoneal fibrosis is an uncommon disease that is characterized by fibrotic tissue deposition.[5] Benign retroperitoneal neoplasms are more rare than malignancies. The cause remains unknown in most patients. Malignant tumors consist of lymphoma, liposarcoma, fibrosarcoma, teratoma, lymphangioma, leiomyosarcoma, and mesothelioma.[1,2]

Clinical symptoms for both primary and secondary retroperitoneal malignancies can encompass those for general carcinoma, such as unexplained weight loss, malaise, and a palpable mass. However, the symptoms can be vague, so that pinpointing the pathology to the retroperitoneum may be difficult. Benign neoplasms may be asymptomatic, unless they gain a larger size and cause pain or other symptoms as a result of pressure. Retroperitoneal fibrosis often encapsulates vessels and portions of the urinary tract, producing related symptoms such as hypertension and dysuria or anuria. The typical patient is a man over the age of 60.

The sonographic appearance of retroperitoneal neoplasms and metastasis can range from hypoechoic to hyperechoic and complex. If these masses attain a large size, it may be difficult to establish their retroperitoneal origin. Large masses are also susceptible to necrosis and hemorrhage. Retroperitoneal fibrosis usually visualizes as a hypoechoic mass or as a sheet of tissue around blood vessels, the ureter, or renal pelvis. This is where anatomic knowledge plays an important role. The sonographer should look for anterior displacement of other retroperitoneal organs, such as the kidney, adrenal gland, or pancreas (Fig. 7-15). For right upper quadrant masses, the direction of the retroperitoneal fat displacement can narrow the differential diagnosis of the organ of origin. Generally if the mass is retroperitoneal, it will displace the fat plane anteriorly.[6] If the mass is peritoneal in origin, it will displace the fat plane posteriorly. For smaller masses the sonographer must demonstrate their relationship to surrounding retroperitoneal structures and define which potential space contains the mass.

Retroperitoneal Hematomas and Abscesses

Hematomas will develop after the hemorrhage of a vessel or organ. This can occur as a result of postsurgical complications, patients receiving anticoagulent therapy, and blunt or sharp trauma to the abdomen. The psoas muscles are a prime area for hematoma involvement.

Abscesses are pockets of purulent material usually found in the presence of systemic or local infection. Causes include postsurgical complications, complications from renal infection, and trauma. The anterior pararenal space is most frequently involved with abscess formation. Retroperitoneal abscesses can prove difficult to document because of their deep position in relation to the bowel. Other techniques, such as CT, can provide a more detailed analysis of these areas.

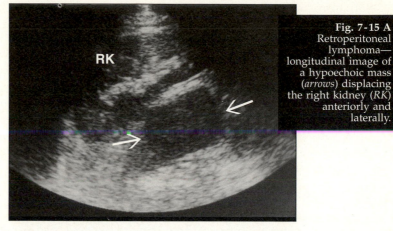

Fig. 7-15 A Retroperitoneal lymphoma—longitudinal image of a hypoechoic mass (*arrows*) displacing the right kidney (*RK*) anteriorly and laterally.

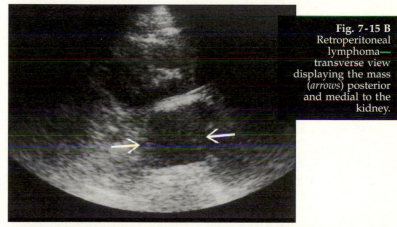

Fig. 7-15 B Retroperitoneal lymphoma—transverse view displaying the mass (*arrows*) posterior and medial to the kidney.

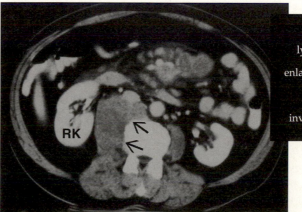

Fig. 7-15 C Retroperitoneal lymphoma—a CT scan reveals an enlarged right psoas muscle (*arrows*) caused by lymphomatous invasion. *RK*, Right kidney.

Both hematomas and abscesses may present as palpable masses. With hematomas the patient may have a decreased RBC count and show signs of anemia. In the presence of an abscess the patient may have a spiking temperature and an elevated WBC count, or the patient may have a low-grade fever of unknown origin and exhibit very subtle signs of a chronic infectious process.

Sonographically, retroperitoneal hematomas and abscesses can appear as cystic, solid, or complex masses, depending on their evolutionary stage.[7,8] Again the sonographer should look for anterior displacement of adjacent organs, such as the kidney, IVC, and pancreas, to determine their retroperitoneal origin. Because of the relative lack of anatomic barriers in the retroperitoneal cavity, all other retroperitoneal spaces should be evaluated if pathology is found.

Lymphadenopathy

The retroperitoneal lymph nodes, normally unidentifiable on sonography, enlarge in the presence of infection, inflammation, hyperplasia, and malignancy. Primary lymphatic carcinomas include lymphoma and Hodgkin's disease. Patients with acquired immunodeficiency syndrome (AIDS) have developed these two types of malignancies.[10] The incidence of non-Hodgkin's lymphoma in this patient group is significantly higher than in the general population. The lymphatic system provides one of the most common pathways of metastatic spread for a wide variety of primary malignancies.

The primary symptoms of lymphoma and Hodgkin's disease are fever, weight loss, excessive sweating, fatigue, and pruritus. Usually the cervical lymph nodes are the first to enlarge and present clinically as firm, nontender palpable masses. The WBC count is decreased or, in advanced cases, totally absent. Patients with metastatic lymph node involvement may have an increased WBC count. Periaortic lymph node involvement sometimes transmits the pulsations of the aorta further toward the right or left of the aorta's normal position.

The classic sonographic pattern for lymphadenopathy is a mass or a series of cystic to hypoechoic or rounded to ovoid-shaped masses that lie posterior, lateral, or anterior to the prevertebral vessels (Fig. 7-16). Nodal enlargement relative to infection tends to retain the more characteristic flat shape of normal lymph nodes and may display a hyperechoic central area.[9] Lymphadenopathy in patients with AIDS typically presents with diffuse involvement of the retroperitoneal nodes with extension into the viscerla nodes.[10] Again, these nodes often displace surrounding organs anteriorly and may be initially misidentified as vascular structures. The use of color-flow or pulsed Doppler can help differentiate vascular from nonvascular structures. In the presence of retroperitoneal lymphadenopathy, the sonographer should scan the adjacent visceral nodes to document the extent of the disease.

TECHNICAL PITFALLS

The most common technical pitfall for the abdominal aorta is failure to use the proper longitudinal plane to demonstrate the entire length of the aorta. The only definitive method to verify an aneurysm is to show its continuity with the normal aorta. The novice sonographer may initially misidentify the IVC as the aorta on longitudinal scans. Verifying through the use of transverse scans and the use of color-flow or pulsed Doppler and noting the variability of the IVC diameter with respirations can alleviate this problem. The main technical pitfall is failure to demonstrate mural thrombi in an aneurysm and therefore failure to identify the true lumen. The gain must be increased to demonstrate these low-level echoes. Also, changing the scanning angle relative to the aortic diameter on transverse scans will allow better visualization of the thrombus throughout the lumen.

The primary technical pitfall during retroperitoneal sonography is mistaking a collapsed bowel for lymphadenopathy and a fluid-filled or stool-filled bowel for tumors and/or abscesses. The sonographer should look for signs of peristalsis and a change in the sonographic pattern. Occasionally the patient may need a repeat examination 4 to 24 hours later. Again, the sonographer should not mistake an ectopic organ for a pathologic mass.

SUMMARY

The sonographic examination of the retroperitoneal cavity can present a challenge to the sonographer. The use of various patient positions can improve the quality of the examination. Not ing the anterior displacement of surrounding organs and structures often allows the interpreting physician to narrow the source of the pathology to the retroperitoneal cavity. Table 7-1 contains a summary of the pertinent clinical laboratory test data for pathology in the retroperitoneal cavity.

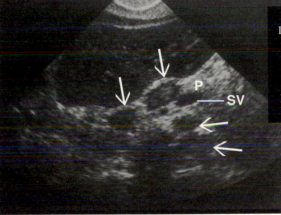

Fig. 7-16 A Lymphadenopathy—transverse image at the level of the pancreas (*P*) showing enlarged lymph nodes (*arrows*).

Fig. 7-16 B Lymphadenopathy—longitudinal scan of enlarged lymph nodes (*arrows*) along the course of the celiac vessels. *P,* Pancreas; *SV,* splenic vein.

TABLE 7-1 CLINICAL LABORATORY TEST VALUES – RETROPERITONEAL CAVITY		
	WBC	*RBC/HEMATOCRIT*
LEAKING AORTIC ANEURYSM	Normal	Decrease
MALIGNANCY	Normal Decrease	Normal
HEMATOMA	Normal Increase	Decrease
ABSCESS	Increase	Normal
PRIMARY LYMPHOMA	Decrease	Normal
METASTASES, LYMPH NODES	Increase	Normal

WBC, White blood cell count; *RBC*, red blood cell count.

REFERENCES

1. Chung WM, Ting YM, Gagliardi RA: Ultrasonic diagnosis of retroperitoneal liposarcoma, *J Clin Ultrasound* 6:266, 1978.
2. Davidson AJ, Hartman DS: Lymphangioma of the retroperitoneum: CT and sonographic characteristics, *Radiology* 175:507, 1990.
3. Davidson AJ, Hartman DS, Goldman SM: Mature teratoma of the retroperitoneum: radiologic, pathologic, and clinical correlation, *Radiology* 172:421, 1989.
4. Dodds WJ, Darweesh RMA, et al: The retroperitoneal spaces revisited, *AJR* 147:1155, 1986.
5. Fagan CJ, Amparo EG, Davis M: Retroperitoneal fibrosis, *Semin Ultrasound CT MR* 3:123, 1982.
6. Gore RM, Callen PW, Filly RA: Displaced retroperitoneal fat: sonographic guide to right upper quadrant mass localization, *Radiology* 142:701, 1982.
7. Graif M, Martinovitz U, et al: Sonographic localization of hematomas in hemophiliac patients with positive iliopsoas sign, *AJR* 148:121, 1987.
8. Hoffer FA, Shamberger RC, Teele RL: Ilio-psoas abscess: diagnosis and management. *Pediatr Radiol* 17:23, 1987.
9. Rubaltelli L, Proto E, et al: Sonography of abnormal lymph nodes in vitro: correlation of sonographic and histologic findings, *AJR* 155:1241, 1990.
10. Townsend RR, Laing FC, et al: Abdominal lymphoma in AIDS: evaluation with US, *Radiology* 171:719, 1989.

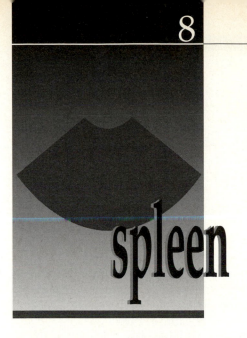

8

spleen

INSTRUCTIONAL OBJECTIVES

At the completion of this chapter, the reader will be able to:

1. Describe the clinical problems that are typical reasons for splenic sonography.
2. Identify on transverse and longitudinal/coronal illustrations and sonograms the major anatomic structures of the spleen, including the splenic capsule, the hilum of the spleen, and the splenic artery and vein.
3. Describe the basic scanning protocol for sonography of the spleen.
4. Describe the clinical laboratory tests used for evaluating splenic function, including the white and red blood cell counts and hematocrit.
5. Describe the clinical symptoms and pathologic basis for the disease processes of the spleen, including infectious processes, splenomegaly, simple cysts, primary benign and malignant neoplasms, metastasis, infarcts, and splenic rupture.
6. Identify on sectional sonograms the above-mentioned disease processes of the spleen, based on their sonographic pattern, the clinical history, and the results of other diagnostic procedures.
7. List several technical pitfalls associated with splenic sonography.

THE CLINICAL PROBLEM

Although the spleen is not essential for life, it plays an important role in the body's defense mechanisms against infection by producing nongranular leukocytes and plasma cells. The reticuloendothelial cells remove microorganisms from the circulatory system. The spleen also breaks down old red blood cells and platelets and returns the hemoglobin and other reusable components to the liver via the splenic vein. Because of these varied functions, numerous systemic disease processes can affect the spleen, such as cirrhosis, hepatitis, hemolytic anemias, and lymphomas. In many patients the first clinical sign of splenic involvement in these pathologic processes is splenomegaly. If the clinician has diagnosed the systemic disease, he or she should document the extent of splenic enlargement to determine further restrictions or treatment. For example, an enlarged spleen may increase the patient's susceptibility to rupture, and the physical activities of the patient may need to be restricted. In some patients a splenectomy may be the treatment of choice. If splenomegaly was the first clinical abnormality detected, the clinician must begin a more extensive clinical workup to determine the cause of the condition. Sonography has proved useful in determining splenomegaly and in narrowing the differential diagnosis of the cause of the condition. The sonographer must understand the various types of disease states that affect the spleen in order to examine other areas and organs, such as the liver, and thus provide the most useful information to the referring physician.

NORMAL ANATOMY

The spleen lies in the posterior aspect of the left upper quadrant and is bordered superiorly by the diaphragm, anteriorly by the stomach and splenic flexure of the colon, and medially by the left kidney and tail of the pancreas. The hilum of the spleen, the entry and exit point for the splenic vessels, is located on its anteromedial surface (Fig. 8-1). The large, tortuous splenic artery provides numerous tributaries, which enter the splenic hilum and further divide into small branches that supply the splenic cells. The tributaries of the splenic vein, which do not accompany their arterial counterparts, merge to form several large tributaries that converge at the hilum to form the splenic vein. The splenic capsule surrounds the organ, which is located in the peritoneal cavity.

CLINICAL LABORATORY TESTS

The primary clinical laboratory tests used for evaluating splenic pathologic conditions are the **white and red blood cell counts.** These tests are covered in detail in Chapter 6. With infections such as hepatitis and mononucleosis, the white blood cell (WBC) count is elevated. With malignancy the WBC count may be increased. Hodgkin's and non-Hodgkin's lymphoma often produce decreased values.

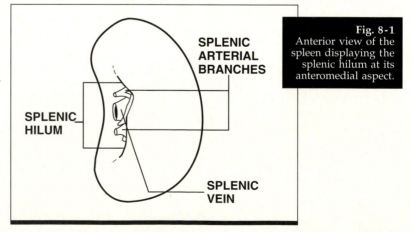

SPLENIC ARTERIAL BRANCHES

SPLENIC HILUM

SPLENIC VEIN

Fig. 8-1 Anterior view of the spleen displaying the splenic hilum at its anteromedial aspect.

Hemolytic anemias are associated with a decreased red blood cell (RBC) count. Polycythemia vera produces an elevated RBC count. Splenic rupture with moderate to severe hemorrhage can produce a decreased RBC count and hematocrit.

RELATED IMAGING PROCEDURES

Plain-Film Radiograph

The plain-film radiograph can provide some information regarding splenic size by outlining the splenic silhouette, particularly in cases of splenomegaly. However, bowel and stomach air can obscure the splenic borders. Splenic calcifications can also be visualized on this examination.

Arteriography

Retrograde filling of the splenic artery with an iodinated contrast medium outlines the splenic vascular system. Arteriography can assist in the differentiation of benign from malignant neoplasms and is occasionally used for evaluating splenic hemorrhage.

Nuclear Medicine Imaging

After the venous injection of ^{99m}Tc-sulfur colloid, nuclear imaging of the spleen allows visualization of both the liver and spleen. It can provide information on splenic size and the presence of accessory spleens, and it can evaluate splenic function. Diffuse or focal areas of decreased radioactive uptake indicate abnormal function. However, the specificity of the type of pathology causing the "cold spot" is not always high. Cysts and benign and malignant neoplasms can produce similar patterns. With minimum risk to the patient, this examination is also useful in determining the presence and extent of splenic trauma.

Computed Tomography

Computed tomography (CT) examination of the spleen can provide specific and detailed information on splenic pathology. The status of surrounding organs and lymph nodes are evaluated during the same examination. This examination can usually distinguish between solid and cystic masses and evaluate splenic size.

SCANNING PROTOCOLS AND TECHNIQUES

The routine scanning protocol for splenic sonography consists of sequential transverse and longitudinal/coronal images through the entire organ. An example of a protocol is listed in the box on this page.

Figs. 8-2 through 8-6 illustrate the splenic scanning protocol.

BASIC SCANNING PROTOCOL

Transverse
- Superior, adjacent to the left hemidiaphragm
- Midportion, at the level of the splenic hilum
- Inferior, at the level of the left kidney

Longitudinal/Coronal
- Medial, at the level of the splenic hilum
- Spleen-diaphragm interface
- Spleen-left kidney interface

Because of the spleen's posterosuperior position, an intercostal scanning approach with the patient in the right lateral position constitutes the standard scanning protocol for the normal spleen. Instructing the patient to place the left arm above the head will enlarge the intercostal spaces. Another technique to accomplish the same objective is to place a folded pillow or foam wedge under the patient's side, from the iliac crest to the costal margin. A midaxillary or posterior intercostal scanning window will avoid the more anteriorly positioned stomach and bowel. For some patients, images of the spleen will prove adequate with the patient in the supine position while still using a posterior intercostal window. In the presence of splenomegaly, supine scans using an anterior subcostal approach will demonstrate the spleen. A 3.5 MHz transducer will adequately image the spleen in average-size patients. The overall acoustic power and gain, as well as time gain compensation (TGC) controls, initally should be set using the liver, with further adjustment during survey scans of the spleen.

NORMAL SONOGRAPHIC PATTERNS

The normal spleen presents a homogeneous parenchymal pattern, isoechoic to slightly hyperechoic in comparison with the normal liver pattern at identical gain settings. The normal renal cortex is isoechoic to hypoechoic when compared with the normal splenic parenchyma (Fig. 8-6). Recognizing minimal spleno-

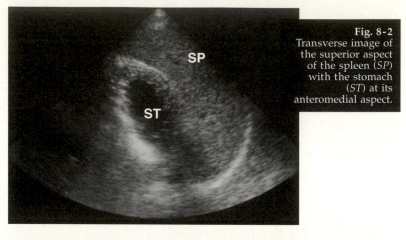

Fig. 8-2
Transverse image of the superior aspect of the spleen (*SP*) with the stomach (*ST*) at its anteromedial aspect.

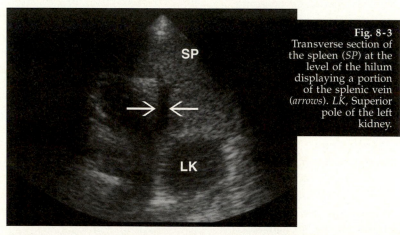

Fig. 8-3
Transverse section of the spleen (*SP*) at the level of the hilum displaying a portion of the splenic vein (*arrows*). *LK*, Superior pole of the left kidney.

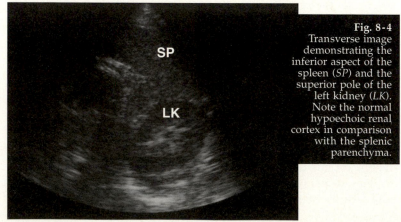

Fig. 8-4
Transverse image demonstrating the inferior aspect of the spleen (*SP*) and the superior pole of the left kidney (*LK*). Note the normal hypoechoic renal cortex in comparison with the splenic parenchyma.

megaly can present a challenge for the sonographer. The normal spleen measures approximately 11 cm in length, 5 cm in width lateromedial, and 4 cm in thickness posteroanterior.[1] Several studies have proposed various methods for determining minimal splenomegaly, including grading systems.[6] The sonographer should obtain the length measurement from the diaphragm to the inferior aspect in a longitudinal/coronal view, close to the midaxillary plane. The lateromedial measurement is obtained by rotating 90 degrees from the length measurement and placing the calipers from capsule interface to capsule interface at the widest dimension. The sonographer should also look for **Asher's sign**, which suggests splenomegaly when the splenic parenchyma protrudes more than 2 cm anterior to the aorta on a supine scan.[1]

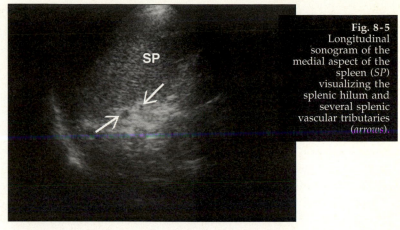

Fig. 8-5 Longitudinal sonogram of the medial aspect of the spleen (*SP*) visualizing the splenic hilum and several splenic vascular tributaries (*arrows*).

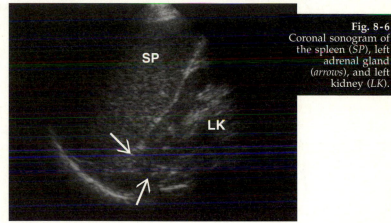

Fig. 8-6 Coronal sonogram of the spleen (*SP*), left adrenal gland (*arrows*), and left kidney (*LK*).

CONGENITAL ANOMALIES

Agenesis of the spleen is rare and is usually associated with other congenital anomalies.

Abnormal anatomic configurations and lobulations do occur, such as a "wandering" spleen and a prominent medial or inferior lobe. A "wandering" spleen refers to an atypical splenic position, such as inferiorly in the pelvis.[7] An **accessory spleen** is a more common anomaly and may be located in various sites in the abdomen, including adjacent to the splenic hilum, in the gastrosplenic ligament, or in the omentum.[14] Sonography may not detect accessory spleens located close to the bowel, which may obscure their pattern. Those accessory spleens located close to the splenic hilum may be detected as a smooth, homogeneous mass, isoechoic to the normal splenic parenchyma (Fig. 8-7). However, this pattern may appear similar to lymphadenopathy and other pathologic processes, and other diagnostic tests such as nuclear medicine may be necessary to verify the diagnosis.

Another congenital condition is the **epidermoid cyst,** which has a wall that is made up of epithelial tissue and contains a varying amount of sebum. This substance can be thick and appear as a hypoechoic pattern on sonography. The walls may also appear irregular, so that sonographic diagnosis of a benign cyst may be difficult.[11]

PATHOLOGIC PROCESSES OF THE SPLEEN

Splenic Cysts

Splenic cysts are rare and are subdivided into several groups: (1) parasitic cysts, usually resulting from echinococcal infections; (2) neoplastic cysts, including dermoid and epithelial cysts; (3) congenital cysts (mentioned previously), including the epidermoid cyst; and (4) pseudocysts that are associated with adult polycystic kidney disease and pseudocysts that may form after occult splenic rupture.

Splenic cysts are usually asymptomatic and cause no laboratory test abnormalities. However, large cysts may cause symptoms related to pressure exerted on adjacent organs or in the spleen itself.

Splenic cysts generally display the three sonographic criteria for a cyst— through transmission, regular borders, and distal acoustic enhancement (Fig. 8-8). Pseudocysts may present with irregular borders and contain debris. Rarely, a splenic abscess may mimic this pattern, although the patient may have symptoms of infection.

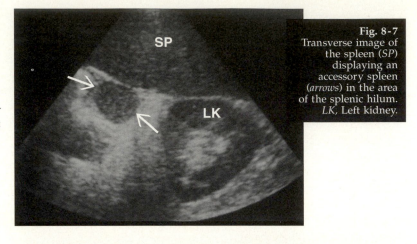

Fig. 8-7 Transverse image of the spleen (*SP*) displaying an accessory spleen (*arrows*) in the area of the splenic hilum. *LK*, Left kidney.

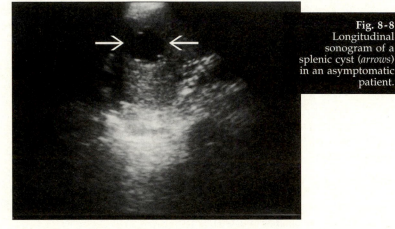

Fig. 8-8 Longitudinal sonogram of a splenic cyst (*arrows*) in an asymptomatic patient.

Splenomegaly

Most cases of splenic enlargement result from systemic disease processes and rarely from primary splenic pathology. Because the spleen is the largest part of the reticuloendothelial system, it is often effected by general infections, inflammatory processes, and general reticuloendothelial diseases, including mononucleosis, lymphomas, chronic lymphocytic leukemia, and hemolytic anemias.

Congestive splenomegaly may be caused by passive venous congestion, which is most commonly the result of portal hypertension secondary to cirrhosis of the liver. Other causes of congestive splenomegaly include thrombosis or a tumor in the portal vein and congestive heart failure.

The clinical symptoms of moderate to marked splenomegaly include an enlarged, palpable spleen extending below the costal margin, possible left upper quadrant pain, and indigestion caused by pressure exerted on the gastrointestinal tract. The WBC count may be increased or decreased, depending on the cause of the splenomegaly. The RBC count and hematocrit may be decreased, except in the case of polycythemia vera, in which these parameters are increased.

Regardless of the cause of the splenomegaly, the main sonographic characteristic is an enlarged spleen with a homogeneous parenchymal pattern (Fig. 8-9). The sonographer should identify the cause by examining the retroperitoneal lymph nodes to rule out lymphomatous invasion and by examining the liver and portal system to rule out cirrhosis. Other causes of splenomegaly may not be apparent on sonography.

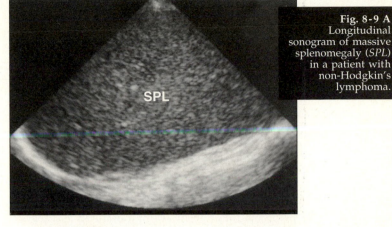

Fig. 8-9 A Longitudinal sonogram of massive splenomegaly (*SPL*) in a patient with non-Hodgkin's lymphoma.

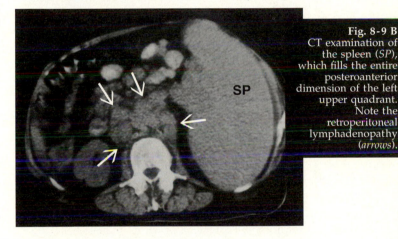

Fig. 8-9 B CT examination of the spleen (*SP*), which fills the entire posteroanterior dimension of the left upper quadrant. Note the retroperitoneal lymphadenopathy (*arrows*).

Primary and Secondary Splenic Neoplasms

Primary splenic neoplasms are rare and include benign osteomas, fibromas, and chondromas. Lymphangioma and hemangioma are more common but still are rare. Malignant primary tumors include lymphoma and hemangiosarcoma.

Although still not classified as common, splenic metastasis occurs more frequently than primary neoplasms and is associated with Hodgkin's and non-Hodgkin's lymphomas, melanoma, bronchogenic carcinoma, and carcinoma of the stomach and breast. Except for lymphomas, usually splenic metastasis only occurs with widespread, diffuse metastasis from the primary tumor.[12]

The clinical symptoms for splenic neoplasms range from asymptomatic for benign entities to left upper quadrant pain, splenomegaly, weakness, and weight loss for the malignant tumors. Clinical laboratory tests may reveal an elevated WBC count in the case of malignancy and a decreased WBC count in the case of anemias. The RBC count may be decreased.

The sonographic pattern for splenic hemangiomas, the most common primary neoplasm, ranges from solid to complex and is related to the clotting stage, since these are vascular tumors. Because this pattern is not specific, color-flow Doppler may prove beneficial, since one study determined that the color-coded vascularity decreases or disappears during compression and reappears after compression is released.[9] The pattern for primary Hodgkin's and non-Hodgkin's lymphoma varies from diffuse invasion, which may cause splenomegaly, to focal hypoechoic masses that vary from less than 1 cm to greater than 3 cm. The rarest pattern is hyperechoic.[4] Splenic metastasis may present as diffuse infiltration or focal masses ranging from hypoechoic (the "bull's eye" sign), to hyperechoic, to complex[3] (Fig. 8-10). The sonographer should always scan the retroperitoneal and splenic lymph nodes and the liver to further define the extent of the disease.

Splenic Infarction

Splenic infarction or localized hemorrhage can occur with several different pathologic processes, such as bacterial endocarditis, leukemias, and anemias, including sickle cell disease. Clinical symptoms range from asymptomatic to sudden left upper quadrant pain or more generalized abdominal pain. The typical sonographic appearance of a recent infarct is a wedge-shaped, hypoechoic area extending from the splenic capsule into the parenchyma.[2] An old infarct that has healed has a more typical hyperechoic pattern. The size may vary and can occur as a solitary mass or in multiples.

Splenic Rupture

Splenic rupture occurs when the splenic vascular supply, parenchyma, or capsule has been disrupted. This condition can be caused by blunt or penetrating abdominal or thoracic trauma or by surgical trauma, or it can occur spontaneously in patients with hematologic diseases. There are three classifications of splenic rupture. The first is **subcapsular hematoma,** in which the splenic capsule remains intact with a hematoma developing between it and the splenic parenchyma. The second type occurs when the splenic capsule is ruptured and a **peritoneal** or **retroperitoneal hematoma** develops. The third type is an **intraparenchymal rupture** that causes the formation of an intrasplenic hematoma.

The clinical symptoms of splenic rupture vary, depending on the severity of the hemorrhage. These symptoms may include left upper quadrant or generalized abdominal pain, tachycardia, a palpable mass, or an area of dull compression. Clinical laboratory data may include a decreased hematocrit and an elevated WBC count.

In the case of a subcapsular hematoma, the sonographic appearance ranges from a cystic, hypoechoic mass to a complex area in the periphery of the splenic parenchyma[8] (Fig. 8-11). A splenic rupture that disrupts the capsule may cause the development of peritoneal or retro-

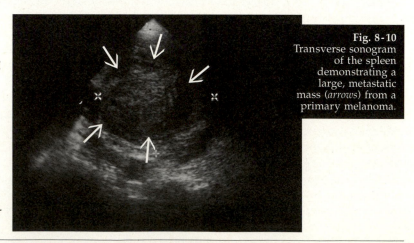

Fig. 8-10
Transverse sonogram of the spleen demonstrating a large, metastatic mass (*arrows*) from a primary melanoma.

peritoneal fluid collections or hematomas.[5] An intraparenchymal hematoma may appear as a solid, complex, or cystic mass, depending on the maturation stage of the hematoma (Fig. 8-12).

Splenic Infection and Abscess

A common infection that may affect the spleen is **histoplasmosis,** which is caused by a mold found in the soil of the central and eastern United States, Canada, and a number of other wide geographic locations. The spores are usually inhaled and phagocytized in the lungs. In some patients the spores will proliferate and travel to other organs via the circulatory system. The typical symptoms range from asymptomatic to flu-like symptoms for 1 to 4 days. When this disease affects the spleen, it can lead to fibrin or granulomatous deposition in the splenic parenchyma. This produces a characteristic hyperechoic pattern that may exhibit acoustic shadowing (Fig. 8-13). Although this is usually an incidental finding and requires no clinical intervention, this pattern in the AIDS patient may represent further infection by **pneumocystis carinii,** which initially affects the lungs.[13] The sonographer should scan the liver and kidneys for a similar granulomatous pattern.

Although uncommon, **splenic abscesses** stem from bacterial or fungal infections. Bacterial infections are more common and usually develop at a distant site and later contaminate the

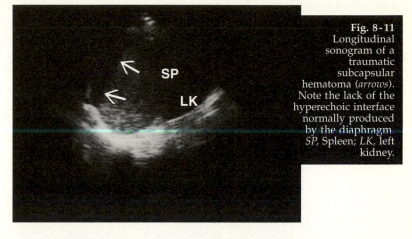

Fig. 8-11 Longitudinal sonogram of a traumatic subcapsular hematoma (*arrows*). Note the lack of the hyperechoic interface normally produced by the diaphragm. *SP,* Spleen; *LK,* left kidney.

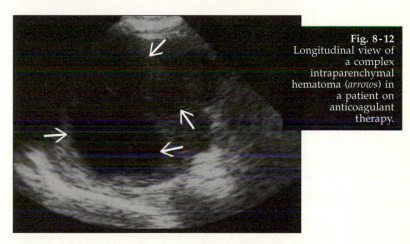

Fig. 8-12 Longitudinal view of a complex intraparenchymal hematoma (*arrows*) in a patient on anticoagulant therapy.

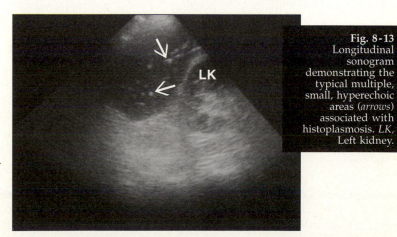

Fig. 8-13 Longitudinal sonogram demonstrating the typical multiple, small, hyperechoic areas (*arrows*) associated with histoplasmosis. *LK,* Left kidney.

spleen.[10] Clinical symptoms range from asymptomatic to the classic signs of fever, an elevated WBC count, and often left upper quadrant pain. The sonographic patterns vary from cystic, complex, or solid, depending on the cause and the evolution of the abscess. Since these often arise from other body areas, the sonographer should perform a survey scan of the abdominal organs and potential peritoneal and retroperitoneal spaces for further infection and abscess development.

TECHNICAL PITFALLS

The most common technical pitfall in splenic sonography is improper gain settings, particularly the TGC adjustment for the near field. If the near field is excessively dampened, the resulting image could mimic a subcapsular hematoma. A diagnosis based on these findings could be a very serious error if surgery is performed. If in doubt, the original near field should be placed in the focal zone of the transducer by changing the patient's position or the location of the scanning window. If the defect is reproduced, the diagnosis of a subcapsular hematoma can be made more confidently.

Another common problem is failure to visualize the spleen, particularly in elderly patients. This is often caused by the use of an intercostal space that is too anterior in relation to the spleen and that interacts with the bowel. The use of the lateral patient position and posterior scanning window will allow adequate visualization. With an atrophic spleen, the sonographer may only be able to obtain a few images of the smaller than normal organ.

SUMMARY

Sonography of the spleen allows the diagnosis of many pathologic and anomalous conditions. Splenomegaly is one of the most common types of pathology that the sonographer will see. The sonographer must remember that many different diseases

TABLE 8-1 CLINICAL LABORATORY TEST VALUES – SPLEEN			
	WBC	**RBC/HEMATOCRIT**	*Other Tests*
CYST	Normal	Normal	
PORTAL HYPERTENSION	Increase	Normal Decreased	Increased Liver Function Tests
LYMPHOMA	Decrease		
POLYCYTHEMIA VERA	Increase	Increase	
HEPATITIS	Increase	Normal	Increased Liver Function Tests
PRIMARY MALIGNANCY	Increase	Normal	
ANEMIAS	Decrease	Decrease	
HEMATOMA	Normal Increase	Decrease	
ABSCESS	Increase	Normal	

WBC, White blood cell count; *RBC*, red blood cell count.

can produce splenomegaly, and therefore the clinical history and laboratory test results are important to the differential diagnosis. The sonographer must scan other anatomic areas, which may provide additional information and refine the sonographic diagnosis. Table 8-1 contains a summary of pertinent clinical laboratory tests that will provide information on splenic pathology.

REFERENCES

1. Craig M: *Pocket guide to ultrasound measurements*, Philadelphia, 1988, JB Lippincott.
2. Georg C, Schwerk WB: Splenic infarction: sonographic patterns, diagnosis, follow-up, and complications, *Radiology* 174:803, 1990.
3. Goerg C, Schwerk WB, Goerg K: Sonography of focal lesions of the spleen, *AJR* 156:949, 1991.
4. Goerg C, Schwerk WB, et al: Sonographic patterns of the affected spleen in malignant lymphoma, *J Clin Ultrasound* 18:569, 1990.
5. Goodman LR, Aprahamaian C: Changes in splenic size after abdominal trauma, *Radiology* 176:629, 1990.
6. Ishibashi H, Higuchi N, et al: Sonographic assessment of grading of spleen size, *J Clin Ultrasound* 19:21, 1991.
7. Kinori I, Rifkin MD: A truly wandering spleen, *J Ultrasound Med* 7:101, 1988.
8. Lupien C, Sauerbrei EE: Healing in the traumatized spleen: sonographic investigation, *Radiology* 151:181, 1984.
9. Niizawa M, Ishida H, et al: Color Doppler sonography in a case of splenic hemangioma: value of compressing the tumor, *AJR* 157:965, 1991.
10. Pawar S, Kay CJ, et al: Sonography of splenic abscess, *AJR* 11138:259, 1982.
11. Ragozzino MW, Singletary H, Patrick R: Familial splenic epidermoid cyst, *AJR* 155:1233, 1990.
12. Siniluoto T, Paivansalo M, Lahde, S: Ultrasonography of splenic metastases, *Acta Radiol* 30:463, 1989.
13. Spouge AR, Wilson SR, et al: Extrapulmonary pneumocystis carinii in a patient with AIDS: sonographic findings, *AJR* 155:76, 1990.
14. Subramanyam BR, Balthazar EJ, Horii SC: Sonography of the accessory spleen, *AJR* 143:47, 1984.

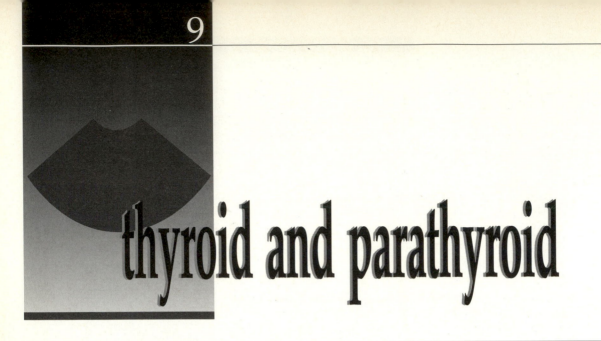

9

thyroid and parathyroid

INSTRUCTIONAL OBJECTIVES

At the completion of this chapter, the reader will be able to:

1. Describe the clinical problems that are typical reasons for sonography of the thyroid and parathyroid.
2. Identify on transverse and longitudinal illustrations and sonograms the major anatomic structures of the thyroid and parathyroid, including the lobes and isthmus of the thyroid, the location of the parathyroid glands, and the surrounding anatomic structures, such as the carotid artery, jugular vein, and neck muscles.
3. Describe the basic scanning protocol for sonography of the thyroid and parathyroid glands.
4. Describe the clinical laboratory tests used for evaluating the function of the thyroid and parathyroid glands, including triiodothyronine and thyroxine, and thyroid-stimulating hormone stimulation test and serum calcium tests.
5. Describe the clinical symptoms and pathologic basis for the disease processes of the thyroid and parathyroid glands, including cysts, goiter, thyroiditis, Grave's disease, benign and malignant neoplasms, and hyperplasia.
6. Identify on sectional sonograms the above-mentioned disease processes of the thyroid and parathyroid, based on the sonographic appearance, the clinical history, and the results of other diagnostic procedures.
7. List several technical pitfalls associated with sonography of the thyroid and parathyroid.

THE CLINICAL PROBLEM

The clinical management of a patient with a palpable thyroid mass usually includes several clinical laboratory tests, nuclear medicine imaging, and sonographic evaluation. Although nuclear medicine imaging excels at verifying whether the thyroid mass is functional and absorbing the radioactive material or dysfunctional with little or no uptake of radioactivity, usually this examination cannot distinguish whether the mass is cystic or solid, benign or malignant. Sonography plays a crucial role in the evaluation of the consistency of thyroid masses. Although the differential diagnosis of benign versus malignant neoplasm is still difficult, the sonographic examination allows the clinician to determine whether a biopsy procedure is required. One of the common symptoms for parathyroid dysfunction is abnormal serum calcium levels. Although the normal parathyroid glands are difficult to visualize with sonography, the examination can rule out parathyroid enlargement or masses and therefore allow the clinician to narrow the differential diagnosis and proceed to evaluate other organs, such as the pituitary gland.

NORMAL ANATOMY

The thyroid gland lies in the anterior region of the neck, just inferior to the larynx (Fig. 9-1). It is divided into three anatomic areas: a **right** and a **left lobe,** located on either side of the trachea, usually joined at the inferior poles by the thin **isthmus,** which drapes across the anterior aspect of the trachea. The size and exact location of the isthmus varies and in some patients is totally absent. Occasionally an accessory lobe, called a **pyramidal lobe,** projects superiorly from the isthmus or the right or left lobe. The apex or superior aspect of each lobe is bordered by the sternothyroid and inferior constrictor muscles of the pharynx. The **sternocleidomastoid muscle** serves as the primary lateral border of each lobe. At the posterolateral aspect, the **jugular vein** and **carotid artery** provide additional landmarks, with the carotid medial to the jugular vein. The **trachea** serves as the medial border for each lobe. The **longus coli muscle** courses posterior to each lobe. The entire gland is covered by a thin fibrous capsule.

The **parathyroid glands** usually consist of four separate structures located at the medial and posterior borders of the thyroid (Fig. 9-1). Two glands are typically located posterior to the right lobe, and the remaining two are located posterior to the left lobe. Masses demonstrated at the posterior aspect of the thyroid may indicate parathyroid rather than thyroid involvement. Fig. 9-2 demonstrates the thyroid and parathyroid with related anatomy in the transverse plane.

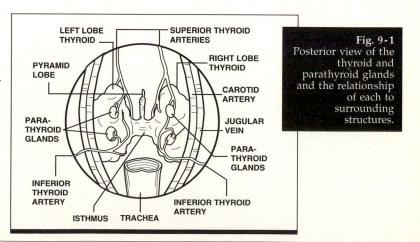

Fig. 9-1 Posterior view of the thyroid and parathyroid glands and the relationship of each to surrounding structures.

LEFT LOBE THYROID

SUPERIOR THYROID ARTERIES

PYRAMID LOBE

RIGHT LOBE THYROID

CAROTID ARTERY

JUGULAR VEIN

PARA-THYROID GLANDS

PARA-THYROID GLANDS

INFERIOR THYROID ARTERY

ISTHMUS   TRACHEA

INFERIOR THYROID ARTERY

NORMAL PHYSIOLOGY

The thyroid consists of numerous follicles, called **acini,** which are the functional and structural units of the gland. Each follicle contains a cavity filled with colloid, a homogeneous substance that collects the secretions of the follicles.

The thyroid, an endocrine gland, secretes **thyroxine** and **triiodothyronine,** the primary thyroid hormones. Both hormones are also stored in the thyroid. They increase the metabolic rate and help regulate the rate of growth and type and rate of tissue differentiation.

Calcitonin, another thyroid hormone, is secreted by the parafollicular cells that are located between the follicles. This hormone inhibits the resorption of calcium in bones, causing the serum calcium levels to decrease and thus assisting in the short-term control of serum calcium levels.

The primary function of the parathyroid glands is the secretion of parathyrin, or **parathyroid hormone** (PTH), by the chief cells. This hormone regulates long-term serum calcium levels. Calcium homeostasis is crucial to normal metabolic activity, particularly to muscle function.

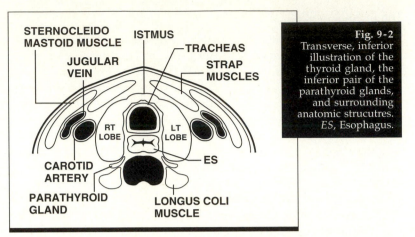

Fig. 9-2
Transverse, inferior illustration of the thyroid gland, the inferior pair of the parathyroid glands, and surrounding anatomic strucutres. *ES,* Esophagus.

CLINICAL LABORATORY TESTS

Triiodothyronine and Thyroxine

The serum levels of triiodothyronine (T_3) and thyroxine (T_4) are measured indirectly by radioimmunoassay. A venous blood sample is "tagged" with a radioactive substance that specifically binds with T_3 or T_4. By measuring the amount of radioactivity, the amount of thyroid hormone can be indirectly determined. Normal thyroid function is termed **euthyroid.** Decreased function is called **hypothyroid,** and an overactive condition is termed **hyperthyroid.** Elevated T_3 levels are found with hyperthyroidism, whereas decreased levels are associated with hypothyroidism. T_4 levels are elevated in hyperthyroidism and decreased in myxedema.

Thyroid-Stimulating Hormone

Produced by the pituitary gland, thyroid-stimulating hormone (TSH) controls the serum levels of the thyroid hormones through a negative feedback mechanism. This test differentiates between primary hypothyroidism, caused by intrinsic thyroid disease, and secondary hypothyroidism, which is caused by insufficient stimulation by the pituitary gland.

A baseline radioactive iodine (RAI) uptake test is performed, after which an intramuscular injection of TSH is administered. Venous blood samples are obtained at certain time intervals, and TSH levels are monitored using radioimmunoassay techniques. TSH levels are increased in primary hypothyroidism and normal in secondary hypothyroidism.

Parathyroid Hormone Assay

As previously mentioned, PTH plays a crucial role in calcium regulation in extracellular fluid. A decreased level of ionized calcium stimulates the secretion of PTH, whereas increased levels should inhibit PTH secretion. In hyperparathyroidism the PTH will be abnormally high compared with the calcium levels. One cause of secondary parathyroidism is chronic renal failure. To aid in the differential diagnosis, renal function tests are obtained along with the PTH test.

Calcium Tests

The amount of urinary calcium excretion provides additional information concerning parathyroid function. A 24-hour urine collection is obtained, and the calcium level is determined. The PTH levels increase with hyperparathyroidism, which results in an increased calcium excretion rate. Hypoparathyroidism causes a decreased calcium excretion rate.

The total serum calcium is an additional evaluative tool. In both hyperparathyroidism and malignancies, the serum calcium levels are increased, which is termed hypercalcemia. Because of the secretion of calcitonin by the thyroid, hyperthyroidism may also cause elevation of the serum calcium levels. Hypocalcemia, or decreased calcium levels, is rarely caused by primary hypoparathyroidism, but this condition can occur with the accidental removal of the parathyroids during thyroid surgery or after irradiation.

RELATED IMAGING PROCEDURES

Nuclear Medicine Imaging

Nuclear imaging of the thyroid using ^{99m}Tc and ^{131}I has been widely used for over 20 years in the evaluation of thyroid function and pathologic conditions. ^{131}I imaging takes advantage of the thyroid's great ability to "trap" iodine. The normal thyroid traps the iodine evenly, resulting in a fairly homogeneous pattern. Nonfunctioning or abnormal cells that have lost this trapping ability visualize as decreased areas of radioactive uptake. Areas that have an enhanced trapping capability, such as autonomous nodules, demonstrate as "hot spots" or areas of increased radioactive uptake. Scans using ^{99m}Tc display similar patterns. These examinations have a high sensitivity for distinguishing normal from abnormal function but have difficulty in differentiating cystic, benign, and malignant processes.

Parathyroid evaluation is performed with the simultaneous injection of ^{201}thallium and ^{99m}Tc, as well as using subtraction techniques to isolate parathyroid activity.[5] This examination may show one or more parathyroid glands that demonstrate as areas of increased radioactive uptake.

Computed Tomography and Magnetic Resonance Imaging

Both computed tomography (CT) and magnetic resonance imaging (MRI) can demonstrate thyroid and often parathyroid gland pathologic conditions. The advantage of these procedures compared with sonography is the adequate examination of the mediastinum for extension and spread of disease processes.

SCANNING PROTOCOLS AND TECHNIQUES

For the sonographic examination of the thyroid, the patient is placed in a supine position with a pillow or cushion placed under the shoulders so that the head and neck are moderately extended. This position allows easier access to the thyroid, which can be a challenge to scan because of the irregular and steep contours of the neck. For the normal- to small-size patient, a 7.5 MHz linear array transducer provides adequate penetration with optimum resolution. The focal zone should be placed through the thyroid. Patients with thick necks, large goiters, or other large neck masses may require a lower frequency transducer. Since the gland is superficial, the sonographer should apply very little pressure while scanning in order to avoid tissue compression and the potential to miss small masses. The normal protocol consists of sequential transverse and longitudinal scans through both lobes and the isthmus. For transverse scans, each lobe is usually scanned separately to allow a smaller field of view and thus a larger image of the gland and any small masses. However, several comparative images are included by increasing the imaging depth, which allows both lobes to be demonstrated on one image. Transverse scans are performed sequentially from inferior to superior or superior to inferior, using the trachea for the medial border of each lobe and the carotid artery and jugular vein for the lateral border. Longitudinal scans consist of sequential views of each lobe, starting medially and moving laterally, or vice versa, using the trachea as the medial border and the carotid artery as the lateral border. Magnified views and pulsed Doppler color flow evaluation may provide additional information on the pathologic composition of thyroid masses. The scanning protocol for thyroid sonography is summarized in the box below.

NORMAL SONOGRAPHIC PATTERNS

The normal thyroid measures approximately 4 cm in length, 3 cm in transverse width, and 2 cm in posteroanterior thickness.[1] The gland should demonstrate as a homogeneous, moderately hyperechoic parenchymal pattern. The acoustic power, gain, and time gain compensation (TGC) controls must be adjusted so that the echo amplitude is balanced as a function of depth, and the carotid artery and jugular vein are not filled with echoes (Fig. 9-3). Since air is usually present in the trachea, reverberation artifacts posterior to the isthmus and medial to each lobe are a common occurrence. Sonographically, the esophagus may appear slightly

---

BASIC SCANNING PROTOCOL

FOR EACH THYROID LOBE:
Longitudinal
- ✔ Images of the medial, mid, and lateral aspects, including a length measurement through the midportion of the gland.

Transverse
- ✔ Images of the inferior, mid, and superior aspects, including transverse and posteroanterior measurements through the largest dimension of each lobe. Images of the isthmus and a view displaying both lobes should be obtained for comparison.

to the left and posterior to the trachea as a hypoechoic mass that may contain a hyperechoic central area. The sonographer must not misidentify this normal structure as a pathologic mass. Best seen on longitudinal scans, the longus coli muscles appear as hyperechoic, thin bands of tissue coursing posterior to each lobe and continuing superiorly to their termination (Fig. 9-4).

The normal parathyroid glands measure approximately 4 mm in length, 3 mm in width, and 3 mm in thickness.[5] Because of the small size, normal parathyroid glands are seldom demonstrated sonographically. The sonographer should perform a routine thyroid scan, giving particular attention to the posterior border of the thyroid looking for solid or cystic masses. If a mass is found, its relationship to the thyroid capsule should be documented to determine, if possible, parathyroid origin.

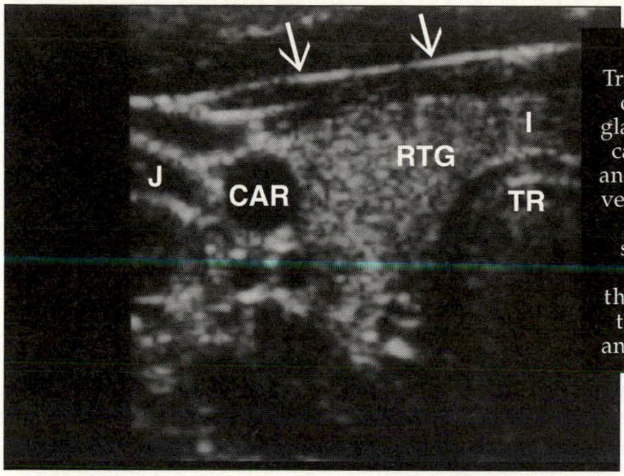

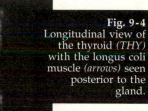

Fig. 9-3 Transverse sonogram of the right thyroid gland *(RTG)* with the carotid artery *(CAR)* and collapsed jugular vein *(J)* seen laterally. The isthmus *(I)* is seen anterior to the trachea *(TR)*. The thin strap muscles of the neck *(arrows)* lie anterior to the gland.

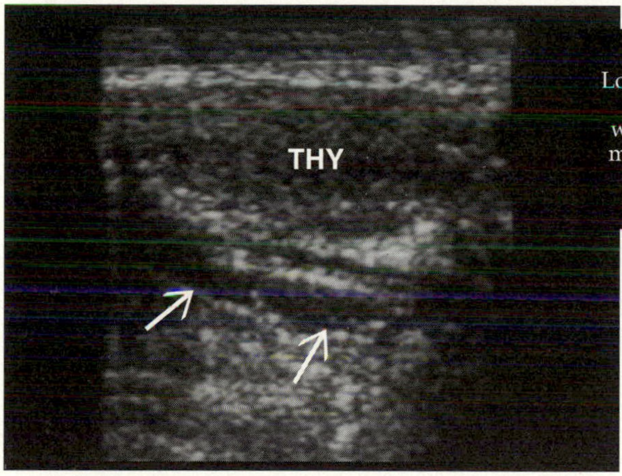

Fig. 9-4 Longitudinal view of the thyroid *(THY)* with the longus coli muscle *(arrows)* seen posterior to the gland.

PATHOLOGIC PROCESSES OF THE THYROID

Thyroid Cysts

Thyroid cysts may occur in the parenchyma of the gland or protrude into surrounding areas. Another type of cyst, called the **thyroglossal cyst,** is typically located at the midline and may extend from the base of the tongue to the isthmus of the thyroid, anterior to the trachea.[2] True thyroid cysts are more common. These cysts are usually asymptomatic, except for a palpable mass. Sonographically, they may meet all criteria for a cyst, or they may demonstrate irregular borders and contain debris as a result of colloidal content or hemorrhage.[2] The sonographer should carefully evaluate for evidence of other thyroid masses, since cystic degeneration of goiterous nodules, adenomas, and malignancies may present a similar sonographic pattern.

Benign Thyroid Neoplasms

Benign thyroid neoplasms include the following types: embryonal, fetal, follicular, Hürthle cell, and papillary adenomas. These entities are usually well encapsulated and surrounded by a thin zone of compressed thyroid tissue. The majority of solitary nodules are benign.

These benign neoplasms are usually asymptomatic and initially present as a palpable mass when larger than 1 cm. They usually present as an area of absent to decreased uptake on nuclear medicine imaging, but occasionally they appear as areas of increased uptake in relation to the surrounding normal tissue.

The classic sonographic appearance of benign thyroid adenomas is a solid, echogenic central area surrounded by a hypoechoic rim of compressed thyroid tissue. Sometimes called the "halo sign," this pattern may also be seen with malignancies. Consequently, this pattern is not a totally specific sonographic sign for a benign tumor.[9] Adenomas may undergo hemorrhage or cystic degeneration and produce a complex appearance (Fig. 9-5). Color Doppler may provide additional information, since the rim of compressed tissue may demonstrate increased vascularity.[4]

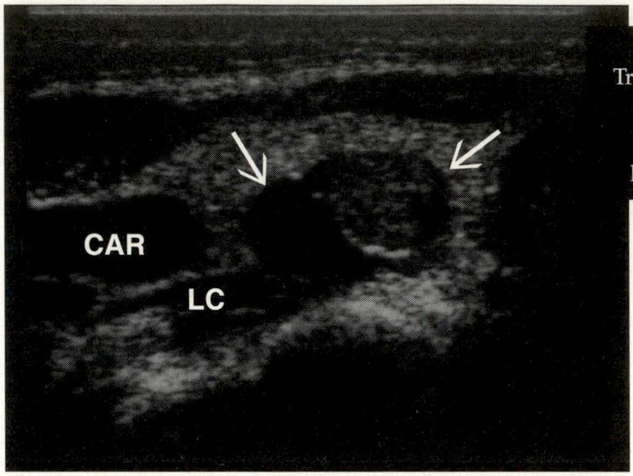

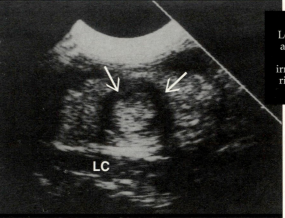

Fig. 9-5
Transverse view of a complex adenoma (*arrows*). *CAR,* Carotid artery; *LC,* longus coli muscle.

Fig. 9-6
Longitudinal scan of a thyroid carcinoma (*arrows*). Note the irregular, hypoechoic rim. *LC,* Longus coli muscle.

Malignant Thyroid Neoplasms

Thyroid carcinoma is two to four times more prevalent in females than in males and can occur at any age. There are four major classifications for thyroid malignancy: papillary, follicular, medullary, and anaplastic adenocarcinoma. Metastasis to the thyroid is associated with lymphosarcoma, and lung, breast, and renal carcinoma.

The main clinical symptom of thyroid carcinoma is a nodular or enlarged thyroid, occasionally with a rapid increase in size. Hoarseness, dysphagia, and dyspnea are later signs. Enlarged cervical lymph nodes may be the presenting symptom, and fixation of the thyroid during swallowing also indicates a localized spread of the malignancy. Typically these patients are euthyroid, and nuclear medicine imaging reveals an area of decreased radioactive uptake.

The typical sonographic appearance for thyroid carcinoma is an isoechoic to hypoechoic mass with irregular borders indicating an incomplete capsule (Fig. 9-6). These masses may contain areas of calcification or degeneration. Small calcifications that measure several millimeters and display acoustic shadowing are particularly suggestive of malignancy.[10] Color Doppler may demonstrate increased vascularity in masses greater than 1 cm.[4] The sonographer should check the cervical lymph nodes located lateral to each thyroid lobe for evidence of lymphadenopathy. Because the sonographic characteristics of benign and malignant thyroid masses are not totally specific, a biopsy procedure is usually performed before surgical intervention.

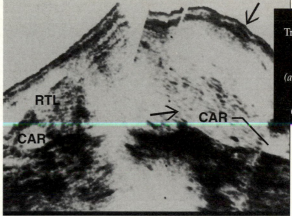

Fig. 9-7
Transverse sonogram of massive enlargement of the left thyroid lobe *(arrows)* as a result of thyroiditis. *RTL,* Right thyroid lobe; *CAR,* carotid artery.

Thyroiditis

Thyroiditis, or inflammation of the thyroid, can be divided into two primary types. The first type, called **subacute thyroiditis,** stems from inflammation. The second type is related to autoimmune responses and includes **Hashimoto's thyroiditis,** which is the most common form of thyroiditis. In the subacute variety the clinical symptoms include an enlarged, tender gland. With Hashimoto's thyroiditis, the thyroid is also enlarged, and the patient may initially develop hyperthyroidism, followed by the development of hypothyroidism.[7]

The sonographic pattern for subacute thyroiditis is an enlarged, hypoechoic gland, which may affect one lobe more than the other[11] (Fig. 9-7). In Hashimoto's thyroiditis the pattern is quite similar, although a multinodular pattern may also appear. Color Doppler may reveal a diffuse increase in vascularity. The sonographer should obtain measurements of the gland, particularly if serial examinations are ordered to monitor the resolution of the disease. In Hashimoto's thyroiditis the gland is usually normal to small as the patient becomes hypothyroid.[7]

Goiter

The term goiter, or multinodular goiter, refers to a benign thyroid enlargement that does not cause thyroid hormone abnormality. Goiter is the most common disease of the thyroid. Most patients are asymptomatic except for an enlarged thyroid or palpable mass(es) in the neck. This enlargement may cause dyspnea by compressing and/or displacing the trachea or dysphagia by exerting pressure on the esophagus. These patients are classically euthyroid. The presence of hyperparathyroidism suggests additional pathologic disorders such as Grave's disease or thyrotoxicosis.

In multinodular goiter the thyroid appears sonographically enlarged, containing multiple nodules that may appear hypoechoic to hyperechoic compared with the surrounding thyroid tissue (Fig. 9-8). These nodules may undergo hemorrhage and cystic degeneration, causing a complex sonographic pattern. Other types of goiter may produce a diffuse enlargement. In all types the enlargement may appear asymmetric. Evaluation with color Doppler may reveal no increase in vascularity.[4] The sonographer should examine any nuclear medicine scan before the sonographic examination and note any discrete areas of decreased or increased radioactive uptake to ensure that these areas are imaged.

Thyrotoxicosis and Grave's Disease

Thyrotoxicosis is a condition related to excessive secretion of thyroid hormones or TSH. It can occur in association with Grave's disease (toxic diffuse goiter) as a single toxic adenoma or as a toxic multinodular goiter. On nuclear medicine scans, these areas may appear as "hot spots" or localized areas of increased radioactive uptake.

The symptoms of Grave's disease consist of goiter, exophthalmos, and thyrotoxicosis. The exophthalmic patient has protruding eyeballs caused by increased intraocular pressure, producing a "wide-eyed" appearance. Clinical laboratory tests reveal marked hyperthyroidism, which can be a life-threatening condition. Treatment includes radioactive iodine therapy or surgery.

The sonographic patterns for thyrotoxicosis and Grave's disease are the same as for nontoxic goiter—glandular enlargement with diffuse pattern changes or discrete solid nodules. The solid nodules may undergo hemorrhage or cystic degeneration, producing a complex pattern.

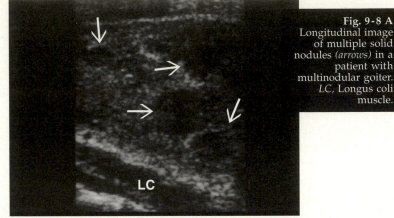

Fig. 9-8 A Longitudinal image of multiple solid nodules *(arrows)* in a patient with multinodular goiter. *LC,* Longus coli muscle.

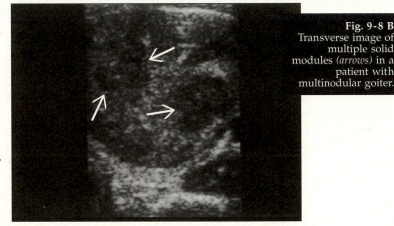

Fig. 9-8 B Transverse image of multiple solid modules *(arrows)* in a patient with multinodular goiter.

PATHOLOGIC PROCESSES OF THE PARATHYROID

The primary clinical indication of parathyroid pathology is the development of parathyroidism, characterized by increased serum and urine calcium and PTH. This condition may be a result of hyperplasia of one or more glands, an adenoma, or carcinoma. Since normal parathyroid glands are not seen sonographically, the primary use of sonography is to identify glandular enlargement. The typical sonographic appearance of an **adenoma** is a round to oval-shaped mass measuring approximately 1 cm with a hypoechoic to anechoic pattern without evidence of acoustic enhancement[8] (Fig. 9-9). Larger adenomas may develop a complex pattern. As mentioned previously, the typical location of the parathyroid glands is posterior to the thyroid or between the thyroid and carotid artery. **Hyperplasia** may be difficult to demonstrate, since enlargement may be minimal or asymmetric. In the latter case the interpreting physician may misinterpret the enlargement for an adenoma. Even the pathologist may experience difficulty differentiating between these two conditions. The same problem arises when differentiating benign from malignant neoplasms. Small **carcinomas** may exhibit the same sonographic characteristics as an adenoma.[3] Larger tumors may develop a complex pattern. A majority of the tumors will demonstrate a hypervascular pattern with color-flow Doppler. Parathyroid **cysts** are rare, and the patient is usually asymptomatic. Usually these cysts fulfill all sonographic criteria for a cystic structure. At the current time, sonography attempts to determine whether a parathyroid mass exists and whether further clinical and pathologic correlation is required for a definitive diagnosis.

TECHNICAL PITFALLS

One of the major technical pitfalls of thyroid sonography is improperly decreasing the extreme near field TGC controls and masking the appearance of the most superficial portion of the thyroid. Excessive pressure while scanning can cause the same problem. The use of a standoff pad can alleviate these artifacts. The anterior portion of the sternocleidomastoid muscle and the other anterior strap muscles should be apparent in the image with the proper gain settings and scanning pressure. Another pitfall lies in the differentiation between solid and cystic masses. Often these thyroid

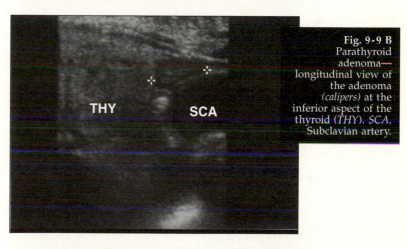

Fig. 9-9 A Parathyroid adenoma—transverse image of the right thyroid gland (*calipers*) demonstrating a small, hypoechoic mass (*arrows*). The thyroid gland (*THY*) is inhomogeneous because of goiter. *CAR*, Carotid artery.

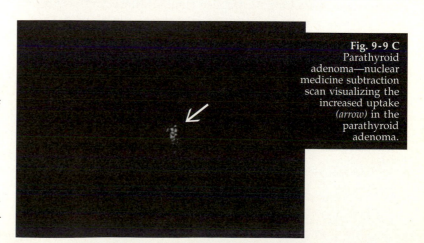

Fig. 9-9 B Parathyroid adenoma— longitudinal view of the adenoma (*calipers*) at the inferior aspect of the thyroid (*THY*). *SCA*, Subclavian artery.

Fig. 9-9 C Parathyroid adenoma—nuclear medicine subtraction scan visualizing the increased uptake (*arrow*) in the parathyroid adenoma.

TABLE 9-1   CLINICAL LABORATORY TEST VALUES – THYROID AND PARATHYROID

	T_3	T_4	TSH	PTH	CALCIUM
THYROID CYST	Normal	Normal	Normal		
THYROID NEOPLASM	Normal	Normal	Normal	Normal	
HASHIMOTO'S THYROIDITIS	Decrease	Decrease	Increase		
SUBACUTE THYROIDITIS	Increase	Increase			
GOITER	Normal	Normal	Normal		
GRAVE'S DISEASE	Increase	Increase			
PARATHYROIDISM				Increase	Increase

T_3, Triiodthyronine; T_4, thyroxine; *TSH*, thyroid-stimulating hormone; *PTH*, parathyroid hormone.

masses are less than 1 cm, so that visualization and determination of the sonographic characteristics depend on the beam width of the selected transducer. Higher frequency transducers usually have a more narrow beam width and therefore better resolution. The acoustic enhancement distal to a cyst can be difficult to appreciate. Because of the shallow depth of soft tissue imaging before meeting highly reflective interfaces, such as the trachea, there is often very little soft tissue distal to a cyst to exhibit acoustic enhancement. Changing the scanning approach so that more soft tissue lies distal to the cyst can alleviate this problem.

SUMMARY

Although sonography cannot always distinguish benign from malignant thyroid and parathyroid neoplasms, the current research with color Doppler holds promise in providing a more definitive interpretation in a number of cases. As in all sonographic examinations, obtaining a complete clinical history and pertinent clinical laboratory test results is of great value to the interpreting physician. Table 9-1 summarizes the clinical laboratory test data for diseases of the thyroid and parathyroid glands.

REFERENCES

1. Berghout Z, Wiersinga WM, et al: Determinants of thyroid volume as measured by ultrasonography in healthy adults in a noniodine deficient area, *Clin Endocrinol* 26:273, 1987.
2. Clark OH, Okerlund MD, et al: Diagnosis and treatment of thyroid, parathyroid, and thyroglossal duct cysts, *J Clin Endocrinol Metab* 48:963, 1979.
3. Edmundson GR, Charboneau JW, et al: Parathyroid carcinoma: high frequency sonographic features, *Radiology* 161:65, 1986.
4. Fobbe F, Finke R, et al: Appearance of thyroid diseases using colour-coded duplex sonography, *Eur J Radiol* 9:29, 1989.
5. Gooding GAW, Okerlund MD, et al: Parathyroid imaging: comparison of double tracer (thallium-201, technetium-^{99}m) scintography and high resolution sonography, *Radiology* 161:57, 1986.
6. Gorman B, Charboneau JW, et al: Medullary thyroid carcinoma: role of high resolution US, *Radiology* 162:147, 1987.
7. Hayashi N, Tamaki N, et al: Sonography of Hashimoto's thyroiditis, *J Clin Ultrasound* 14:123, 1986.

8. Kinishita Y, Fukase M, et al: Significance of preoperative use of ultrasonography in parathyroid neoplasms: comparison of sonographic textures with histologic findings, *J Clin Ultrasound* 13:457, 1985.
9. Propper RA, Skolnick ML, et al: The non-specificity of the thyroid halo sign, *J Clin Ultrasound* 8:129, 1980.
10. Solbiati L, Arsio B, et al: Microcalcifications: a clue in the diagnosis of thyroid malignancies, *Radiology suppl,* 177:140, 1990.
11. Tokuda Y, Kasagi K, et al: Sonography of subacute thyroiditis: changes in the findings during the course of the disease, *J Clin Ultrasound* 18:21, 1990.

scrotum and prostate

INSTRUCTIONAL OBJECTIVES

At the completion of this chapter, the reader will be able to:

1. Describe the clinical problems that are typical reasons for sonography of the scrotum and prostate.
2. Identify on transverse and longitudinal illustrations and sonograms the major anatomic structures of the male reproductive system, including the scrotum, testes, epididymis, vas deferens, seminal vesicles, prostate, and urethra and their anatomic subdivisions and surrounding anatomic landmarks.
3. Describe the basic scanning protocol for sonography of the scrotum and prostate, including national guidelines, if applicable.
4. Describe the clinical laboratory tests used for evaluating the function of the testes and prostate, including the prostate-specific antigen assay.
5. Describe the clinical symptoms and pathologic basis for the disease processes of the epididymis, testis, and prostate, including inflammatory conditions and benign and malignant neoplasms, as well as varicocele, spermatocele, hydrocele, and testicular torsion.
6. Identify on sectional sonograms the above-mentioned disease processes of the scrotum and prostate, based on their sonographic appearance, the clinical history, and the results of other diagnostic procedures.
7. List several technical pitfalls associated with sonography of the scrotum and prostate.

THE CLINICAL PROBLEM

The use of sonography for the evaluation of the scrotum and prostate has increased during the past 5 years as a result of enhanced resolution capabilities, the advent of color-flow Doppler, and the development of endocavitary transducers. The patient who has a palpable scrotal mass requires further diagnostic procedures, particularly if the physician believes that the mass is intratesticular. The majority of intratesticular solid masses are malignant, whereas most extratesticular masses are benign. In most patients sonography can verify the origin and composition of the palpable mass. Prostate carcinoma remains one of the most frequent malignancies in men and often eludes early diagnosis. The development of the prostate-specific antigen (PSA) radioimmunoassay test coupled with sonographic evaluation and localization for biopsy procedures has provided the clinician with the necessary diagnostic tools to evaluate prostatic nodules discovered during the digital rectal examination. With further refinement and research, these diagnostic tools may provide the means to routinely discover and treat prostatic carcinoma in its earliest stages.

NORMAL ANATOMY OF THE MALE REPRODUCTIVE SYSTEM

The pelvic cavity is bordered superiorly by the pelvic brim and inferiorly by the levator ani muscles (Fig. 10-1). It contains various segments of the small bowel and colon, the rectum, and the anus. The pelvis also contains the urinary bladder, distal ureters, and seminal vesicles, the distal vas deferens, ejaculatory ducts, and prostate gland. The **urinary bladder** is located posterior to the pubic symphysis. The **ureters** join the urinary bladder at the posterosuperior aspect of the bladder floor (the trigone). At the anterior apex of the trigone, the **urethra** leaves the bladder, courses through the posterior portion of the prostate gland, and continues through the penis to its external orifice. The doughnut-shaped **prostate gland** lies just inferior to the bladder. The gland is an accessory male sex organ that secretes a milky substance that increases sperm motility. The **seminal vesicles** are almond-shaped bilateral structures that are each composed of a single coiled tubule and are situated at the posterosuperior aspect of the prostate gland. The **rectum** lies posterior to the bladder, and various segments of small bowel and colon lie anterior, lateral, and superior to the collapsed urinary bladder.

Scrotum

The scrotum is a continuation of the abdominal wall and consists of skin and an incomplete layer of smooth muscle called the dartos muscle. The inferior position of the scrotum allows the maintenance of a 3° to 5° F temperature below the normal internal body temperature, which is necessary for the survival and normal motility of the sperm. The scrotal septum divides the scrotum into two sacs, each contain-

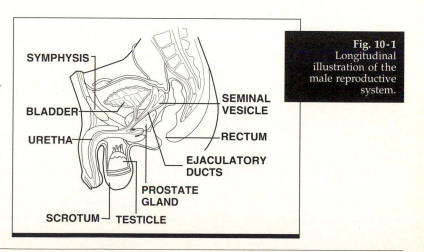

SYMPHYSIS

BLADDER

URETHA

SCROTUM — TESTICLE

SEMINAL VESICLE

RECTUM

EJACULATORY DUCTS

PROSTATE GLAND

Fig. 10-1 Longitudinal illustration of the male reproductive system.

ing a testis and epididymis. Each testicle measures 4 to 5 cm in length, 3 cm in width, and 3 cm in the posteroanterior dimension. Each sac contains a double lining called the **tunica vaginalis,** which creates a potential space that contains a small amount of fluid that prevents friction between the scrotal structures (Fig. 10-2). The **tunica albuginea** is composed of dense connective tissue and encases each testis. The tunica albuginea extends inward at its posterior aspect to

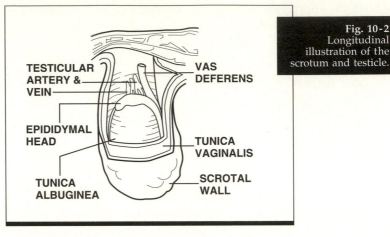

Fig. 10-2
Longitudinal illustration of the scrotum and testicle.

form an incomplete vertical septum, called the **mediastinum testis,** which further divides to form 250 to 400 wedge-shaped lobules. Each lobule contains one to three **seminiferous tubules,** which house sperm cells in various stages of development. In the testicular parenchyma, **Sartoli's cells** support and nourish the spermatozoa, whereas the **interstitial cells of Leydig** secrete androgens, primarily testosterone. The seminiferous tubules join to form a series of straight ducts, called **tubuli recti,** which then merge to form the **rete testis** that is located at the posterosuperior border of each testis. From the rete testis, the sperm pass through the ductuli efferentes and into the **epididymis.** The epididymis consists of three anatomic divisions: the tail and body, located posterior to each testis, and the head, located at the superior border. The epididymal tail merges with the **vas deferens,** which courses superiorly along the spermatic cord and enters the pelvic cavity through the inguinal canal.

The **spermatic cord** contains the testicular, deferential, and cremasteric arteries; the pampiniform plexus of veins, lymphatics, and nerves; and the vas deferens. The **testicular arteries** arise from the abdominal aorta just inferior to the renal arteries. The spermatic cord is attached to the testis at the mediastinum testis. At this location the testicular artery divides into numerous branches that course along the periphery of the testis and are called the **capsular arteries.** These tributaries give rise to the **centripetal branches,** which travel through the testicular parenchyma and course toward the mediastinum testis. The **deferential artery** supplies the vas deferens and the epididymis, whereas the **cremasteric artery** supplies the scrotal wall and muscle. The testicular venous branches within the scrotal sac, and the **pampiniform plexus** accompanies the testicular artery in the spermatic cord located superior to the testis. The **left testicular vein** drains into the left renal vein, whereas the **right testicular vein** empties directly into the inferior vena cava.

Prostate

The prostate gland measures approximately 3 cm in length, 5 cm tranversely at the base, and 3 cm in the posteroanterior dimension. The gland is roughly triangular with the base located superiorly and the narrow apex located at its inferior aspect, adjacent to the urogenital diaphragm. The prostate borders the anterior rectal wall posteriorly, separated by **Denonvillier's fascia.** The seminal vesicles lie at its posterosuperior aspect. The trigone of the urinary bladder forms the anterosuperior border. The levator ani and obturator internus muscles form the lateral borders. The anterior portion of the gland is in contact with a collection of vessels, fascia, and fat that is called the **anterior prostatic fat.** The ejaculatory ducts course from the seminal vesicles, through the prostatic tissue just lateral to midline, and drain into the prostatic urethra near the **verumontanum** at the prostatic utricle. The urethra courses through the midportion of the gland, parallel to the rectum.

The prostate is covered by a fibrous capsule that is composed of a muscular and fibrous layer. Histologically the prostate consists of two major areas: the prostatic glandular zones and the periurethral area. The **central zone** surrounds the ejaculatory ducts throughout their course in the prostate. The **transition zone,** which is roughly 5% of the glandular prostate, surrounds the proximal urethra between the verumontanum and neck of the bladder (Fig. 10-3). The **peripheral zone** accounts for approximately 75% of the glandular tissue and surrounds the central zone along its posterior and lateral aspects and includes all of the apex. The **surgical capsule** divides the central zone from the periph-

eral zone. The **periurethral glandular tissue** is a continuation of the ductal system of the peripheral and transition zones and courses from the verumontanum to the bladder neck. The **anterior fibromuscular stroma,** located anterior to the urethra, is composed of smooth muscle that is continuous with the muscles of the anterior bladder wall, adjacent to the neck of the bladder. It reaches its thickest dimension just inferior to the verumontanum and progressively narrows as it courses toward the apex.

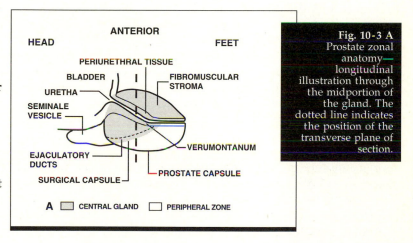

Fig. 10-3 A Prostate zonal anatomy— longitudinal illustration through the midportion of the gland. The dotted line indicates the position of the transverse plane of section.

CLINICAL LABORATORY TESTS

PSA is an enzyme normally produced by the prostate. The normal PSA values vary with age, and the values for men under 40 years of age range from 0 to 2.7 ng/ml, whereas the values for men over 40 range from 0 to 4.0 ng/ml.[6,21] Both benign prostatic hypertrophy and carcinoma will increase the PSA levels. A digital rectal examination or biopsy procedure may also cause an eleva-

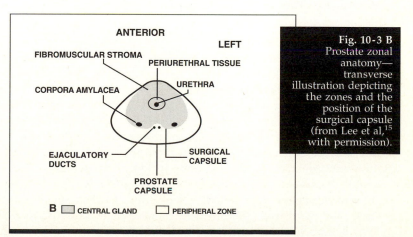

Fig. 10-3 B Prostate zonal anatomy— transverse illustration depicting the zones and the position of the surgical capsule (from Lee et al,[15] with permission).

tion. In patients with verified prostatic carcinoma, the PSA levels should decrease and fall in the normal range if treatment has effectively destroyed the malignancy. Evaluating for both PSA and prostate acid phosphatase (PAP) levels enhances the detection of early-stage carcinomas, as well as the monitoring for recurrence of the malignancy. The role of PSA by itself in screening for early-stage prostate carcinoma remains controversial, since the discriminatory zone between benign prostatic hypertrophy and early malignancy is not precise.[18] In these cases clinicians usually order a sonographic examination and biopsy procedure or request follow-up PSA levels.

Clinical laboratory tests are not always useful in determining pathologic processes of the testes. Certain neoplasms may cause increased secretion of testosterone. The choriocarcinoma may cause the secretion of female sex hormones, such as human chorionic gonadotropin. Infectious processes may elevate the white blood cell count.

RELATED IMAGING PROCEDURES

Sonography currently provides the most cost-effective method for evaluating scrotal and prostate pathologic disorders. Other diagnostic procedures can provide correlation and additional information on metastatic spread in cases of malignant neoplasms.

Computed Tomography

Computed tomography (CT) can provide additional information on metastasis from testicular and prostate primary carcinomas. This information is used in determining the patient's course of radiation or chemotherapy. A small primary carcinoma may be difficult to differentiate with this method.

Nuclear Medicine

Nuclear medicine procedures are also used to document the extent of metastasis with prostate and testicular carcinomas. Bone scans performed with ^{99m}Tc allow the diagnosis of bone metastasis, which often occurs with late-stage prostate carcinoma. For testicular torsion, a flow scan with ^{99m}Tc can diagnose decreased or absent flow to the affected testicle. The use of color-flow Doppler has enabled sonography to also document abnormal testicular flow conditions.

SCANNING PROTOCOLS AND TECHNIQUES

Scrotum

The standard scanning protocol for scrotal sonography consists of transverse and longitudinal scans performed sequentially through each scrotal sac. The box appearing on the following page is a sample protocol for scrotal sonography.

Coronal scans may prove useful to demonstrate medial scrotal masses and comparative views of the testes. Proper positioning of the scrotum usually entails the placement of a rolled towel between the patient's legs, which supports the scrotum. Another towel is placed behind the penis; the patient holds the ends of the towel and pulls the penis superiorly toward the abdominal wall, revealing the anterior wall of the scrotum. Since the scrotal contents are only loosely attached in the scrotum, the sonographer may need to reposition the scrotum to obtain true transverse and longitudinal images of each testicle. For all scans, the imaging depth is adjusted so that the testis and epididymis fill the image frame, and all scans are correctly labeled as the right or left scrotal sac. Usually a 7.5 MHz linear array transducer provides adequate penetration with optimum resolution. The sonographer should adjust the acoustic power and gain controls so that the homogeneous testicular parenchyma is displayed. These controls should remain the same for both testicles to allow comparison of the sonographic patterns. Scrotal sonography requires very little scanning pressure, since undue pressure may distort the parenchymal pattern and mask the pathologic condition.

Prostate

Transabdominal sonography provides a general survey of the pelvis, including the superior portion of the prostate, and assists in the identification of the

---

BASIC SCANNING PROTOCOL OF THE SCROTUM

Longitudinal
- ✔ Medial aspect of the testicle
- ✔ Midline image of the testicle (measurements, when appropriate)
- ✔ Lateral aspect of the testicle
- ✔ Epididymal head in relation to the testicle

Transverse
- ✔ Epididymal head
- ✔ Superior aspect of the testicle
- ✔ Midportion of the testicle (measurements, when appropriate)
- ✔ Inferior aspect of the testicle
- ✔ At least one image demonstrating both testes for pattern comparison

---

cause and severity of obstructive uropathy. The scanning protocol consists of transverse and longitudinal scans with a full urinary bladder. Transverse scans should proceed sequentially from either the superior aspect of the bladder or the inferior aspect at the level of the symphysis. Since a large portion of the prostate lies inferior to the symphysis, a caudal angulation may demonstrate more of the gland. When proceeding superiorly, the sonographer should try to identify the distal ureters and seminal vesicles. Longitudinal scans should proceed sequentially from midline to the left lateral aspect of the urinary bladder and repeat the sequence for the right side. Again, the sonographer should try to demonstrate the prostate gland, seminal vesicles, and the area of the distal ureters.

Endorectal sonography is the method of choice for the evaluation of prostate pathology. Patient preparation consists of cleansing enemas 1 hour before the examination. Antibiotics are routinely administered before a biopsy procedure. The patient is placed in either the right or left lateral position, and the endocavitary transducer is slowly inserted while the sonographer watches the image monitor until the prostate appears. The sonographer must avoid advancing the transducer too superiorly to decrease the risk of injury to the colon. The transducer must be properly prepared according to the manufacturer's instructions, which usually require the use of two sterile or aseptic sleeves or condoms. The outer sleeve connects to a catheter, which attaches to a syringe of water. Once the transducer is inserted, the sonographer injects a small amount of water in order to place a water path between the transducer and rectal wall, which allows better resolution of the posterior portion of the prostate. A 3.5 MHz transducer provides adequate penetration for patients with enlarged prostates. A higher frequency may also provide adequate penetration. The scanning protocol consists of sequential transverse and longitudinal images. The box appearing on the following page is a sample protocol for endorectal prostatic sonography.

Transverse scans should proceed sequentially from either the inferior aspect of the apex or the superior border of the seminal vesicles. To change the scanning plane, the sonographer should slowly move the transducer either superiorly or inferiorly in the rectum. Longitudinal scans should proceed sequentially from the midline to the right lateral aspect of the prostate and then repeat the sequence for the left side. The transducer is moved slowly in a lateromedial orientation in the rectum.

NORMAL SONOGRAPHIC PATTERNS

Scrotum

The normal testicle demonstrates a homogeneous, fine, moderately hyperechoic sonographic pattern. The tunica albuginea normally produces a fine hyperechoic outline around the testis. Along the posterior aspect of the testis, the tunica albuginea invaginates into the testis as the **mediastinum testis,** which appears sonographically as a hyperechoic linear area, best seen on transverse scans (Fig. 10-4); although it may also appear as a linear structure on longitudinal scans.[13] The potential space surrounding each testicle, the **tunica vaginalis propria testis,** normally contains a few millimeters of fluid and

---

BASIC SCANNING PROTOCOL OF THE PROSTATE

Transverse
- Inferior aspect of the apex
- Area of the verumontanum
- Midportion of the gland
- Superior aspect of the prostate
- Seminal vesicles

Longitudinal
- Midline of the prostate (prostatic urethra may be seen in inferior aspect)
- Area of right and left ejaculatory ducts
- Lateral aspect of the gland bilaterally
- Seminal vesicles in relation to the superior portion of the prostate

---

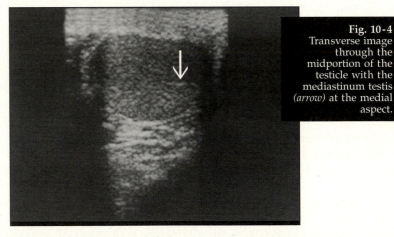

Fig. 10-4 Transverse image through the midportion of the testicle with the mediastinum testis *(arrow)* at the medial aspect.

---

should not be mistaken for a hydrocele or other pathology.[3] The body and tail of the epididymis courses along the posterior aspect of the testicle, whereas the head lies at the superior aspect. The normal epididymis possesses a courser pattern than the testicle and appears isoechoic to hyperechoic when compared with the normal testis (Fig. 10-5).

The use of color-flow Doppler has enhanced the diagnosis of scrotal pathologic disorders. The capsular and centripetal arterial branches are demonstrated with a color-flow system capable of detecting slow flow. These tributaries demonstrate a low resistance pattern with a high level of diastolic flow indicating decreased vascular resistance. The typical resistive index for the intratesticular arteries is 0.48 to 0.78 with a mean of 0.66. The typical resistive index for the capsular arteries is 0.46 to 0.78 with a mean of 0.62.[14] The supratesticular branches that supply the epididymis, scrotal wall, and muscles have a higher resistive index in the range of 0.63 to 1.00, which indicates that they feed a higher resistance vascular bed. Color flow does not normally detect intratesticular venous flow.[20] The pampiniform plexus of veins will normally demonstrate some flow.

Prostate

The normal prostate should appear symmetric. The appearance of the prostatic capsule varies from well defined to merging with the surrounding fascia. The sonographic pattern of the zones varies somewhat with age. The anterior fibromuscular stroma and periurethral tissues usually appear hypoechoic (Fig. 10-6). The central zone appears slightly to moderately hypoechoic when compared with the peripheral zone.[11] With state-of-the-art equipment, the sonographer can distinguish the hypoechoic band that separates the central and peripheral zones and corresponds to the surgical capsule. The area of the verumontanum appears slightly hyperechoic to the surrounding parenchyma. The seminal vesicles, located at the superior and posterior borders of the prostate, typically demonstrate a hypoechoic pattern when compared with the prostate and are surrounded by a

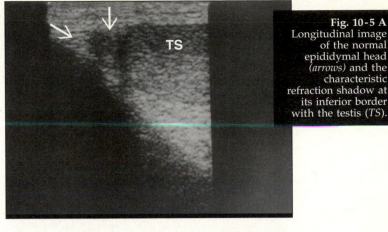

Fig. 10-5 A Longitudinal image of the normal epididymal head *(arrows)* and the characteristic refraction shadow at its inferior border with the testis *(TS)*.

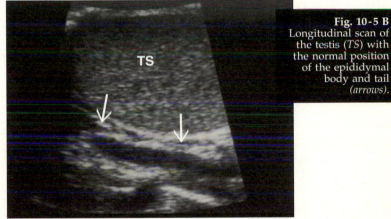

Fig. 10-5 B Longitudinal scan of the testis *(TS)* with the normal position of the epididymal body and tail *(arrows)*.

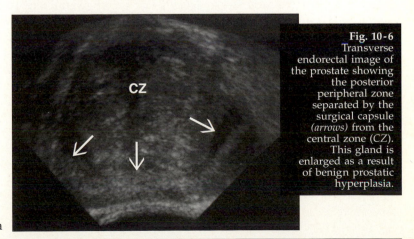

Fig. 10-6 Transverse endorectal image of the prostate showing the posterior peripheral zone separated by the surgical capsule *(arrows)* from the central zone *(CZ)*. This gland is enlarged as a result of benign prostatic hyperplasia.

variable amount of adipose tissue[1] (Fig. 10-7). The angle formed between each seminal vesicle and the prostate should be symmetric. The normal prostatic urethra may appear as a hyperechoic linear structure coursing through the middle of the gland, inferior to the ejaculatory ducts. The ejaculatory ducts may also appear as hyperechoic lines coursing from the seminal vesicles lateral to midline, approaching the midline of the gland as they merge with the prostatic urethra.

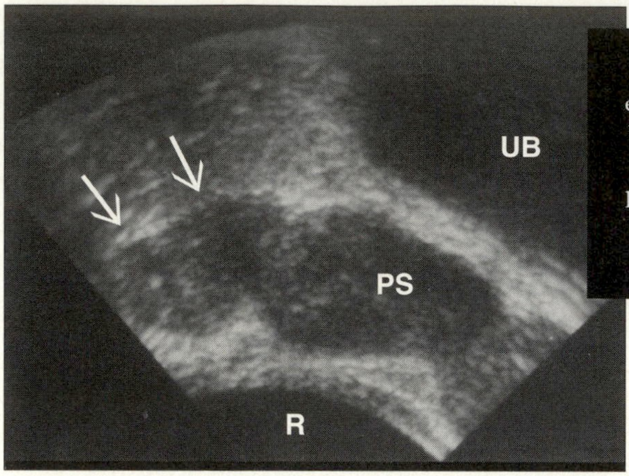

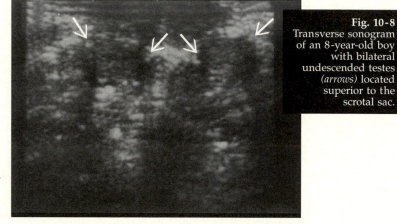

Fig. 10-7 Longitudinal endorectal image of the normal seminal vesicle *(arrows)* superior to the lateral aspect of the prostate *(PS).UB* Urinary bladder; *R* rectum.

Fig. 10-8 Transverse sonogram of an 8-year-old boy with bilateral undescended testes *(arrows)* located superior to the scrotal sac.

PATHOLOGIC PROCESSES OF THE SCROTUM

Undescended Testis

Until the seventh month of embryologic development, both the male and female gonads lie in the abdominal cavity. The testes descend through the inguinal canal into the scrotal sac in response to the stimulation of testosterone and pituitary hormones. The ligament gubernaculum extends through the inguinal canal and connects the testis to the scrotal wall. This ligament does not grow as the fetus continues to develop and therefore gradually pulls the testis into the scrotum. Later this ligament undergoes atrophy and disappears. The failure of one or both testes to descend into the scrotum is termed **cryptorchidism** and may be a developmental anomaly or associated with a number of genetic syndromes. In approximately 70% of cases the testis remains in the inguinal canal. The common clinical presentation consists of manual palpation of the scrotal sac and the lack of one or both testicles. An undescended testicle increases the patient's risk for the development of testicular carcinoma, as well as infertility problems, since the increased testicular temperature causes atrophy.

The typical sonographic pattern is an ovoid or elliptic mass in the area of the inguinal canal, which demonstrates the normal homogeneous testicular pattern.[23] The sonographer should also perform a standard scrotal sonographic examination to verify the presence of the descended testicle and to look for the affected testicle in the superior recesses of the scrotal sac (Fig. 10-8).

Hydrocele

A hydrocele, an abnormal collection of fluid between the visceral and parietal layers of the tunica vaginalis, has numerous causes. It may be congenital as a result of direct communication with the abdominal cavity. Secondary hydroceles may develop as a result of epididymitis/orchitis, chronic or missed torsion, scrotal trauma, or testicular neoplasms. Many are classified as idiopathic, which means that neither the clinical history nor the sonographic examination can determine a cause. The primary clinical symptom is scrotal swelling.

Sonographically, hydroceles typically present as a unilocular fluid collection surrounding the testis (Fig. 10-9). A moderate amount of fluid will allow the demonstration of the posterior attachment of the testis to the epididymis. Septations are associated with chronic infection or hemorrhage (Fig. 10-10). The sonographer must obtain a complete clinical history and check for abnormal patterns in the epididymis and testis in order to allow a specific diagnosis regarding the cause of the hydrocele.

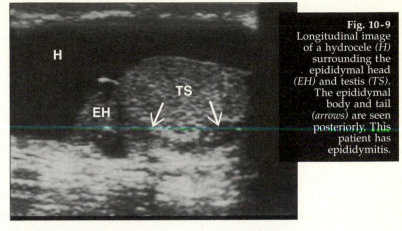

Fig. 10-9 Longitudinal image of a hydrocele (*H*) surrounding the epididymal head (*EH*) and testis (*TS*). The epididymal body and tail (*arrows*) are seen posteriorly. This patient has epididymitis.

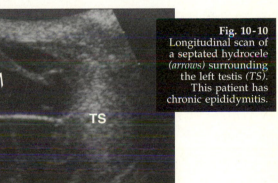

Fig. 10-10 Longitudinal scan of a septated hydrocele (*arrows*) surrounding the left testis (*TS*). This patient has chronic epididymitis.

Testicular Torsion

Testicular torsion, or torsion of the spermatic cord, typically occurs in prepubertal boys but may occur at a later age. This condition causes strangulation or decreased vascular supply to the testis, which in turn causes edema of the testicle and cord, up to the point of occlusion. The most common clinical symptom is scrotal pain. However, the differential diagnosis associated with this symptom includes epididymitis/orchitis, strangulated hernia, and neoplasm. Because of this wide differential diagnosis, sonography plays a crucial role in the evaluation of scrotal pain. The clinical diagnosis of testicular torsion is correct in only 50% of patients. Torsion produces testicular damage in only 4 hours and is thus treated as a surgical emergency. The salvage rate of the affected testicle ranges from 80% to 100% when surgery is performed within 5 hours of the onset of symptoms and drops to less than 20% if surgery is delayed by more than 20 hours.[16]

The sonographic pattern for testicular torsion varies according to the severity of the torsion and the amount of time that has elapsed from the onset of clinical symptoms. The pattern ranges from an enlarged, hypoechoic testicle to an inhomogeneous pattern. The sonographer may note the presence of a reactive hydrocele, a thickening of the scrotal wall, and an enlarged epididymis with an inhomogeneous parenchymal pattern. These patterns are associated with other types of pathologic disorders, but the color-flow Doppler results are distinctive. With torsion, Doppler reveals total absence of flow in the affected testicle with the normal testicle serving as the control, since it should demonstrate the normal vascular intratesticular and extratesticular patterns. If the torsion occurred between 1 and 10 days before the examination, which is called a **missed torsion,** flow in the affected testicle remains absent, but there may be increased flow in the peritesticular tissues.[12] Incomplete torsion may demonstrate some flow, and these patients may require a nuclear medicine flow study to verify the diagnosis.

Epididymitis and Orchitis

Epididymitis usually occurs secondary to a bacterial infection most commonly from the urinary tract. Common clinical symptoms include scrotal pain, an enlarged scrotum, and a fever. Orchitis typically develops secondary to epididymitis as a result of direct spread of the infection. Less than 20% of patients with epididymitis have coexisting orchitis.[22] The typical treatment is antibiotic therapy.

The sonographic pattern for epididymitis consists of an enlarged epididymal head, body, and/or tail with a hypoechoic parenchymal pattern (Fig. 10-11). The sonographer may also find scrotal wall edema and a reactive hydrocele. Color-flow Doppler can enhance the diagnosis by demonstrating increased flow in the affected epididymis, again using the unaffected side as the control, since the normal epididymis exhibits very little flow.[17] This may occur before any gray scale pattern change. Focal hypoechoic areas may suggest the possibility of early abscess formation. Chronic epididymitis may cause the development of a hyperechoic pattern. The sonographer should always evaluate the testis for signs of infection or ischemia caused by epididymal edema and the consequent compression of the testicular venous outflow. Typically, orchitis presents as a hypoechoic, peripheral intratesticular mass (Fig. 10-12), which exhibits increased flow on color Doppler.[20] However, this pattern is also associated with testicular neoplasms, so that clinical correlation and a follow-up sonographic examination are usually necessary. The infection may also cause testicular enlargement with

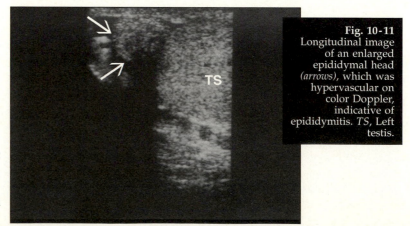

Fig. 10-11 Longitudinal image of an enlarged epididymal head *(arrows)*, which was hypervascular on color Doppler, indicative of epididymitis. *TS,* Left testis.

a diffuse hypoechoic pattern change, requiring comparative views of the unaffected testis at the same gain settings to verify the diagnosis.

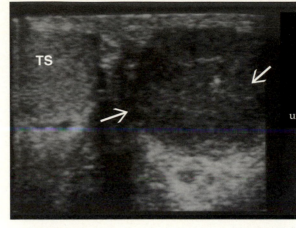

Fig. 10-12 Transverse view of orchitis of the left testicle *(arrows)*, producing an enlargement and a hypoechoic pattern compared with the unaffected testis *(TS)*.

Primary Neoplasms

Extratesticular masses are most likely a result of inflammation, trauma, or benign neoplasms. Intratesticular masses are considered malignant until proven otherwise. The most common benign epididymal tumor is the **adenoma.** The **spermatocele is** a retention cyst stemming from the small tubules in the epididymis and usually effects the head. These may be unilateral or bilateral, unilocular or multilocular. These often form as a result of previous infection, and the frequency increases with age. Primary neoplasms may also arise from the spermatic cord or tunica albuginea.

Testicular neoplasms typically occur between the ages of 25 and 35 and 97.6% are malignant germ-cell tumors. **Seminoma** is the most common germ-cell tumor and accounts for 40% to 50% of all testicular neoplasms. Other types of testicular malignancies include the **embryonal cell, teratoma, and choriocarcinoma.**[2] On histologic examination, many of these tumors have a mixed composition. The clinical symptoms may include swelling, a palpable lump, and secondary hemorrhage. Most of these neoplasms remain confined to the testicular tissue, although the embryonal carcinoma tends to invade the tunica albuginea and the epididymis. **Testicular cysts** can occur and increase in frequency with age. Small calcifications in the testicular parenchyma can occur in normal patients or in association with inflammatory changes or primary neoplasms.

Spermatoceles usually exhibit the three sonographic criteria of a cyst; regular borders, anechoic interior, and distal enhancement (Fig. 10-13). An adenoma of the epididymis typically presents as a discrete hyperechoic extratesticular mass. Since sonography cannot distinguish between benign and malignant neoplasms, the primary role of sonography is to demonstrate whether the mass is extratesticular or intratesticular. Testicular cysts may display the sonographic criteria of a cyst or may appear as a complex mass[10] (Fig. 10-14). The typical sonographic pattern for testicular neoplasms consists of a round-to-oval hypoechoic mass (Fig. 10-15) or masses. Embryonal cell carcinoma presents as an inhomogeneous mass as a result of necrosis and hemorrhage and may contain calcifications. Choriocarcinoma, the rarest type, is highly malignant with widespread distant metastasis. Primary neoplasms that may metastasize to the testes include bronchogenic, lymphoma, renal, prostate, urinary, melanoma, and gastrointestinal. Color Doppler can provide additional information, but the differentiation between malignancy and other pathologic processes is difficult. The degree of vascularity is related to size, with tumors less than 1.5 cm appearing hypovascular and those over 1.5 cm demonstrating a hypervascular pattern in relation to the normal testicular parenchyma.[17] Benign neoplasms may also present a hypervascular pattern. Currently the use of color-flow Doppler does not assist in specifying the type of intratesticular mass.

Varicocele

Variococeles are caused by incompetent valves in the testicular veins leading to dilatation in the pampiniform plexus, usually in the left scrotal sac. This condition may develop in association with increased pressure as a result of an enlarged liver or spleen, pronounced hydronephrosis, muscle strain, or abdominal tumors. They may be idiopathic. Varicoceles also cause infertility.

Sonography reveals dilated tubular structures in the scrotal sac (Fig. 10-16). The use of the upright position or the Valsalva maneuver will increase the diameter of the veins. Color Doppler will typically reveal increased flow during the Valsalva maneuver or when scanning the patient in the upright position (Fig. 10-17).

Scrotal Trauma

Scrotal trauma can occur with a blunt or sharp traumatic injury to the scrotal sac. The sonographic pattern for a scrotal wall hematoma depends on the location and the elapsed time from the injury. Before 48 hours the wall usually appears thickened. After 48 to 72 hours the sonographer may see hypoechoic areas in the wall. Intratesticular hematomas usually appear as inhomogeneous hypoechoic areas in the testis.[22] The sonographer must evaluate the integrity of

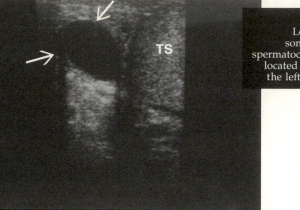

Fig. 10-13 Longitudinal sonogram of a spermatocele *(arrows)* located superior to the left testis *(TS)*.

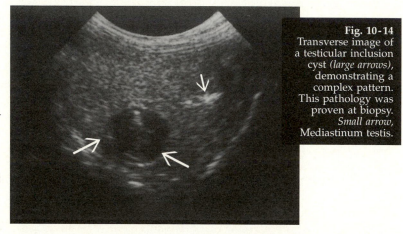

Fig. 10-14 Transverse image of a testicular inclusion cyst *(large arrows)*, demonstrating a complex pattern. This pathology was proven at biopsy. *Small arrow,* Mediastinum testis.

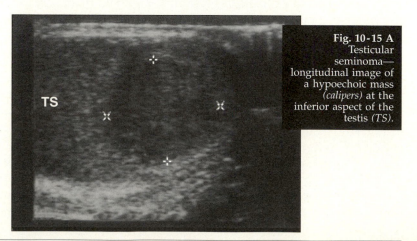

Fig. 10-15 A Testicular seminoma—longitudinal image of a hypoechoic mass *(calipers)* at the inferior aspect of the testis *(TS)*.

the tunica albuginea. A rupture of the tunica albuginea allows the protrusion of testicular tissue into the scrotal sac and presents as an irregular contour and pattern. A hematocele may also develop, causing a complex pattern in the scrotal sac (Fig. 10-18). Color flow may provide additional information regarding the vascular supply to the testis and whether the testicle can be saved.

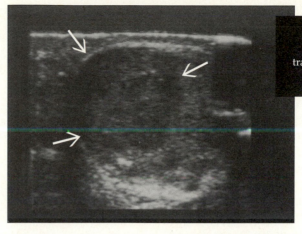

Fig. 10-15 B Testicular seminoma—transverse image of the seminoma *(arrows)*.

PATHOLOGIC PROCESSES OF THE PROSTATE

Benign Prostatic Hyperplasia

Benign prostatic hyperplasia (BPH), the most common disease of the prostate, originates in the transitional and periurethral zones. The clinical symptoms consist of urinary frequency, nocturia, and urgency. Surgical indications for prostatectomy include overflow incontinence, recurrent urinary tract infections, acute urinary tract retention, and severe hematuria.

Sonographically, BPH causes a symmetric diffuse enlargement or a discrete nodular appearance in the central portion of the prostate[5] (Fig. 10-19). Additional signs include retention cysts and areas of calcification (Fig. 10-20). The sonographer should also evaluate the size of the prostatic urethra and look for other evidence of urinary obstruction. A patient who has had a previous transurethral prostatic resection may demonstrate a prominent urethra.

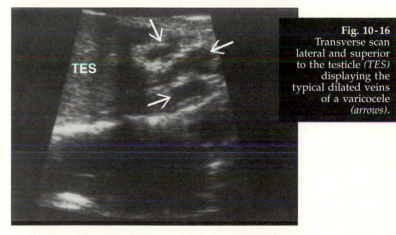

TES

Fig. 10-16 Transverse scan lateral and superior to the testicle *(TES)* displaying the typical dilated veins of a varicocele *(arrows)*.

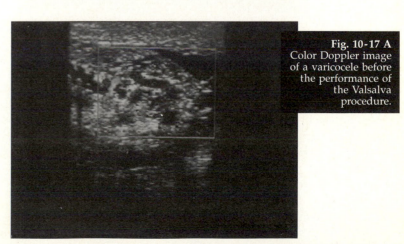

Fig. 10-17 A Color Doppler image of a varicocele before the performance of the Valsalva procedure.

Prostatic Carcinoma

Many patients with early prostatic carcinoma have no clinical symptoms or exhibit symptoms that are indistinguishable from benign prostatic hypertrophy. A clinical examination typically reveals an enlarged prostate containing a hard nodule. Autopsy studies have shown that up to 70% of men in their 80s have prostate carcinoma, although only 6% to 8% of men display the clinical symptoms.[14] PSA levels increase with prostatic carcinoma, with marked increases seen in more advanced grades. The most common grading system used in sonography was developed by Lee, Littrup, et. al.[14] This system classifies the sonographic pattern in relation to the extent of involvement in the prostate and surrounding structures. In stage U*A the carcinoma measures less than 1 cm and is confined in the prostate. In stage U*B the tumor measures greater than 1 cm but is still confined to the prostate. Stage U*C denotes extension beyond the prostate or in the seminal vesicles (Fig. 10-21). This classification is crucial in the selection of the method of treatment. Most of these carcinomas appear to originate in the peripheral zone, but they may also arise in the central and transition zones.

The classic sonographic pattern for stage U*A tumors is a hypoechoic mass in the peripheral zone (Fig. 10-22). Other pathologic processes may mimic this pattern, such as prostatitis and hyperplasia. Additional signs of malignancy include irregular margins, a capsular bulge, asymmetry of the peripheral zone, and a change in the

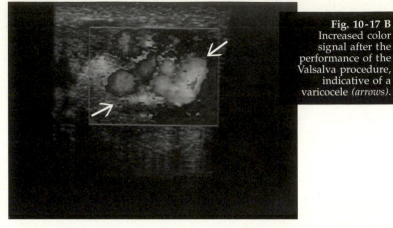

Fig. 10-17 B Increased color signal after the performance of the Valsalva procedure, indicative of a varicocele *(arrows)*.

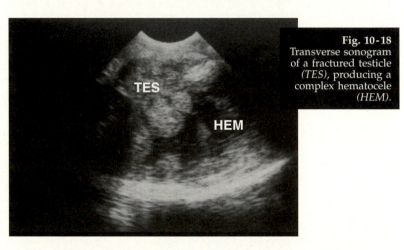

Fig. 10-18 Transverse sonogram of a fractured testicle *(TES)*, producing a complex hematocele *(HEM)*.

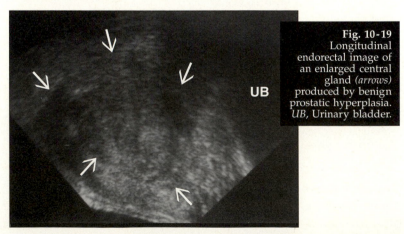

Fig. 10-19 Longitudinal endorectal image of an enlarged central gland *(arrows)* produced by benign prostatic hyperplasia. *UB*, Urinary bladder.

seminal vesicle/prostatic angle corresponding to seminal vesicle extension.[9] Isoechoic tumors are the most difficult to demonstrate. More advanced carcinomas may appear hypoechoic, hyperechoic, or mixed. They may contain focal hyperechoic areas or calcifications.[8] Since none of these patterns are totally specific for malignancy, usually a biopsy is ordered to verify the diagnosis.

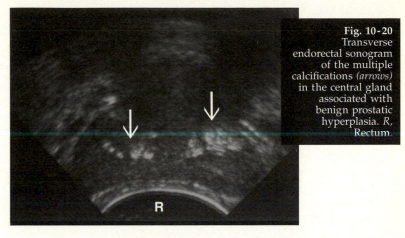

Fig. 10-20 Transverse endorectal sonogram of the multiple calcifications *(arrows)* in the central gland associated with benign prostatic hyperplasia. *R*, Rectum.

Prostatitis

Prostatitis, or inflammation of the prostate, has several causes that include acute bacterial prostatitis, chronic prostatitis, and prostatodynia. Patients with acute bacterial prostatitis often have a fever, chills, dysuria, urinary frequency, and back pain. The rectal examination reveals a swollen, very tender prostate. The patient has positive urine cultures and increased numbers of white blood cells in the prostate secretions. The symptoms for chronic prostatitis are less obvious and may include urinary frequency. The prostate may feel normal or slightly enlarged on rectal examination. Again, there are increased numbers of white blood cells in the prostatic secretions. With prostatodynia, the patient shows no clinical signs of bacterial infection, although he may complain of urinary symptoms or perineal pain. The patient may show signs of pain on rectal examination.[7]

The sonographic pattern for acute or bacterial prostatitis usually consists of an enlarged

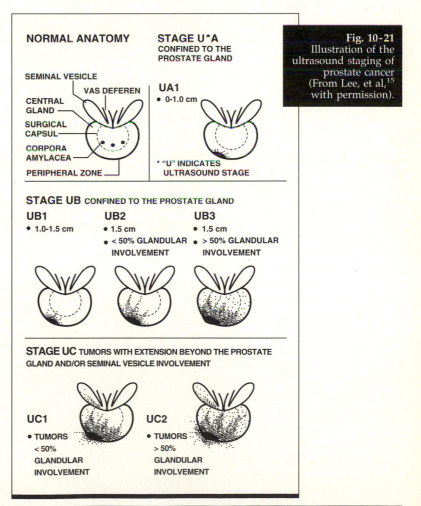

Fig. 10-21 Illustration of the ultrasound staging of prostate cancer (From Lee, et al,[15] with permission).

NORMAL ANATOMY

SEMINAL VESICLE
VAS DEFEREN
CENTRAL GLAND
SURGICAL CAPSUL
CORPORA AMYLACEA
PERIPHERAL ZONE

STAGE U*A CONFINED TO THE PROSTATE GLAND

UA1
● 0-1.0 cm

* "U" INDICATES ULTRASOUND STAGE

STAGE UB CONFINED TO THE PROSTATE GLAND

UB1
● 1.0-1.5 cm

UB2
● 1.5 cm
● < 50% GLANDULAR INVOLVEMENT

UB3
● 1.5 cm
● > 50% GLANDULAR INVOLVEMENT

STAGE UC TUMORS WITH EXTENSION BEYOND THE PROSTATE GLAND AND/OR SEMINAL VESICLE INVOLVEMENT

UC1
● TUMORS < 50% GLANDULAR INVOLVEMENT

UC2
● TUMORS > 50% GLANDULAR INVOLVEMENT

gland with inhomogeneous hypoechoic pattern changes[4] (Fig. 10-23). Patients may develop an abscess that should appear as a more discrete mass with a complex pattern. In chronic prostatitis, the sonographic pattern is again inhomogeneous, except that areas of calcification may cause acoustic shadowing to occur. The sonographer should also check for signs of dilated veins surrounding the prostate and enlarged, hypoechoic seminal vesicles.

TECHNICAL PITFALLS

The most common pitfall in scrotal sonography is applying too much pressure while scanning and thus distorting the testicular shape and sonographic pattern. Another problem occurs when the testicles are not properly positioned. To obtain a true longitudinal and transverse scanning plane, the scrotum must be repositioned so that the correct anatomic relationships are apparent. The most common gain-related errors are the near-field reverberation artifacts and the use of excessive system gain or acoustic power. Since many testicular neoplasms are small and subtly hypoechoic, this error could lead to the misdiagnosis of a normal testicular pattern.

Endorectal sonography of the prostate requires careful transducer preparation. Any air in the transducer covers can cause reverberation artifacts or a general degradation of image quality. The sonographer must introduce enough water so that the posterior portion of the pros-

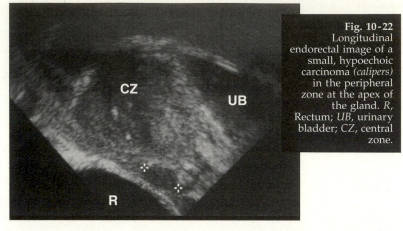

Fig. 10-22 Longitudinal endorectal image of a small, hypoechoic carcinoma *(calipers)* in the peripheral zone at the apex of the gland. *R,* Rectum; *UB,* urinary bladder; *CZ,* central zone.

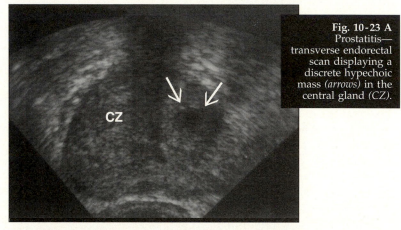

Fig. 10-23 A Prostatitis— transverse endorectal scan displaying a discrete hypoechoic mass *(arrows)* in the central gland *(CZ).*

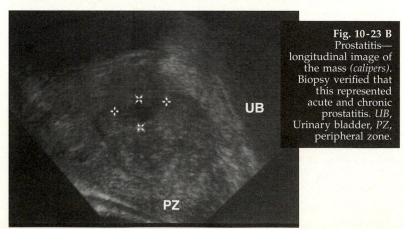

Fig. 10-23 B Prostatitis— longitudinal image of the mass *(calipers).* Biopsy verified that this represented acute and chronic prostatitis. *UB,* Urinary bladder, *PZ,* peripheral zone.

TABLE 10-1   CLINICAL LABORATORY TEST VALUES – SCROTUM AND PROSTATE

	WBC	AFP	hCG	PSA
EPIDIDYMITIS	Increase	Normal	Normal	Normal
EMBYONAL CELL CARCINOMA	Normal	Normal to an Increase	Normal	Normal
TERATOMA	Normal	Normal to an Increase	Normal	Normal
CHORIOCARCINOMA	Normal	Normal	Increase	Normal
BPH	Normal	Normal	Normal	Low to Moderate Increase
PROSTATIC CARCINOMA	Normal	Normal	Normal	Moderate to High Increase
PROSTATITIS	Increase	Normal	Normal	Low Increase

WBC, White blood cell count; *AFP,* alpha feto-protein; *hCG,* human chorionic gonadotropin; *PSA,* prostate specific antigen.

tate, which is the peripheral zone, is in the focal zone of the transducer and is imaged free of any artifacts. This is crucial to the diagnosis of prostatic carcinoma, since the majority occur in the peripheral zone. Because many of these small malignancies are isoechoic to hypoechoic, excessive gain or acoustic power settings can lead to the misdiagnosis of a normal peripheral zone. On the other hand, too much water can cause compression of the tissue and again mask the appearance of abnormal areas.

SUMMARY

Scrotal and prostate sonography allow the diagnosis of many types of pathologic conditions. The sonographer must obtain a complete clinical history and the results of other diagnostic tests to refine the differential diagnosis. Table 10-1 contains a summary of the clinical laboratory test data that pertain to scrotal and prostate pathology.

REFERENCES

1. Asch MR, Toi A: Seminal vesicles: imaging and intervention using transrectal ultrasound. *J Ultrasound Med* 10:19, 1991.
2. Benson CB: The role of ultrasound in diagnosing and staging of testicular cancer, *Semin Urol* 6:189, 1988.
3. Benson CB, Doubilet PM, Richie JP: Sonography of the male genital tract, *AJR* 153:705, 1989.
4. Bude R, Bree RL, et al: Transrectal ultrasound appearance of granulomatous prostatitis, *J Ultrasound Med* 9:677, 1990.
5. Burks DD, Drolshagen LF, et al: Transrectal sonography of benign and malignant prostatic lesions, *AJR* 146:1187, 1986.
6. Catalona WJ, Smith DS, et al: Measurement of prostate-specific antigen in serum as a screening test for prostate cancer, *N Engl J Med* 324:1156, 1991.
7. Chantelois AE, Parker SH, et al: Malakoplakia of the prostate sonographically mimicking carcinoma, *Radiology* 177:193, 1990.

8. Doherty FJ, Mullins TL, et al: Testicular microlithiasis: a unique sonographic appearance, *J Ultrasound Med* 6:389, 1987.
9. Griffiths GJ, Clements R, et al: The ultrasound appearances of prostatic cancer with histologic correlation, *Clin Radiol* 38:219, 1987.
10. Hamm B, Fobbe F, Loy V: Testicular cysts: differentiation with ultrasound and clinical findings, *Radiology* 168:19, 1988.
11. Hardt NS, Kaude JV, et al: Sonography of the prostate: in vitro correlation of sonographic and anatomic findings in normal glands, *AJR* 151:955, 1988.
12. Jenson MC, Lac KP, et al: Color Doppler sonography in testicular torsion, *J Clin Ultrasound* 18:446, 1990.
13. Krone KD, Carroll BA: Scrotal ultrasound. *Radiol Clin North Am* 23:121, 1985.
14. Lee F, Littrup PJ, et al: The use of transrectal ultrasound in the diagnosis, guided biopsy, staging and screening of prostate cancer, *Radiographics* 7:627, 1987.
15. Lee F, Siders DB, et al: Prostate cancer: transrectal ultrasound and pathology comparison, *Cancer* 67:1132, 1991.
16. Middleton WD, Siegel BA, et al: Acute scrotal disorders: prospective comparison of color Doppler US and testicular scintigraphy, *Radiology* 177:177, 1990.
17. Middleton WD, Thorne D, Melson GL: Color Doppler ultrasound of the normal testes, *AJR* 152:293, 1989.
18. Palken M, Cobb OE, et al: Prostate cancer: comparison of digital rectal examination and transrectal ultrasound for screening, *J Urol* 145:86, 1991.
19. Rall PW, Jenson MC, et al: Color Doppler sonography in acute epididymitis and orchitis, *J Clin Ultrasound* 18:383, 1990.
20. Rall PW, Larsen D, et al: Color Doppler sonography of the scrotum, *Semin Ultrasound CT MR* 12:109, 1991.
21. Stamey TA, Yang N, et. al.: Prostate specific antigen as a serum marker for adenocarcinoma of the prostate, *N Engl J Med* 317:909, 1987.
22. Tumeh SS, Benson CB, Ritchie JP: Acute diseases of the scrotum, *Semin Ultrasound CT MR* 12:115, 1991.
23. Weiss RM, Carter AR, Rosenfield AT: High resolution real-time ultrasonography in the localization of the undescended testis, *J Urol* 135:936, 1986.

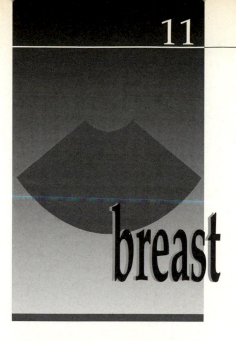

11

breast

INSTRUCTIONAL OBJECTIVES

At the completion of this chapter, the reader will be able to:

1. Describe the clinical problems that are typical reasons for sonography of the breast.
2. Identify on transverse and longitudinal illustrations and sonograms the major anatomic structures of the breast, including the pectoralis major muscles, ribs and intercostal cartilage, Cooper's ligaments, retromammary fat, subcutaneous fat, breast parenchyma, and the ductal system.
3. Describe the basic scanning protocol for sonography of the breast.
4. Describe the clinical symptoms and pathologic basis for the disease processes of the breast, including fibrocystic disease, primary benign neoplasms, and primary and metastatic carcinoma.
5. Identify on sectional sonograms the above-mentioned disease processes of the breast, based on the sonographic appearance, the clinical history, and the results of other diagnostic procedures.
6. List several technical pitfalls associated with sonography of the breast.

THE CLINICAL PROBLEM

Carcinoma of the breast still ranks as one of the most frequent malignancies in women. Although advances in radiographic mammography have allowed the more frequent diagnosis of early malignancies, research continues to strive for a more definitive screening test. Currently, sonography is not considered a screening test for most patients. Clinicians who discover a lump will usually order a mammographic examination. The primary role of sonography is to differentiate solid and cystic breast masses seen on mammography. The clinician may order sonography as a screening examination in pregnant patients and in patients under 35 years of age. Sonographically, the differentiation of benign and malignant breast masses is not definitive, and a biopsy procedure is often required to reach a diagnosis.

NORMAL ANATOMY

Each breast consists of several layers or subsections of tissue: the skin and nipple, the subcutaneous layer, and the mammary and retromammary layers. The subcutaneous layer consists of fatty tissue divided by thin septae of connective tissue. The mammary or parenchymal layer consists of 15 to 20 lobes and is divided by **Cooper's ligaments,** which consist of connective tissue. Each lobe opens to the surface of the nipple through a **lactiferous duct.** The retromammary layer consists of loose areolar tissue. The pectoralis major muscle and the ribs and intercostal cartilage lie posterior to the retromammary layer. The amount of fat in the subcutaneous, mammary, and retromammary layers will vary from patient to patient. Postmenopausal breasts tend to contain more fatty and fibrous tissue, whereas the breasts in the premenopausal group tend to have more glandular tissue.

RELATED IMAGING PROCEDURES

Currently, radiographic mammography serves as the primary method for both screening and differentiating breast pathologic conditions. Cysts typically appear as opaque, smooth, well-defined masses on mammography. The dense pattern associated with fibrocystic disease can obscure these radiographic characteristics. A fibroadenoma usually visualizes as a discrete mass with well-defined borders. Both cysts and fibroadenomas can have atypical characteristics, such as irregular shapes and less distinct borders. On mammography, the classic sign for smaller malignant lesions is the presence of microcalcifications and a spiculated border. However, malignant neoplasms can appear similar to cysts and fibroadenomas; consequently, a biopsy is performed if the mass has a questionable appearance on mammography.

SCANNING PROTOCOLS AND TECHNIQUES

In most departments a hand-held, real-time transducer is used for sonography of the breast. The automated water-path system provides a more regimented sequential examination of the breast with a more accurate positioning for serial examinations. Either a 5.0 or 7.5 MHz linear array transducer is used, depending on the size of the breast and the amount of attenuation. The gain and acoustic power controls must be adjusted so that the near field is not overly amplified and so that the amplification rate is correct throughout the imaging depth. The sonographer must employ a light scanning touch to avoid tissue compression. The imaging depth should be adjusted according to the maximum depth of the pectoralis muscle. The patient is usually placed in the right posterior oblique position for the left breast and in the left posterior oblique position for the right breast.[2] This position allows good transducer contact and visualization, particularly for the outer quadrants of the breast. The patient's arm on the side being examined is placed above the head. For pendulous breasts, the patient is placed supine for a more adequate visualization of the inner quadrants, or the patient is placed in the right posterior oblique position for the right breast and in the left posterior oblique position for the left breast. The scanning protocol consists of transverse and longitudinal scans of the four quadrants: superior outer, superior inner, inferior outer, and inferior inner, with the nipple serving as the primary landmark (Fig. 11-1). The sonographer must make very subtle scanning movements to demonstrate small breast masses. Additional transverse and longitudinal scans, including measurements, are usually required for any mass.

Another scanning method for breast sonography is the "clock" method, where 12:00 to 3:00, 3:00 to 6:00, 6:00 to 9:00, and 9:00 to 12:00 mark the four quadrants (Fig. 11-2). Some interpreting physicians prefer this method for a survey of the breast. Any mass requires standard transverse and longitudinal views with measurements. Examples of scanning protocols are listed in the box on the following page.

NORMAL SONOGRAPHIC PATTERNS

The normal sonographic pattern of the breast varies with the patient's age and the amount of adipose and fibrous tissue. The near-field resolution should allow adequate visualization of the skin and subcutaneous layers. The nipple usually causes acoustic shadowing, and the larger lactiferous ducts may be visualized posteriorly. The skin should appear as a hyperechoic line, with the more posterior subcutaneous layer visualizing as hypoechoic fat layers separated by hyperechoic Cooper's ligaments.[2] If more fibrous tissue is present in this layer, it may appear more hyperechoic, and the ligaments may appear less distinct. The sonographic pattern of the mammary layer varies. In premeno-

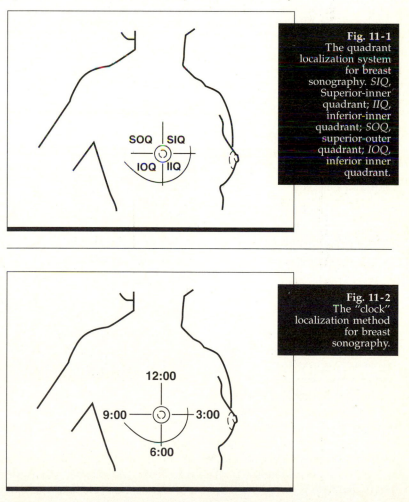

Fig. 11-1
The quadrant localization system for breast sonography. *SIQ,* Superior-inner quadrant; *IIQ,* inferior-inner quadrant; *SOQ,* superior-outer quadrant; *IOQ,* inferior inner quadrant.

Fig. 11-2
The "clock" localization method for breast sonography.

pausal women, the breast contains more glandular tissue, which exhibits a moderately hyperechoic parenchymal pattern. Fat lobules appear as hypoechoic areas with thin Cooper's ligaments coursing between the functional and fatty lobes (Fig. 11-3). In the postmenopausal patient functional breast tissue is replaced by fatty and fibrous tissue. Breasts containing a large amount of fibrous tissue may cause excessive attenuation and compromise the quality of the examination. Predominantly fatty deposition may cause a homogeneous hypoechoic pattern throughout the breast layers, separated by Cooper's ligaments. The retromammary fat layer typically displays as a hypoechoic pattern. The pectoralis muscle appears as a moderately hyperechoic layer posterior to the retromammary fat, with the ribs and intercostal cartilage often indenting this layer and causing acoustic shadowing.

PATHOLOGIC PROCESSES OF THE BREAST

Fibrocystic Disease

Fibrocystic disease, or mammary dysplasia, is the most frequent disease of the breast. It appears to be related to hormonal activity, since it is most common in women between 30 and 50 years of age and is rare in the postmenopausal group. The patho-

---

BREAST SCANNING PROTOCOL

The "Clock" Method:

✔ Starting at 12:00, the sonographer should perform a survey scan, preceding around the clock face. The correct scan orientation should always be verified. For each visualized mass, detailed views in the transverse and longitudinal planes should be obtained with measurements in three dimensions.

The Quadrant Method:

✔ The sonographer should obtain transverse and longitudinal images of each quadrant. For each visualized mass, detailed views in the transverse and longitudinal planes should be obtained with measurements in three dimensions.

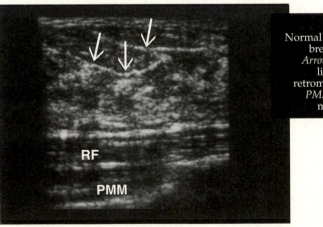

Fig. 11-3
Normal sonographic breast anatomy. *Arrows,* Copper's ligaments; *RF,* retromammary fat; *PMM,* pectoralis major muscle.

---

logic findings include microscopic and macroscopic cysts, ductal epithelial hyperplasia, adenosis, and papillomatosis.[8] The clinical symptoms of this typically bilateral process consist of painful masses in the breast, rapid fluctuation in the size of the masses, and occasionally a discharge from the nipple. Often the pain occurs or increases during the premenstrual portion of the cycle, and the mass or masses may enlarge. Some types of fibrocystic disease may increase the patient's risk for the development of malignancy. If a mass does not fluctuate in size or disappear, it requires further clinical investigation.

The typical sonographic pattern for fibrocystic disease is solitary (Fig. 11-4) or multiple cysts in one or both breasts (Fig. 11-5). The sonographer must demonstrate all three sonographic criteria of a cyst: smooth regular borders, anechoic interior, and acoustic enhancement. This requires proper gain settings and placement of the focal zone to coincide with the cyst. Small cysts may require a higher frequency transducer to demonstrate these characteristics. The sonographer should correlate all masses and cysts with the clinical palpation findings and mammographic location.

Carcinoma of the Breast

Breast cancer ranks second to lung cancer as the most common malignancy that causes death in women, and the breast is the most common site for cancer. The risk of developing breast cancer increases with advancing age, with the median age being between 60 and 61 years.[4] Risk factors include a history of breast carcinoma in the mother or a sister, a previous history of endometrial cancer or cancer in the other breast, early menarche before the age of 12, late menopause after the age of 50, nulliparity, or a late first pregnancy. The typical presenting symptom is the discovery of a single, firm,

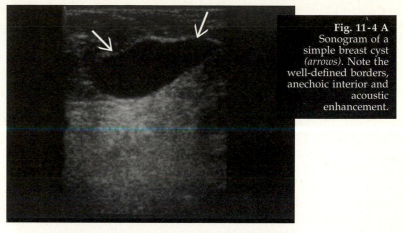

Fig. 11-4 A Sonogram of a simple breast cyst *(arrows)*. Note the well-defined borders, anechoic interior and acoustic enhancement.

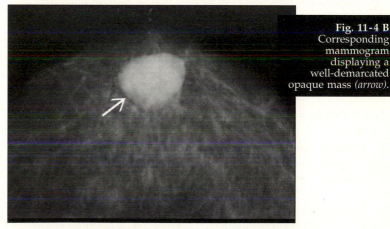

Fig. 11-4 B Corresponding mammogram displaying a well-demarcated opaque mass *(arrow)*.

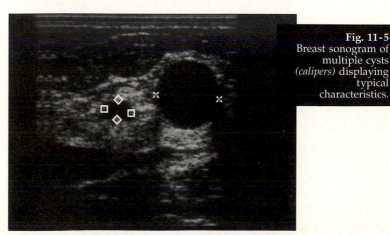

Fig. 11-5 Breast sonogram of multiple cysts *(calipers)* displaying typical characteristics.

mass that has ill-defined borders and is not tender. Later symptoms include a retraction of the skin or nipple as a result of fixation of the malignancy, nipple discharge, and palpable axillary or supraclavicular nodes.

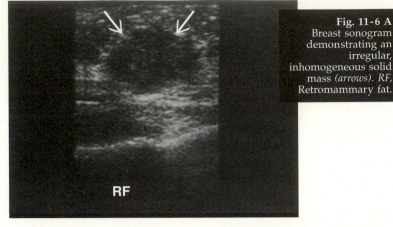

Fig. 11-6 A Breast sonogram demonstrating an irregular, inhomogeneous solid mass *(arrows)*. *RF,* Retromammary fat.

Breast cancer consists of two main types. The first, termed intraductal, arises from the epithelial lining of the larger ducts and accounts for 70% to 80% of all breast malignancies. The second, termed lobular, arises from the epithelium of the terminal ducts in the breast lobules. Other classifications, such as medullary and scirrhous, are subclassifications of ductal carcinoma. Most ductal carcinomas are invasive, whereas lobular carcinomas may be invasive or remain localized.

The classic sonographic pattern for breast carcinoma is an irregularly shaped mass containing an inhomogeneous sonographic pattern, including hyperechoic areas with acoustic shadowing (Fig. 11-6). However, malignancies may have regular borders and display a homogeneous sonographic pattern. A

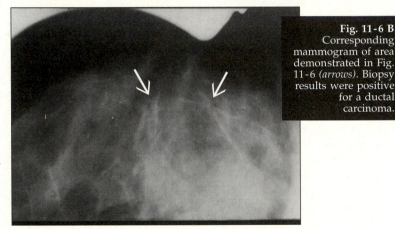

Fig. 11-6 B Corresponding mammogram of area demonstrated in Fig. 11-6 *(arrows).* Biopsy results were positive for a ductal carcinoma.

rare pattern consists of a cyst containing a solid projection or debris. Color-flow Doppler may reveal increased vascularity.[1] Pulsed Doppler may reveal an increased systolic frequency compared with the contralateral mirror image, but this technique requires further refinement before it can provide reliable and accurate information.[6] Because of these variable patterns, the sonographic documentation of a complex or solid mass requires further clinical evaluation, often including a biopsy procedure.

Benign Neoplasms

The **fibroadenoma** is the most common benign neoplasm of the breast and occurs most frequently in younger women. This tumor is usually discovered as a firm, discrete, rather movable palpable mass measuring 1 to 5 cm. This presentation becomes more complicated in the presence of fibrocystic disease. The fibroadenoma usually appears sonographically as a well-defined hypoechoic mass with regular borders that may display acoustic enhancement[5] (Fig. 11-7). These tumors can meld into the adjacent adipose tissue, and the sonographer may have a difficult time identifying this neoplasm. If sonography fails to reveal a cystic or solid mass in the area consistent with the palpable mass or radiographic abnormality, further clinical investigation, including biopsy, may be necessary.

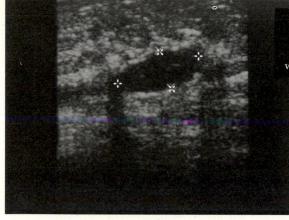

Fig. 11-7
Classic pattern of a fibroadenoma *(calipers)*. Note the well-defined borders.

Fat necrosis is a rare process in the breast, but it may mimic the symptoms of carcinoma, such as a palpable mass and skin or nipple retraction. Experts presume that the cause is trauma of the breast, although only half of the patients will give a history of breast trauma.[8] Sonographic patterns include an ill-defined hypoechoic mass that may or may not cause acoustic shadowing and skin retraction. Since this pattern can be similar to carcinoma, a biopsy procedure is usually required to reach a definitive diagnosis.

Abscess

Breast abscesses, although not common, typically occur in the lactating patient. The initial symptoms include localized tenderness and redness and swelling of the affected breast. Early treatment consists of antibiotic therapy. Occasionally the infection advances and forms a localized abscess that causes more widespread signs of infection. The patient should not nurse, and the abscess should be drained.

Depending on the evolutionary stage of the abscess, the sonographic pattern ranges from a discrete hypoechoic to complex to cystic mass. Clinical correlation and needle aspiration will allow a more definitive diagnosis.

In the **augmented breast,** patients may develop pain and hardening of the implants. Leakage of silicone into the adjacent tissues causes additional complications. In the postoperative patient, an abscess may develop adjacent to the implant. Later, leaks may also cause this complication. An abscess may appear sonographically as a cystic or complex mass adjacent to the implant. The leak itself will disrupt the hyperechoic pattern of the implant surface. A fibrotic reaction to the implant or leak will distort the shape or contour of the implant.[4]

TECHNICAL PITFALLS

The most common technical pitfall in breast sonography is the use of excessive gain and acoustic power setttings, which can mask the appearance of solid breast lesions and make cystic masses appear solid. The sonographer should adjust the gain so that the breast parenchymal pattern is demonstrated and the hyperechoic structures, such as Cooper's ligaments, are not excessively hyperechoic. The near-field gain should be decreased to reduce the artifacts in this region. A stand-off pad can also alleviate this problem. The use of a higher frequency, such as 7.5 MHz, will also decrease the artifact production and allow better visualization of the first several centimeters of breast tissue.[7] The use of too much pressure during scanning will also cause increased near-field artifact production and may cause enough tissue compression to mask the appearance of both cystic and solid masses. The sonographer may initially misidentify a normal breast lobule surrounded by Cooper's ligaments as a breast mass. The lobules are ovoid or elliptical, which becomes apparent when the transducer scanning plane is changed. Also, the size, shape, and pattern are similar to those of the surrounding breast lobules. The patient should always be asked to identify the location of the palpable mass, or the sonographer should look at the mammogram to accurately localize the area of interest. If the mammogram was not performed in the same department, the patient should be instructed to bring a copy of the mammogram with her.

SUMMARY

Breast sonography plays a valuable role in the further documentation of breast masses by differentiating between cystic and solid lesions. The continuing advances in pulsed and color Doppler may allow sonography to distinguish between benign and malignant neoplasms.

REFERENCES

1. Adler DD, Carson PL, et al: Doppler ultrasound color flow imaging in the study of breast cancer: preliminary findings, *Ultrasound Med Biol* 16:553, 1990.
2. Bassett LW, Kimme-Smith C: Breast sonography: technique, equipment, and normal anatomy, *Semin US CT MR* 10:82, 1989.
3. Cole-Beuglet C, Schwartz G, et al: Ultrasound mammography for the augmented breast, *Radiology* 146:737, 1983.
4. Cole-Beuglet C, Soriano RZ, et al: Ultrasound analysis of 104 primary breast carcinomas classified according to histopathologic type, *Radiology*, 147:191, 1983.
5. Jackson VP, Rothschild PA, et al: The spectrum of sonographic findings of fibroadenoma of the breast, *Invest Radiol* 21:34, 1986.
6. Jackson VP: Duplex sonography of the breast, *Ultrasound Med Bio* (suppl 1) 14:131, 1988.
7. Kimme-Smith C, Rothschild PA, et al: Ultrasound artifacts affecting the diagnosis of breast masses, *Ultrasound Med Biol*, (suppl 1) 14:203, 1988.
8. Sickles EA, Filly RA, Callen PW: Benign breast lesions: ultrasound detection and diagnosis, *Radiology* 151:467, 1984.

12

gynecologic anatomy and physiology

INSTRUCTIONAL OBJECTIVES

At the completion of this chapter, the reader will be able to:

1. Identify on coronal, transverse, and longitudinal illustrations and sonograms the major anatomic structures of the female pelvis, including the pelvic bony landmarks, the pelvic muscles, the uterus and its major anatomic divisions, the suspensory ligaments of the uterus, the ovaries and their major anatomic divisions and structures, the suspensory ligaments of the ovaries, the fallopian tubes and their major anatomic divisions and suspensory ligaments, the potential peritoneal spaces of the pelvis, and the vascular supply of the female reproductive system.
2. Describe the phases and events that occur in the ovarian and menstrual cycles and the actions of the female steroid hormones.
3. Describe the basic scanning protocol for transabdominal sonography of the female reproductive system according to national guidelines.
4. Describe the basic scanning protocol for endovaginal sonography of the female reproductive system.
5. List several technical pitfalls associated with transabdominal and endovaginal sonography of the female reproductive system.

NORMAL ANATOMY

Pelvic Cavity

The pelvic cavity is bordered superiorly by the pelvic brim, inferiorly by the levator ani muscles, and laterally by the abdominal walls. The pelvis contains various segments of small bowel and colon, the rectum and anus, the urinary bladder, and the distal ureters (Fig. 12-1). The bony pelvis is divided into the greater, or **false pelvis,** and the lesser, or **true pelvis.** The greater pelvis consists of the expanded portion located superior and anterior to the pelvic brim and primarily contains loops of bowel. The lesser pelvis, located inferior to the pelvic brim, is continuous with the greater pelvis, but its bony walls are more complete. The true pelvis contains the female reproductive system, urinary bladder, and distal ureters. Measurements of the true pelvis are important in obstetrics. The superior circumference is formed by the pelvic brim. The enclosed area is called the superior aperture, or **pelvic inlet.** The inferior circumference, or **pelvic outlet,** is bordered posteriorly by the sacrum and coccyx, laterally by the ischial tuberosities, and anteriorly by the pubic arcuate ligament and the inferior rami of the pubic bones (Fig. 12-2).

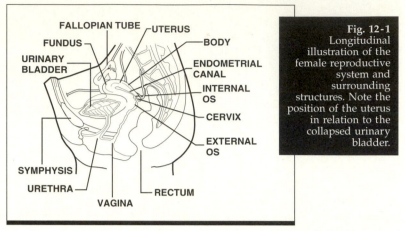

Fig. 12-1 Longitudinal illustration of the female reproductive system and surrounding structures. Note the position of the uterus in relation to the collapsed urinary bladder.

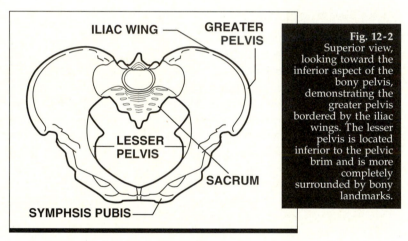

Fig. 12-2 Superior view, looking toward the inferior aspect of the bony pelvis, demonstrating the greater pelvis bordered by the iliac wings. The lesser pelvis is located inferior to the pelvic brim and is more completely surrounded by bony landmarks.

Pelvic Muscles

Many of the pelvic muscles serve as anatomic landmarks in gynecologic sonography. The paired **psoas major** muscles are large, triangular muscles that arise from the lumbar transverse processes and the body and disks from the twelfth thoracic through the second lumbar vertebrae.[4] The muscles descend through the false pelvis on the anterior aspect of the pelvic sidewall and exit posteriorly to the inguinal ligament, where they converge with the iliacus muscle to form a tendon that attaches to the lesser trochanter of the femur. The **iliacus muscle** arises from the concavity of the upper two thirds of the iliac fossa. In the false pelvis the iliopsoas muscles are medial and slightly anterior to the iliacus muscles. The iliac wings are posterior and lateral to the iliopsoas muscles. In the true pelvis the iliacus and psoas muscles are separated by a fascial plane, which is continuous with the psoas tendon. This results in the typical "bull's eye" sonographic appearance of this muscle (Fig. 12-3).

The paired **piriformis muscles** arise from the sacrum between the pelvic sacral foramina and the gluteal surface of the ilium. Along with the sacrum and coccyx, these muscles form the posterior border of the true pelvis. These muscles are typically located posterior to the ovaries (Fig. 12-4). The paired **obturator internus muscles** arise from the anterolateral pelvic wall and surround the obturator foramen. They course through the lesser sciatic foramen and attach to the greater trochanter. These muscles form a portion of the lateral border of the true pelvis. On transverse sonograms these muscles are seen at the posteromedial aspect of the ovaries and are also seen adjacent to the lateral walls of the urinary bladder (Fig. 12-5).

The paired **levator ani muscles** consist of two components; the pubococcygeus and the iliococcygeus. These muscles form the inferior aspect of the pelvic cavity, also called the pelvic floor. The levator ani muscles contribute to the sphincteric actions of the anal canal and vagina. These muscles are demonstrated on inferior transverse images, posterior and lateral to the vagina (Fig. 12-6).

Peritoneal Spaces
Reflections of the thin peritoneum form two major potential

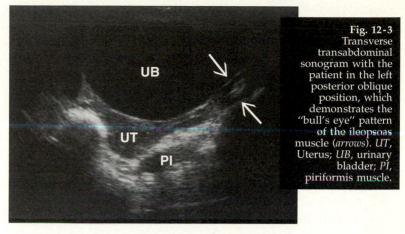

Fig. 12-3 Transverse transabdominal sonogram with the patient in the left posterior oblique position, which demonstrates the "bull's eye" pattern of the ileopsoas muscle (*arrows*). *UT*, Uterus; *UB*, urinary bladder; *PI*, piriformis muscle.

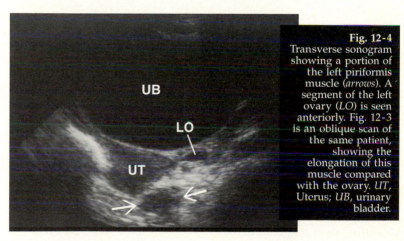

Fig. 12-4 Transverse sonogram showing a portion of the left piriformis muscle (*arrows*). A segment of the left ovary (*LO*) is seen anteriorly. Fig. 12-3 is an oblique scan of the same patient, showing the elongation of this muscle compared with the ovary. *UT*, Uterus; *UB*, urinary bladder.

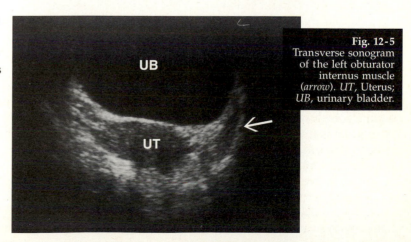

Fig. 12-5 Transverse sonogram of the left obturator internus muscle (*arrow*). *UT*, Uterus; *UB*, urinary bladder.

spaces in the female pelvic cavity.[4] The **anterior cul-de-sac,** or the **uterovesical space,** is located posterior to the urinary bladder and anterior to the uterine body and fundus (Fig. 12-7). When the uterus is positioned normally, this space is compact and empty. With a retroflexed or retroverted uterus, the anterior cul-de-sac often contains loops of bowel. The **posterior cul-de-sac,** also called the **pouch of Douglas** or the **rectouterine space,** is located posterior to the uterus and the upper third of the vagina and lies anterior to the rectum. This space is the most dependent portion of the peritoneal cavity in the supine patient.

The **space of Retzius,** also called the **prevesical** or **retropubic space,** lies between the transversalis fascia of the abdominal wall and the umbilical prevesical fascia. Pathologic processes located in this potential space displace the urinary bladder posteriorly.

Vascular Anatomy

The **common iliac arteries** arise from the distal aorta and course anteriorly and medially in relation to the psoas muscles. The common iliac arteries bifurcate to form the **external and internal iliac arteries** (Fig. 12-8). The external iliac arteries supply a large portion of the lower extremities. The internal iliac arteries supply the pelvic viscera, pelvic walls, perineum, and gluteal regions. The lumen of the external iliac arteries is larger than the lumen of the internal iliac arteries. The ureters, ovaries, and fimbriated

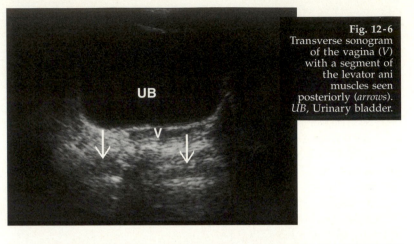

Fig. 12-6 Transverse sonogram of the vagina (*V*) with a segment of the levator ani muscles seen posteriorly (*arrows*). *UB,* Urinary bladder.

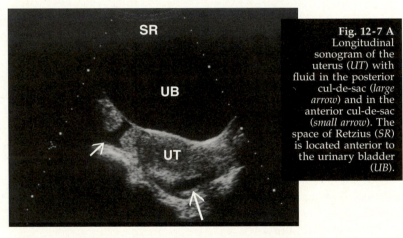

Fig. 12-7 A Longitudinal sonogram of the uterus (*UT*) with fluid in the posterior cul-de-sac (*large arrow*) and in the anterior cul-de-sac (*small arrow*). The space of Retzius (*SR*) is located anterior to the urinary bladder (*UB*).

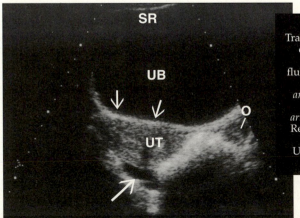

Fig. 12-7 B Transverse sonogram demonstrating the uterus (*UT*) with fluid in the posterior cul-de-sac (*large arrow*). The anterior cul-de-sac (*small arrows*) and space of Retzius (*SR*) contain no structures. *UB,* Urinary bladder; *O,* left ovary.

ends of the fallopian tubes are located anterior to the internal iliac arteries. The **right common iliac vein** ascends posteriorly and then laterally to the right common iliac artery. The **left common iliac vein** ascends medially and then posteriorly to the left common iliac artery. The right and left common iliac veins merge to form the **inferior vena cava.**[4]

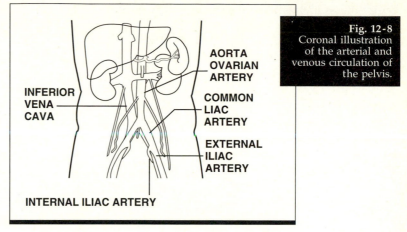

AORTA
OVARIAN ARTERY

INFERIOR VENA CAVA

COMMON LIAC ARTERY

EXTERNAL ILIAC ARTERY

INTERNAL ILIAC ARTERY

Fig. 12-8
Coronal illustration of the arterial and venous circulation of the pelvis.

The internal iliac arteries divide into the **anterior and posterior trunks.** The **uterine artery,** a branch of the anterior trunk, courses medially on the levator ani to the cervix, where it crosses superiorly and anteriorly to the ureter. It then ascends lateral to the uterus in the broad ligament to the junction of the fallopian tubes and the uterus. From the uterine cornua, the uterine artery then courses laterally to reach the hilum of the ovary, where it terminates by joining the ovarian artery. The uterine arteries join each other across the midline through the anterior and posterior **arcuate arteries,** which run through the broad ligament and then enter the myometrium. The uterine plexus of veins, or the **arcuate veins,** accompany the arcuate arteries. These veins are larger than the arteries and are frequently demonstrated with both transabdominal and endovaginal sonography.

The **ovarian arteries** arise from the lateral margin of the aorta, slightly inferior to the renal arteries. At the pelvic brim they cross the external iliac artery and vein and course medially in the suspensory ligament of the ovary. They then pass posteriorly in the mesovarium and divide into branches. The **right ovarian vein** empties into the inferior vena cava, just inferior to the renal vein. The **left ovarian vein** empties into the left renal vein.

Uterus

The uterus, located in the true pelvis, is bordered by the urinary bladder anteriorly and by the rectosigmoid colon posteriorly. The uterine position changes with various degrees of bladder and rectosigmoid distension. The uterus consists of three layers. The outer layer, the **perimetrium,** forms a capsule around the uterus. The middle layer, the **myometrium,** consists of smooth muscle and forms the thickest layer. The **endometrium,** the inner layer, lines the **endometrial cavity** (EMC), and its thickness varies in response to estrogen and progesterone serum levels.[2] The EMC is flat and triangular with the apex pointing toward the cervix. The uterus has four anatomic subdivisions: the superior **fundus,** the **body** (or corpus), the **isthmus** (or lower uterine segment), and the **cervix.** The isthmus joins the cervix at the **internal cervical os.** The cervix joins the vagina at the **external cervical os** (Fig. 12-9). The prepubertal uterus measures approximately 3 cm in length, 1 cm in the posteroanterior plane, and 1 cm in the transverse plane. The cervix constitutes two thirds of the total uterine length, and the posteroanterior diameter of the cervix is twice the diameter of the body. The postpubertal uterus measures a maximum of 7 cm in length, 2 cm in the posteroanterior plane, and 4 cm in the transverse dimension. Multiparity increases all uterine measurements by approximately 1 to 2 cm. In the postmenopausal group, the uterus experiences atrophy and is approximately 1 to 2 cm thick and 3 to 7 cm long.[1]

In the postpubertal group the fundus is larger and longer than the cervix. Normally the uterus is flexed between the body and cervix, with the body lying over the superior surface of the collapsed urinary bladder and pointing inferiorly and slightly posterior. (Fig. 12-10). The cervix points inferiorly and posteriorly from the point of flexion, joining the vagina at approximately a 90-degree angle. There are several uterine positional anomalies. In **retroflexion** the body of the uterus bends posteriorly in relation to the cervix, and the angle between the cervix and vagina is variable. In **retroversion** the entire uterus is positioned more posteriorly than normal, without a change in the relationship to the cervix.[3]

Suspensory Ligaments

A number of ligaments suspend the uterus in the peritoneal cavity. The paired **broad ligaments** contain double folds of peritoneum that extend from the lateral aspect of the uterus to the lateral pelvic sidewalls (Fig. 12-11). The area of the broad ligament is called the adnexal area. The portion of the broad ligament immediately adjacent to

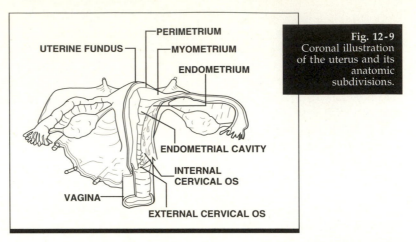

Fig. 12-9 Coronal illustration of the uterus and its anatomic subdivisions.

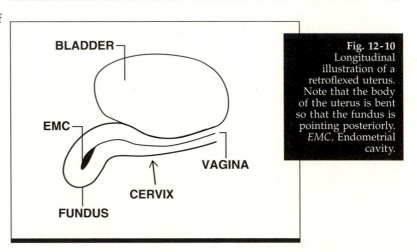

Fig. 12-10 Longitudinal illustration of a retroflexed uterus. Note that the body of the uterus is bent so that the fundus is pointing posteriorly. *EMC*, Endometrial cavity.

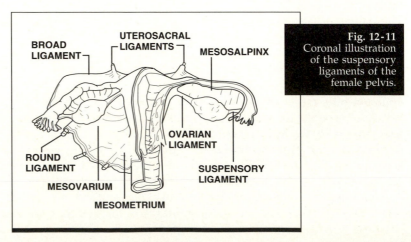

Fig. 12-11 Coronal illustration of the suspensory ligaments of the female pelvis.

the uterus is termed the **mesometrium.** The free border of this sheetlike ligament contains the fallopian tubes. The portion of the broad ligament between each fallopian tube and the ovarian ligament is called the **mesosalpinx.**[4] The portion of the broad ligament adjacent to the ovary is called the **mesovarium.** The ovary is attached to the posterior layer of the broad ligament by the mesovarium. The portion of the broad ligament that extends from the infundibulum of the fallopian tube, the superior portion of the ovary, and the pelvic sidewall is called the **suspensory ligament of the ovary.** The uterine portion of this ligament includes a narrow, cordlike structure, the **ovarian ligament,** which attaches to the laterosuperior border of the uterus, just posterior to each fallopian tube.

The paired **round ligaments** arise in the uterine cornua, anterior to the fallopian tubes, and extend anterolaterally, where they course posterior to the inguinal ligament and insert into the fascia of the labia majora. The paired **uterosacral ligaments** attach the posterior surface of the uterus to the sacrum. The single **posterior ligament** extends from the posterior surface of the uterus to the rectum. The single **anterior ligament** attaches the anterior surface of the uterus to the posterior aspect of the urinary bladder.[3] These ligaments are not routinely visualized with sonography.

Fallopian Tubes

The fallopian tubes are trumpet-shaped muscular canals that extend from the superior angles of the uterine fundus to the ovary and course in the free margin of the broad ligament. Each tube measures an average of 10 cm in length.[4] The walls of the fallopian tubes are made up of three layers: the outer serous, the middle muscular, and the inner mucous layers. The inner layer is contiguous with the uterine endometrium and consists of ciliated columnar epithelium. A combination of muscular contraction and the wavelike movement of the cilia propels the ovum through the tube. Each tube consists of four sections: the interstitial, isthmus, ampulla, and infundibulum (Fig. 12-12). The interstitial is a short segment that passes through the uterine wall. The isthmus is the constricted portion adjacent to the uterus. The ampulla is the widest portion that curves over the ovary. The infundibulum, with its abdominal ostium or opening, is surrounded by fimbriae. One of the fimbria, the **ovarian fimbria,** or primum ostium, is attached to the ovary.[3] Frequently one or more small, pedunculated vesicles are connected to the fimbriae or to the adjacent broad ligament. These vesicles are called **hydatids of Morgagni** or **appendices vesiculosae,** which are vestigial remnants of the mesonephric ducts.[3] Although usually microscopic, these ducts may develop a larger cystic component and constitute one type of paraovarian cyst. The sonographer should remember that the fallopian tubes open directly into

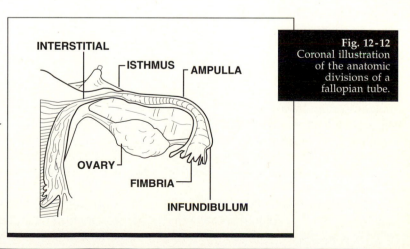

INTERSTITIAL
ISTHMUS **AMPULLA**
OVARY
FIMBRIA
INFUNDIBULUM

Fig. 12-12
Coronal illustration of the anatomic divisions of a fallopian tube.

the peritoneal cavity, and therefore microorganisms have a direct route from the vagina into the abdominal cavity.

Ovaries

In the nulliparous woman the ellipsoid ovaries lie in the ovarian fossa, called the **fossa of Waldeyer,** which is positioned on the lateral pelvic wall and is bordered anteriorly by the obliterated umbilical artery; posteriorly by the ureter, internal iliac artery, and piriformis muscle; laterally by the obturator internus muscle; and superiorly by the external iliac vein. Ovarian size varies with age. In the prepubertal stage each ovary is 1 cm long, 1 cm wide, and 1 cm thick, with an average volume of 0.46 cm^3. One formula for calculating a prolate ellipse is length times width times thickness times 0.532.[2] During the reproductive years the ovaries measure approximately 3 cm in length, 2 cm in width, and 1 cm in posteroanterior thickness. The ovarian volume ranges from 1.8 cm^3 to 5.7 cm^3. The postmenopausal ovary measures up to 2 cm in length and 0.5 cm in posteroanterior thickness. The ovarian volume should be less than 4 ml.[1]

Each ovary contains two tissue layers, the cortex and the medulla. The medulla contains connective tissue and blood vessels, whereas the cortex consists of glandular tissue. The cortex contains follicles and also produces estrogen and progesterone. The size of the follicles varies with the menstrual cycle. In the follicular or proliferative phase, the follicle size ranges from 5 to 10 mm. In the late follicular phase just before ovulation, the dominant follicle size ranges from 18 to 25 mm.[1]

NORMAL PHYSIOLOGY

Ovarian Cycle

The ovaries produce two types of female steroid hormones, estrogen and progesterone. Estrogen is secreted primarily by the graafian follicles and by the placenta during pregnancy. Progesterone is primarily secreted by the corpus luteum in the nongravida state and by the corpus luteum and later by the placenta during pregnancy. Estrogen performs several functions. In the early phase of the menstrual cycle, it promotes the regeneration of the endometrium after menses. During the preovulatory phase, estrogen causes the endometrium to thicken. It also affects electrolyte and fluid metabolism, with a tendency to produce salt and water retention, especially in the endometrium. Estrogen also promotes myometrial contraction during normal menstruation and especially during labor and delivery. High serum concentrations of estrogen inhibit the secretion of follicle-stimulating hormone (FSH) by the anterior lobe of the pituitary gland, thus preventing pregnancy.[3]

Progesterone also serves several functions. It acts on the estrogen-primed endometrium and converts it to the secretory type of endometrium. This produces a thick, vascular endometrial layer in preparation for implantation. Progesterone decreases myometrial contractions. When implantation occurs, the corpus luteum of pregnancy vigorously secretes progesterone. These elevated serum progesterone levels with the excess spilled into the urine form the basis for the clinical laboratory tests to determine pregnancy.

The **graafian follicle** is the structure in the cortex of the ovary that contains the immature ova. The follicle supports the growth and maturation of the ovum. At birth each ovary contains approximately 400,000 immature follicles.[3] During the reproductive years, one follicle a month usually reaches maturation. The follicular cells begin to proliferate and secrete estrogen along with small amounts of progesterone. The anterior pituitary gland secretes FSH, which stimulates the ovarian follicles to develop and stimulates the secretion of estrogen by the ovaries. During this period the oocyte undergoes meiosis, which produces a haploid chromosomal complement. A clear membrane, the **zona pellucida,** forms around the ovum. The follicular cells grow in number and size and arrange themselves in layers around the ovum. Fluid collects inside the follicle, causing a substantial increase in the size of the follicle. Luteinizing hormone (LH), also secreted by the anterior pituitary, works with FSH to cause the final maturation of the follicle and to trigger its rupture. In response to this hormonal stimulation, the follicle ruptures, propelling the ovum toward the fallopian tube, which is termed **ovulation.** After ovulation, the ruptured follicle collapses and fills with blood and serous fluid (corpus hemorrhagicum). At this point the entire follicle becomes the **corpus luteum,** which secretes estrogen and progesterone. The secretion of luteotropic hormone (LTH) by the anterior pituitary stimulates these hormonal secretions. If the ovum is not fertilized, the corpus luteum reaches its maximum development approximately 7 days after ovulation and then degenerates into a mass of fibrous tissue, called the **corpus albicans.** If fertilization occurs, the corpus luteum continues to grow and to secrete hormones, reaching maximum development during the second month of pregnancy. It then gradually regresses as the placenta matures and takes over its endocrine function (Fig. 12-13).

Menstrual Cycle

The menstrual cycle begins with the first day of menstrual flow. During menses, or the **menstrual phase,** approximately day 1 through day 5, portions of the endometrial layer undergo necrosis as a result of sudden vaso-contriction. The sloughing of the endometrium is usually a controlled process with moderate bleeding (Fig. 12-13). Serum levels of estrogen and progesterone are reduced. The **proliferative** or **follicular phase** begins on ap-

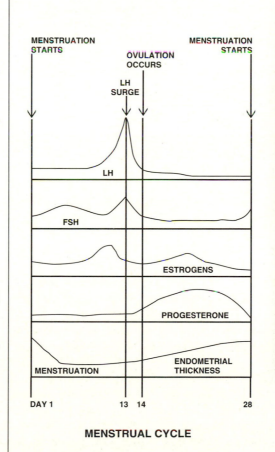

Fig. 12-13 Graph depicting the hormonal events associated with the normal menstrual and ovarian cycles. Luteinizing hormone (LH) normally peaks 24 to 36 hours before ovulation and is called the LH surge. Levels of follicle-stimulating hormones (FSH) reach their maximum at the time of the LH surge. Estrogen levels attain their maximum value just before the LH surge. Progesterone levels coincide with the development of the corpus luteum and reach their highest levels after ovulation. The endometrium lining is the thickest after ovulation, in preparation for possible implantation.

proximately day 5 of a 28-day cycle and extends to about day 14. The endometrium thickens in preparation for ovulation. If the menstrual cycle is irregular, this phase is either longer or shorter. The serum estrogen levels increase during this phase, and ovulation occurs on day 14 of a 28-day cycle. The **secretory, postovulatory** or **luteal phase** occurs from day 14 through day 28. During this phase the endometrium continues to thicken in preparation for possible implantation of an embryo. The superficial layer becomes vascular and edematous, and the serum progesterone levels rise and peak in synchronization with the development of the corpus luteum. Estrogen levels also peak during this phase. If the ovum is not fertilized, or if implantation does not occur, the corpus luteum regresses, and the declining serum levels of ovarian hormones cause vasocontriction of the arterioles in the endometrium, which triggers necrosis and the start of menses.[3]

SCANNING PROTOCOLS AND TECHNIQUES

Transabdominal Technique

Transabdominal pelvic sonography requires a distended urinary bladder in order to displace the surrounding bowel and to allow adequate visualization of the uterus and ovaries. This typically requires that the patient drink 24 to 32 ounces of clear liquids over a 15- to 20-minute period 1 hour before the ultrasound examination. The patient must be instructed not to void once she starts drinking the liquids. Patients receiving intravenous fluids who cannot drink any liquids should be instructed not to void approximately 2 hours before the examination. Patients requiring emergency pelvic examinations may need urethral catheterization and retrofilling of the bladder with 400 to 600 ml of sterile water. To decrease the risk of infection, the sonographer must ensure that proper sterile precautions are maintained with this procedure. Although tempting, the sonographer should never perform the examination with an inadequately filled urinary bladder, since the misidentification of both normal anatomy and pathologic processes may occur.

Usually a 3.5 MHz transducer provides adequate penetration with optimum resolution for the average-size patient. A 5.0 MHz transducer may prove adequate for thin patients, whereas a 2.25 MHz transducer is usually required for obese patients. Because of the posterior location of the uterus and ovaries, the sonographer must place the focal zone deep in the image field. The system acoustic power and gain controls, as well as the time gain compensation (TGC), must be set so that the parenchymal pattern of the uterus and ovaries is homogeneous and adequately demonstrated. Because of the acoustic enhancement distal to the urinary bladder, the gain controls are typically decreased to allow depiction of the sonographic patterns.

The standard scanning protocol usually consists of transverse and longitudinal views through the true pelvis. Longitudinal scans begin at the anatomic midline, which corresponds to a line connecting the midpoint of the symphysis and the umbilicus. The transducer must be positioned inferiorly, close to the symphysis, and angled superiorly to use the urinary bladder as an acoustic window for the entire uterus. Sequential scans begin from the midline and proceed to the right lateral aspect of the urinary bladder. The transducer is then repositioned at the midline, and sequential scans are obtained through the left lateral aspect of the urinary bladder. Because of the variable position of the uterus and ovaries, oblique scans may be necessary to demonstrate their true longitudinal dimensions. Since the vagina is a rather stable structure and therefore usually at the midline, the sonographer should localize the vagina and then angle obliquely until the vagina, cervix, corpus, and fundus are demonstrated. The EMC and the vaginal canal typically produce a hyperechoic line that allows the sonographer to know when the scan plane coincides with the true anatomic midline of these structures. This view should be used for longitudinal and posteroanterior measurements of the uterus and for the posteroanterior measurement of the EMC. Since the cervix is a portion of the uterus, the calipers should be positioned from the most superior portion of the uterus to the level of the external cervical os (Fig. 12-14). The ovaries are usually located just lateral to the uterine fundus. To use the urinary bladder as an acoustic window, the sonographer should move the transducer to the left of midline and angle back toward the right ovary, and then move to the right of midline and angle back toward the left ovary. The presence of follicles in the ovary and the posterior location of the internal iliac artery and vein are the most consistent anatomic landmarks for accurate ovarian identification. The right posterior oblique position for the right ovary and the left posterior oblique position for the left ovary also allow use of the bladder as a scanning window and may allow better separation of the ovary from the surrounding bowel and soft tissue. An image demonstrating the mid-longitudinal plane of the ovary is used to measure the ovarian length. The sonographer should verify the ovarian position on survey transverse scans if unsure of the ovarian position on initial longitudinal scans. The sonographer should always scan superior to the uterus and lateral to the urinary bladder to avoid missing ovarian cysts or other pathologic conditions.

Transverse scans may start inferiorly at the level of the symphysis or superiorly at the top of the urinary bladder. Starting inferiorly provides more anatomic landmarks for accurate identification of the uterus, adnexal structures, and cystic or solid pathologic disorders. Initial scans should be performed in sequence demonstrating the vagina, cervix, isthmus, corpus, and fundus of the uterus. This often requires a superior angulation in order to use the bladder as a scanning window. An image coinciding with the largest dimension of the fundus is used for obtaining the posteroanterior and transverse measurements. If the EMC echo complex is demonstrated, the sonographer may obtain a posteroanterior measurement. For transverse scans of the ovaries, the same techniques required for longitudinal scans are necessary; that is, the patient is placed in the oblique positions and the sonographer scans from the opposite side of the urinary bladder. On an image corresponding to the largest transverse dimension of the ovary, the sonographer measures the posteroanterior and transverse dimensions of the ovary.

The typical scanning protocol for transabdominal pelvic sonography is summarized in the box that appears on the following page.

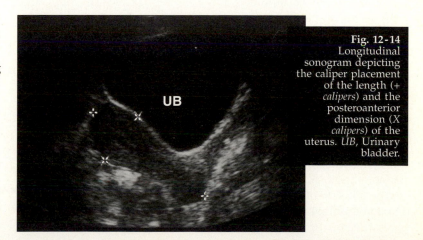

Fig. 12-14 Longitudinal sonogram depicting the caliper placement of the length (+ *calipers*) and the posteroanterior dimension (*X calipers*) of the uterus. *UB*, Urinary bladder.

Figs. 12-15 through 12-20 provide examples of the transabdominal examination.

Endovaginal Technique

For the endovaginal pelvic examination the patient empties her bladder to place the uterus and ovaries in the imaging field of the endovaginal transducer. Most manufacturers currently use a 5.0 to 7.5 MHz transducer to improve resolution. These frequencies allow adequate penetration for most patients, since the transducer is so close to the organs of interest. Many sonographers unfamiliar with this technique are initially disoriented to the anatomic relationships and transducer orientation. The sonographer should remember that a collapsed urinary bladder changes the position of the uterus and ovaries. With the transducer introduced inferiorly in the vagina, the sonographer does not scan in the true transverse body imaging plane but in the coronal imaging plane (see Fig. 12-21**A** on page 217). The coronal plane divides the body into anterior and posterior sections. Because the uterus normally drapes over the collapsed bladder, the sonographer should point the transducer anteriorly to image the body and fundus of the uterus, which typically coincides with the transverse plane of these structures. Image orientation is the same as in transabdominal sonography; that is, the patient's right side is displayed on the left side of the screen. The longitudinal plane does not

---

BASIC SCANNING PROTOCOL OF THE TRANSABDOMINAL PELVIS

Longitudinal Views of the Midline Uterus
✔ Demonstrate the vagina, cervix, corpus, and fundus with EMC. Longitudinal and posteroanterior measurements should be obtained.

Longitudinal Views to the Right of Midline
✔ Demonstrate the lateral aspect of the uterus and the right ovary. Longitudinal measurement of the ovary should be obtained.

Longitudinal Views to the Left of Midline
✔ Demonstrate the lateral aspect of the uterus and the left ovary. Longitudinal measurement of the ovary should be obtained.

Transverse Views from Inferior to Superior or Superior to Inferior
✔ Demonstrate the true transverse plane of the vagina, cervix, isthmus, and corpus with EMC.

Fundus with EMC
✔ Obtain transverse and posteroanterior measurements of the uterus and posteroanterior measurement through the thickest portion of the EMC.

Right Ovary
✔ Obtain transverse and posteroanterior measurements.

Left Ovary
✔ Obtain transverse and posteroanterior measurements. Dominant follicle on ovary(ies) may also be measured.

change with this inferior transducer placement. The orientation
is again the same in that the inferior aspect of the patient is displayed on the right side of the
screen[6] (see Fig. 12-21**B** on
page 217).

Before the examination, the
sonographer should place a
small amount of gel inside a condom and slip it over the transducer, ensuring that no air is
trapped between the condom
and the transducer face. The patient should remove her under-
wear, and the sonographer
should place a sheet over the
pelvis and lower extremities. Depending on the type of transducer, the sonographer may
need to place a thick foam
square or several pillows under
the patient. It is important that
the patient's entire torso be elevated, since elevation of only
the pelvis may cause fluid in the
cul-de-sac to relayer in a more
superior recess. In most cases the
patient is instructed to insert the
tip of the transducer into the
vagina, similar to the insertion of
a tampon. The sonographer
should hand the transducer to
the patient and watch the viewing screen, instructing the patient not to insert the transducer
any farther once the cervix
comes into view. Alternately, the
sonographer may insert the
transducer, always ensuring that
the patient is properly draped
and that the examination room
provides for the patient's pri-
vacy. Male sonographers should
always use a chaperone to avoid
any accusations of impropriety.

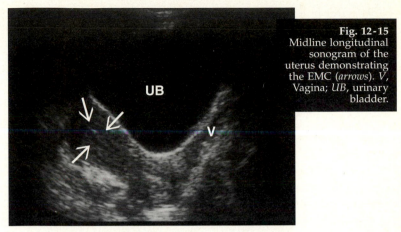

Fig. 12-15
Midline longitudinal
sonogram of the
uterus demonstrating
the EMC (*arrows*). *V*,
Vagina; *UB*, urinary
bladder.

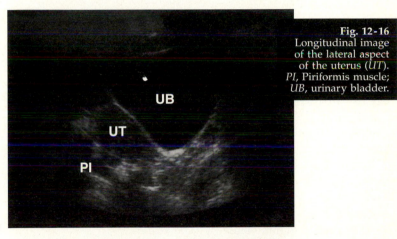

Fig. 12-16
Longitudinal image
of the lateral aspect
of the uterus (*UT*).
PI, Piriformis muscle;
UB, urinary bladder.

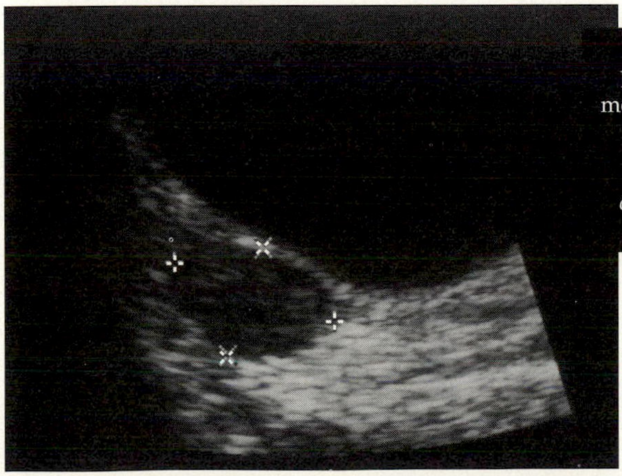

Fig. 12-17
Longitudinal image
measuring the length
(+ *calipers*) and the
posteroanterior
dimensions (*X
calipers*) of the right
ovary.

The scanning protocol for the endovaginal examination consists of sequential images of the uterus and ovaries in the coronal and longitudinal body planes. If the uterus is in the normal position, the sonographer points the transducer anteriorly to bring the uterine corpus and fundus into view. Again, an oblique scanning plane may be necessary in order to demonstrate the corpus and fundus with the EMC in one longitudinal view. To demonstrate the cervix, the sonographer may have to pull the transducer out slightly to place it in a more inferior portion of the vaginal canal and point the transducer more posteriorly. This longitudinal image of the cervix should also demonstrate the posterior cul-de-sac. In the case of a retroverted or retroflexed uterus, usually the transducer must be pointed more posteriorly to display the uterine body and fundus. After obtaining the midline images of the uterus and cervix, the sonographer should obtain images of the right and left lateral aspects of the uterus. Obtaining longitudinal images of the ovaries may prove difficult if they are located adjacent to the lateral pelvic wall. Placing the patient's legs in stirrups or draping the legs over the cart rails can relax the pelvic muscles and may allow a more anteromedial ovarian location.[6]

In the coronal imaging plane the sonographer should obtain anatomic tranverse images of the cervix, isthmus, body, and fundus of the uterus. When the

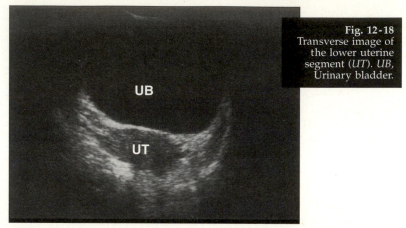

Fig. 12-18
Transverse image of the lower uterine segment (*UT*). *UB*, Urinary bladder.

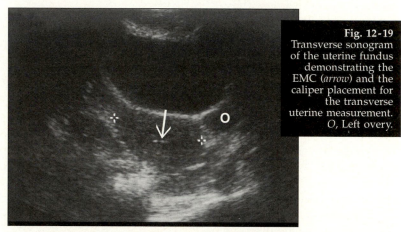

Fig. 12-19
Transverse sonogram of the uterine fundus demonstrating the EMC (*arrow*) and the caliper placement for the transverse uterine measurement. *O*, Left overy.

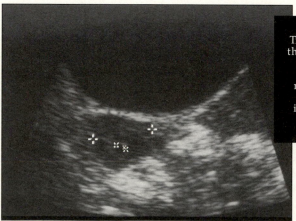

Fig. 12-20
Transverse image of the right ovary with the transverse diameter measurement (*large calipers*). An immature follicle is seen in the cortex (*small calipers*).

uterus is in the normal position, this scanning sequence requires a progressive posterior to anterior movement of the transducer. The transverse view of the cervix should also demonstrate the posterior cul-de-sac. The sonographer should measure the posteroanterior and transverse dimensions of the uterine fundus and the posteroanterior thickness of the EMC. Although the position of the ovaries varies, their typical position is posterior, adjacent to the internal iliac artery and vein. The transducer is pointed toward the patient's right lateral aspect for the right ovary and toward the left lateral aspect for the left ovary. The sonographer should always inform the patient before moving the transducer in this fashion and inquire whether it is causing any pain or severe discomfort. The sonographer should point the transducer posteriorly, looking for the internal iliac artery and vein, and then move anteriorly until the ovary comes into view. As in transabdominal sonography, bowel loops may interfere with the visualization of the ovaries. To assist in locating the ovaries on the endovaginal examination, the sonographer should note the location of the ovaries on the transabdominal examination, particularly if they appear very lateral or superior.

The scanning protocol for the endovaginal pelvic examination is summarized in the box that appears on the following page.

Figs. 12-22 to 12-25 provide examples of the endovaginal protocol.

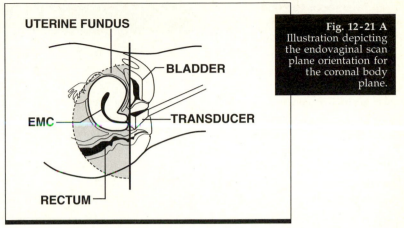

Fig. 12-21 A
Illustration depicting the endovaginal scan plane orientation for the coronal body plane.

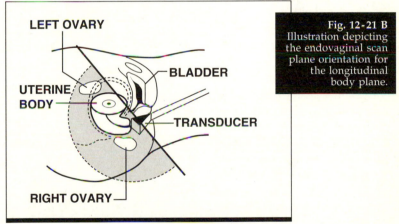

Fig. 12-21 B
Illustration depicting the endovaginal scan plane orientation for the longitudinal body plane.

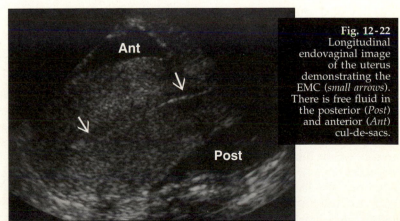

Fig. 12-22
Longitudinal endovaginal image of the uterus demonstrating the EMC (*small arrows*). There is free fluid in the posterior (*Post*) and anterior (*Ant*) cul-de-sacs.

Because of the limited scanning depth of endovaginal transducers, large masses located in the false pelvis may not be demonstrated. Therefore the standard practice generally requires the performance of a transabdominal examination in conjunction with the endovaginal scan. A general exception to this practice is in the case of follicular monitoring in the infertile patient, although a baseline transabdominal scan is often performed during the initial sonographic examination to rule out pelvic pathologic processes.

NORMAL SONOGRAPHIC PATTERNS

On both transabdominal and endovaginal examinations of the uterus, the myometrium appears as a homogeneous, moderately hyperechoic sonographic pattern. The perimetrium or uterine capsule visualizes as a thin, hyperechoic linear pattern surrounding the uterus. Since this structure acts as a specular reflector, it is angle dependent, and the sonographer must attain a scanning angle of approximately 90 degrees to adequately demonstrate this border. The EMC appears as a hyperechoic, elliptic sonographic pattern in the center of the uterine body and fundus, and it reaches its largest diameter during the secretory (or postovulatory) phase, where it may approach 5 mm (Fig. 12-26). During menstruation this pattern may appear inhomogeneous with hypoechoic to cystic areas. In the early proliferative phase the EMC may be difficult to demonstrate because of the preliminary stages of endometrial proliferation.[2] The retroflexed or retroverted uterus provides an imaging challenge for the sonographer. Because the uterine body and fundus lie more posteriorly, the image resolution degrades. The EMC may not adequately visualize as a result of poor resolution and the inability to achieve a proper scanning angle. Attaining a true transverse image of the uterus, especially for measurement purposes, is also a problem. The sonographer

---

BASIC PROTOCOL OF THE ENDOVAGINAL PELVIS

Longitudinal View of the Cervix, Including the Posterior Cul-de-Sac

Longitudinal Views of the Uterine Body and Fundus
✔ Obtain longitudinal measurement.

Longitudinal View of the Right Lateral Aspect of the Uterus

Longitudinal View of the Left Lateral Aspect of the Uterus

Longitudinal Views of the Right and Left Ovaries
✔ Obtain longitudinal measurement. Dominant follicle(s) may be measured.

Transverse View of the Cervix, Including the Cul-de-Sac

Transverse Views of the Uterine Body and Fundus
✔ Obtain posteroanterior and transverse measurements of the fundus and a posteroanterior measurement of the EMC.

Transverse Views of Both Ovaries
✔ Obtain transverse and posteroanterior measurements. Dominant follicle(s) may be measured.

should remember that the perimetrium is a specular reflector and angle dependent. The sonographer must change the scanning angle until the posterior perimetrium is demonstrated and the EMC lies in the central portion of the fundal myometrium. If this view cannot be attained, any transverse measurements should be interpreted very cautiously.[5] Endovaginal sonography provides better resolution of the retroverted or retroflexed uterus.

The ovaries also visualize as moderately hyperechoic elliptic structures containing immature or dominant follicles, depending on the patient's status in the ovarian cycle. Since immature follicles measure less than 2 cm, they may appear indistinct on transabdominal sonography, causing a less echogenic ovarian pattern. The most consistent landmarks for ovarian localization are the ureter and the internal iliac artery and vein that are seen posterior to the ovary, particularly on longitudinal scans (Fig. 12-27). On transverse images, the ovaries typically lie in a plane coinciding with the anterior half of the uterus, close to the posterior bladder wall. In many patients the uterus deviates toward the right or left lateral aspect. Since the ovaries are attached to the uterus via the ovarian ligament, this rotation will also change the ovarian position. If the uterus deviates toward the right, the left ovary often appears more directly posterior to the urinary bladder, whereas the right ovary will

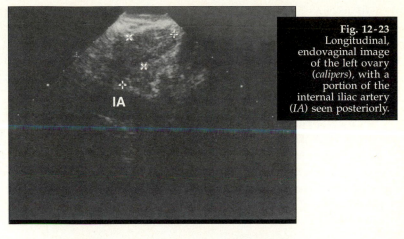

Fig. 12-23 Longitudinal, endovaginal image of the left ovary (*calipers*), with a portion of the internal iliac artery (*IA*) seen posteriorly.

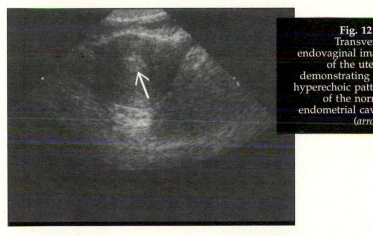

Fig. 12-24 Transverse, endovaginal image of the uterus demonstrating the hyperechoic pattern of the normal endometrial cavity (*arrow*).

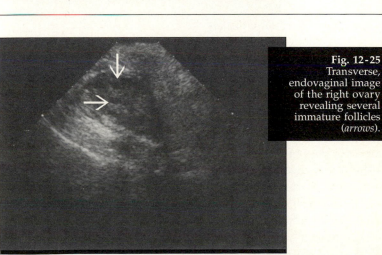

Fig. 12-25 Transverse, endovaginal image of the right ovary revealing several immature follicles (*arrows*).

slide more laterally and anteriorly, or it will move more posteriorly, with a portion of the uterus lying anterior to it. The same process occurs when the uterus deviates toward the left. With a retroflexed uterus the ovaries may appear in their normal position or may lie superior to the uterine fundus. The sonographer must remember all these possible ovarian locations and methodically examine them if the ovary does not visualize in the "normal" location. In endovaginal sonography the ureter and the internal iliac artery and vein again serve as initial landmarks for ovarian localization. Because of enhanced resolution, both immature and dominant follicles are easily demonstrated as cystic structures in the ovarian cortex. However, the arcuate vessels often lie adjacent to the ovary, and the sonographer can mistake circular loops of these vessels for ovarian follicles. The use of color-flow Doppler will help to avoid this problem.

Because of the very small size of the normal fallopian tube, each is not usually visualized on transabdominal sonography. On endovaginal examinations the interstitial portion of the tube may appear on coronal scans of the uterus (Fig. 12-28). Because of the small amount of serous fluid normally present in the peritoneal cavity, the fluid may layer around more distal portions of the tube, allowing its identification. If the tube contains a small amount of fluid, easier identification is allowed.

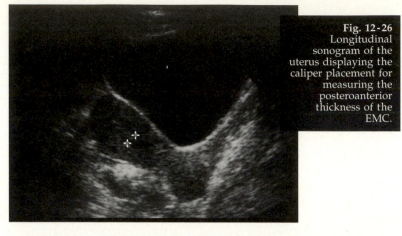

Fig. 12-26 Longitudinal sonogram of the uterus displaying the caliper placement for measuring the posteroanterior thickness of the EMC.

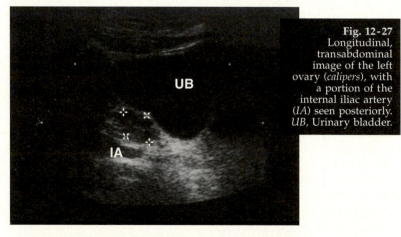

Fig. 12-27 Longitudinal, transabdominal image of the left ovary (*calipers*), with a portion of the internal iliac artery (*IA*) seen posteriorly. *UB*, Urinary bladder.

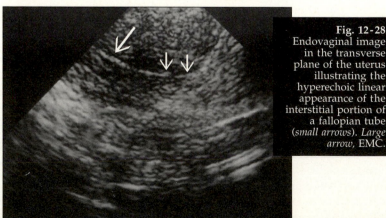

Fig. 12-28 Endovaginal image in the transverse plane of the uterus illustrating the hyperechoic linear appearance of the interstitial portion of a fallopian tube (*small arrows*). *Large arrow*, EMC.

TECHNICAL PITFALLS

The sonographer must avoid numerous pitfalls in gynecologic sonography. In transabdominal sonography, proper bladder distention plays a crucial role in the identification of normal anatomy, as well as in the identification of the sonographic pattern and the organ of origin for pathologic processes. The superior border of the urinary bladder should appear superior to the uterine fundus. This not only allows the use of the bladder as an acoustic window for the uterus, but also provides a good window for the ovaries, even if they lie in a more superior position. However, overdistention of the bladder may compress the uterine tissue, masking pathologic disorders; or overdistention may compress the ovaries and distort their location, making their identification difficult. The patient should be asked to partially void the bladder into a cup, voiding a half or full cup and then emptying it into the toilet. The patient should never be asked to void a little in the toilet, since many will void completely.

The sonographer should always position the imaging depth so that the area of the posterior cul-de-sac is demonstrated. It may take several minutes for any fluid to layer in the cul-de-sac after the patient lies down. The cul-de-sac should always be checked again at the end of the examination to ensure that any fluid is documented. The rectosigmoid colon may mimic a mass or free fluid in the cul-de-sac. The sonographer should always check for signs of peristalsis or for a change in the sonographic pattern. If necessary, the patient may need a water enema, which will distend the rectum and the distal sigmoid, producing the microbubble effect, which allows a more confident diagnosis. A tampon may cause an inhomogeneous, abnormal sonographic pattern in the vagina, cervix, and occasionally in the EMC. When faced with this pattern, the sonographer must always ask the patient if she is wearing a tampon and, if so, to remove it. This may result in a normal sonographic pattern or at least a different pattern.

Student sonographers seem to have the most difficulty in identifying ovaries. One common pitfall is mistaking the piriformis or obturator internus muscles for ovarian tissue. The sonographer should remember that this muscle lies posterior or medial to the ovary and, on longitudinal scans, will appear as a much longer structure than the ovary. The sonographer should always look for follicles in the cortex, using the internal iliac vessels as landmarks. The use of the posterior oblique positions often allows better identification. Scanning in the transverse plane provides more anatomic landmarks as the sonographer scans through the entire adnexal area. With both transabdominal and endovaginal sonography, the arcuate vessels may appear as circular or tubular structures and hypoechoic to anechoic, particularly in multigravida patients. Because of the massive increase in the size of the uterus and hence the vascular supply of these vessels, they may never decrease to their nulliparous size. The sonographer may misidentify these vessels as follicles in the ovary. The use of color-flow Doppler will demonstrate that these vessels are vascular structures.

SUMMARY

Many inexperienced sonographers find the gynecologic sonographic examination a challenge. A thorough knowledge of anatomy, including the adjacent pelvic muscles, allows more accurate identification of the ovaries. Developing the skill of using the urinary bladder as an acoustic window, changing the patient's position to enhance organ definition, and appreciating the position of the uterus and ovaries on an endovaginal examination comes only with experience and a tolerance for some initial frustration.

REFERENCES

1. Craig M: *A pocket guide to ultrasound measurements*, Philadelphia, 1988, pp 84-85.
2. Fleischer AC, Kalemelli GC, et al: Sonographic depiction of normal and abnormal endometrium with histopathologic correlation, *J Ultrasound Med* 5:445-452, 1986.
3. Netter FH, Oppenheimer E, editors: *The CIBA collection of medical illustrations: reproductive system*, West Caldwell, NJ, 1965, Ciba Pharmaceutical.
4. Pernoll M, Benson R, editors: *Current obstetric and gynecologic diagnosis and treatment*, ed 6, Norwalk, Conn, 1987, Appleton and Lange. pp 34-44.
5. Sample WF, Lippe BM, Gyepes MT: Gray scale ultrasonography of the female pelvis, *Radiology* 125:477-483, 1977.
6. Timor-Tritsche IE, Rottem S, Elgali S: How transvaginal sonography is done. In Timor-Tritsch IE, Rottem S, editors: *Transvaginal sonography*, New York, 1988, Elsevier.

uterine pathology

INSTRUCTIONAL OBJECTIVES

At the completion of this chapter, the reader will be able to:

1. Describe the clinical problems that are typical reasons for sonography of the uterus.
2. Describe the clinical laboratory tests used for evaluating uterine pathology, including the white blood cell count.
3. Describe the various types of uterine anomalies, and identify each on sectional sonograms.
4. Describe the various types of intrauterine contraceptive devices, and identify each on sectional sonograms.
5. Describe the clinical symptoms and pathologic basis for the disease processes of the uterus, including myomas, carcinoma, adenomyosis, and pelvic inflammatory disease.
6. Identify on sectional sonograms the above-mentioned disease processes of the uterus, based on the sonographic appearance, the clinical history, and the results of other diagnostic procedures.
7. Describe several technical pitfalls associated with the identification of uterine congenital anomalies and disease processes.

THE CLINICAL PROBLEM

The clinical evaluation of gynecologic disease often poses a challenge to the examining physician. Many of the symptoms are not specific for one type of pathology. The manual pelvic examination performed by a skilled clinician can offer additional information regarding the existence of a palpable mass, its consistency, and whether it arises from the uterus or ovary. However, many factors affect the accuracy of this procedure, including patient obesity and the amount of tenderness and guarding that occurs during the examination. Differentiation of a cystic from a solid ovarian mass is often difficult, and the clinician will order a pelvic sonogram to verify the findings of a mass and to determine whether it is cystic or solid. The primary role of sonography in the evaluation for gynecologic pathology includes determining whether a mass or other abnormality is present and identifying the organ of origin and its sonographic characteristics. With no clinical history, the resulting differential diagnosis can be quite extensive. The sonographer must obtain a complete clinical history to narrow this differential diagnosis. The more common use of endovaginal sonography has also allowed a more accurate classification of the internal consistency of pelvic masses and their organ of origin. A guiding principle in pelvic sonography is that solid masses are more likely to be uterine in origin, whereas predominantly cystic masses tend to originate in the ovaries. The demonstration of a mass directly adjacent to the endometrial cavity (EMC) also points to the uterus as the organ of origin. During transabdominal sonography, the sonographer should remember that the uterus and ovaries are located in the far field. If there is any doubt regarding the sonographic characteristics of the mass, a endovaginal examination should be performed.

OBTAINING THE CLINICAL HISTORY

As previously mentioned, the clinical history plays an important role in gynecologic sonography. The sonographer should obtain the date of the last menstrual period and whether the periods are regular, irregular, heavy, or light. Other important information includes the pregnancy history, the duration and location of pelvic pain, the presence of fever, and whether the patient is experiencing any bloody or creamy vaginal discharge. The patient should be asked whether she uses a contraceptive method, particularly an intrauterine contraceptive device (IUCD), and whether she is aware of any congenital uterine anomalies. The sonographer should obtain the patient's history in relation to gynecologic surgery. An important question is whether the patient has had a recent pelvic examination or a previous pelvic sonogram. Many departments use a standard clinical history sheet that is completed by the patient or the sonographer.

CLINICAL LABORATORY TESTS

The importance of clinical laboratory tests varies according to the preliminary clinical diagnosis. For example, very large uterine myomas may cause urinary tract problems, such as infection and hydronephrosis, and renal function tests may provide useful information. In the case of pelvic inflammatory disease the serum white blood cell (WBC) count may be elevated. These tests are discussed in previous chapters. The results of serum and urine pregnancy tests may also play a role, although they are of primary importance in obstetric sonography. These tests are discussed in Chapter 15.

RELATED IMAGING PROCEDURES

The **plain-film radiograph** can demonstrate calcifications related to uterine fibroids, as well as noncalcified soft tissue masses in the pelvis. In conjunction with an **intravenous pylogram (IVP) examination,** films of the opacified urinary bladder may reveal a mass effect caused by uterine enlargement as a result of fibroids. Hydronephrosis may occasionally occur because of extrinsic pressure from uterine enlargement or pedunculated fibroids.

Hysterosalpingography visualizes the EMC and fallopian tubes. A radiographic contrast medium is introduced via the cervix and outlines the uterine cavity. This procedure can diagnose uterine anomalies, such as a bicornuate uterus or the T-shaped uterus associated with diethylstilbestrol (DES) exposure. Hysterosalpingography can also diagnose tubal patency. The contrast medium normally flows through the fallopian tubes and into the peritoneal cavity. Failure of full visualization of the tubes is indicative of obstruction. However, nonvisualization can occur as a result of tubal spasm.

Computed tomography and **magnetic resonance imaging** can also diagnose uterine pathology. It is most useful in imaging the pelvic and retroperitoneal lymph nodes to look for evidence of lymphadenopathy, which would aid in differentiating benign from malignant uterine pathology.

BASIC SCANNING PROTOCOL

Transabdominal Examination

- **Longitudinal views of the midline uterus,** demonstrating the vagina, cervix, corpus, and fundus with EMC. Longitudinal and posteroanterior measurements should be obtained.
- **Longitudinal views to the right of midline,** demonstrating the lateral aspect of the uterus and the right ovary. Longitudinal measurement of the ovary should be obtained.
- **Longitudinal views to the left of midline,** demonstrating the lateral aspect of the uterus and left ovary. Longitudinal measurement of the ovary should be obtained.
- **Transverse views from inferior to superior or superior to inferior,** demonstrating the true transverse plane of the following structures: vagina, cervix, isthmus, and corpus with EMC.
- **Fundus with EMC,** obtaining transverse and posteroanterior measurements of the uterus and posteroanterior measurement through the thickest portion of the EMC.
- **Right ovary,** obtaining transverse and posteroanterior measurements.
- **Left ovary,** obtaining transverse and posteroanterior measurements. Dominant follicle on ovary(ies) may also be measured.

SCANNING PROTOCOLS AND TECHNIQUES

The scanning protocols and techniques for gynecologic sonography are discussed in Chapter 12. When confronted with a pelvic mass, the sonographer must determine whether the mass is uterine or ovarian in origin or whether the mass is arising from another structure. For uterine pathology, the sonographer should determine if the mass is contiguous to the EMC echo complex. This increases the possibility of a uterine origin. The sonographer should pay attention to the contours of the urinary bladder adjacent to the uterus. The initial clue to small uterine fibroids is often a displacement of the wall of the bladder. Another general guideline is that solid masses are more likely to be uterine in origin. To confirm this, the sonographer must also identify the ovaries and verify that they are not involved. The boxes appearing on this page and on the previous page review the basic scanning protocol for gynecologic sonography.

CONGENITAL ANOMALIES

The uterus derives from the müllerian ducts as two halves that later fuse together. Many of the anomalies relate to incomplete or partial fusion. The rate of uterine anomalies in the general population is less than 1%. Many of

---

BASIC SCANNING PROTOCOL

Endovaginal Examination
- **Longitudinal view of the cervix,** including the posterior cul-de-sac.
- **Longitudinal view of the uterine body and fundus,** obtaining longitudinal measurement.
- **Longitudinal views of the right lateral aspect of the uterus.**
- **Longitudinal views of the left lateral aspect of the uterus.**
- **Longitudinal views of the right and left ovaries,** obtaining longitudinal measurements. Dominant follicle(s) may be measured.
- **Transverse view of the cervix,** including the cul-de-sac.
- **Transverse view of the uterine body and fundus,** obtaining posteroanterior and transverse measurements of the fundus and posteroanterior measurement of the EMC.
- **Transverse views of both ovaries,** obtaining transverse and posteroanterior measurements. Dominant follicle(s) may be measured.

---

these anomalies are asymptomatic and are incidental findings during the bimanual pelvic or sonographic examination. Exposure to DES, a widely prescribed drug during the 1940s through the 1960s to prevent spontaneous abortion, increases the incidence of several uterine anomalies. Exposure may also cause a unique anomaly referred to as the T-shaped uterus.[11] The sonographer must remember that renal anomalies, particularly renal agenesis on the left side, are frequently associated with uterine anomalies and that the kidneys should be examined in all patients with uterine anomalies. Some of these uterine anomalies are difficult to identify on sonography.

Uterine aplasia, or total absence of the uterus, signifies bilateral arrested development and is not common. **Uterus unicornis** occurs when there is unilateral arrested development that causes only one half of the uterus to be present. **Uterus didelphys,** a very rare anomaly, signifies total failure of fusion and produces two separate uterine bodies, two cervices, and two vaginas, all of which function separately. **Uterine bicornis bicollis** is another type of partial fusion that produces one vagina, two cervices, and two uterine bodies. The more common **uterus bicornis unicollis,** also called the **bicornuate uterus,** produces one vagina, one cervix, and two uterine horns.

There are several other more subtle anomalies. In **uterus septus** a septum completely divides the uterine bodies. The thickness of this septum varies depending on the amount of myometrial tissue deposition. **Uterus subseptus** creates a partial septum between the uterine bodies, with a communication in the area of the isthmus or cervix. The last type of anomaly is **uterus arcuatus,** a near complete fusion that results in a depressed, arched fundus.[7]

The primary sonographic criteria for determining these uterine anomalies is the identification of two EMC echo complexes (Fig. 13-1). The initial sonographic finding may consist of a rather prominent solid mass that is isoechoic to the uterine myometrium. The patient may require an endovaginal examination to verify the presence of two EMCs. In uterus didelphys the sonographic examination shows two separate vaginas, cervices, and uterine bodies. Again, longitudinal and transverse scans should demonstrate two separate EMCs (Fig. 13-2). The identification of a complete or partial uterine septum is difficult in the nongravida patient. During the first trimester of pregnancy, the amniotic fluid allows clearer demonstration of the moderately hyperechoic septa[9] (Fig. 13-3). Demonstrating a depression in the central portion of the fundus and the resulting fundal arching associated with uterus arcuatus presents a challenge, since the sonographer must look for these subtle contour abnormalities, often in the

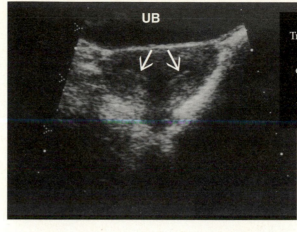

Fig. 13-1 Transverse sonogram of the uterus depicting both endometrial cavities (*arrows*) in a patient with a bicornuate uterus. *UB*, Urinary bladder.

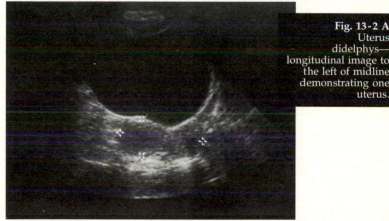

Fig. 13-2 A Uterus didelphys—longitudinal image to the left of midline demonstrating one uterus.

Fig. 13-2 B Uterus didelphys—longitudinal image to the right of midline visualizing a second uterus.

presence of bowel gas. Patients who have been exposed to DES may develop a T-shaped uterus, named for the classic T-shaped EMC on hysterography. Studies have shown that the uterine volume is decreased compared with a controlled population.[11] Sonographically this condition is best displayed on transverse images of the uterus, which demonstrate a smaller than normal fundus with the characteristic T-shape. Again, the sonographer should examine the kidneys for any signs of anomalies, particularly if the current sonographic examination is the initial diagnosis of the uterine anomaly.

PATHOLOGIC PROCESSES OF THE CERVIX

Nabothian Cysts

Nabothian cysts usually occur as a result of cervicitis. During the healing process the epithelium obstructs the drainage of glandular tissue, which produces retention cysts in the cervix. These cysts vary in size and usually cause no symptoms. Although occasionally large enough to visualize on transabdominal examinations, nabothian cysts are typically an incidental finding during endovaginal scans (Fig. 13-4). These cysts usually do not require any treatment.[5]

Cervical Carcinoma

As a result of the widespread use of the Papanicolaou test, or the Pap smear, cervical carcinoma is now the second most frequently diagnosed uterine malignancy after endometrial carci-

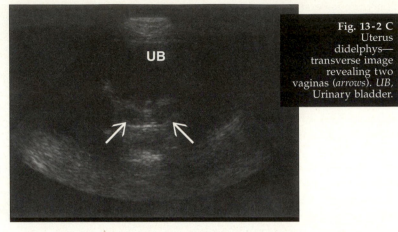

Fig. 13-2 C Uterus didelphys—transverse image revealing two vaginas (arrows). UB, Urinary bladder.

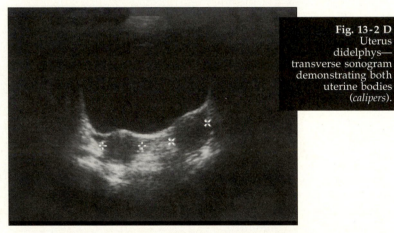

Fig. 13-2 D Uterus didelphys—transverse sonogram demonstrating both uterine bodies (calipers).

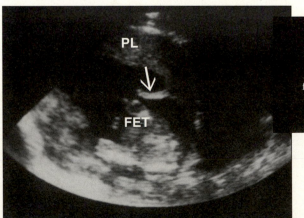

Fig. 13-3 Longitudinal sonogram demonstrating a second trimester fetus (FET) and a partial uterine septum (arrow). (PL), Placenta.

noma. This disease typically occurs in women between the ages of 45 and 55. The most common symptoms consist of metrorrhagia and cervical ulceration. Late symptoms include rectal and bladder dysfunction, pain, and a thick vaginal discharge. Because of the Pap test, most of these malignancies are diagnosed early in the disease. Sonography proves most useful for staging by verifying the size of the mass and the extent of lymphadenopathy.

PATHOLOGIC PROCESSES OF THE UTERUS

Leiomyoma Uteri

Leiomyoma uteri, more commonly known as myomas or fibroids, are the most common tumors of the female pelvis. These benign smooth muscle neoplasms can occur in the uterus, vagina, vulva, ligaments, and fallopian tubes. They typically afflict women over 35 years of age and are more frequently seen in women of African descent. Experts postulate that fibroids occur as a result of an imbalance or excess secretion of ovarian hormones. Although they are usually asymptomatic, approximately half of the patients will complain of profuse and prolonged bleeding. Other symptoms include urinary frequency, infertility, and pelvic fullness. The bimanual pelvic examination usually reveals an enlarged uterus with irregular borders. Myomas rarely develop during the postmenopausal years, and previously existing

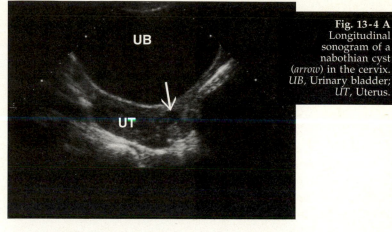

Fig. 13-4 A Longitudinal sonogram of a nabothian cyst (*arrow*) in the cervix. *UB*, Urinary bladder; *UT*, Uterus.

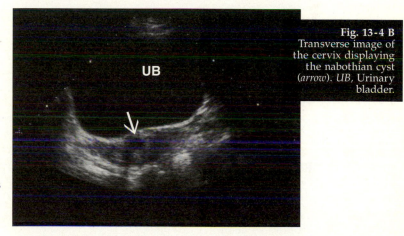

Fig. 13-4 B Transverse image of the cervix displaying the nabothian cyst (*arrow*). *UB*, Urinary bladder.

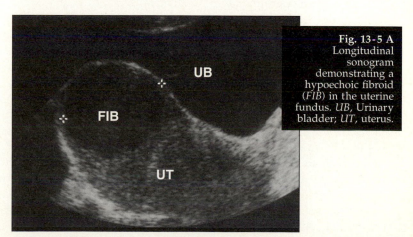

Fig. 13-5 A Longitudinal sonogram demonstrating a hypoechoic fibroid (*FIB*) in the uterine fundus. *UB*, Urinary bladder; *UT*, uterus.

fibroids tend to stabilize or di-
minish in size.

There are several categories
of fibroids, based on their anatomic location in the uterine tissue layers. The **submucosal,** located adjacent to the
endometrium, is the least common type of fibroid but is the
most common variety to become
symptomatic or infected or to
undergo malignant changes. The
intramural, located in the myometrial layer, is the most common variety of fibroid. The **sub-
serosal,** located adjacent to the
perimetrium, can cause contour
irregularities when relatively
small. These fibroids will frequently become pedunculated
and appear as adnexal masses
(intraligamentous) or as a mass
superior to the uterus. Cervical
myomas are rare, but they may
cause fecal impaction when located in the cul-de-sac or cause
dystocia during pregnancy.

The typical sonographic pattern of uterine fibroids includes
an enlarged uterus with irregular
contours and an inhomogeneous
myometrial pattern. Small fi-

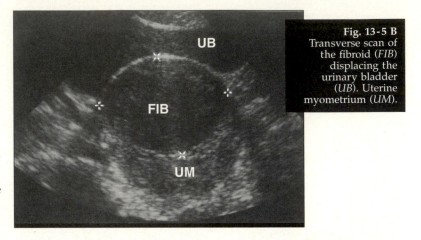

Fig. 13-5 B
Transverse scan of
the fibroid (*FIB*)
displacing the
urinary bladder
(*UB*). Uterine
myometrium (*UM*).

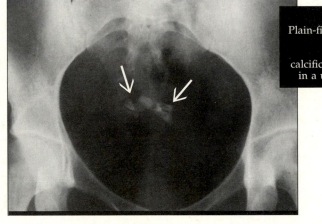

Fig. 13-6
Plain-film radiograph
of the pelvis
depicting
calcifications (*arrows*)
in a uterine fibroid.

broids may appear as rounded, hypoechoic or hyperechoic discrete masses (Fig. 13-5).
However, the sonographic pattern varies considerably and depends on secondary
changes that occur in the myomas. They may experience fatty degeneration and
calcification, causing focal hyperechoic areas and some areas of acoustic shadowing.[6]
In some instances, acoustic shadowing occurs to the extent that the sonographer may
be unsure of the position of the uterine borders or even if the shadowing is related to
the bowel. In these cases a simple plain-film radiograph of the pelvis will provide a
diagnosis (Fig. 13-6). Fibroids may also experience degeneration and produce areas of
necrosis and/or hemorrhage, which appear sonographically as cystic areas. A ligamentous fibroid usually appears as a solid adnexal mass (Fig. 13-7). The sonographer
should try to demonstrate the mass in relation to the uterine EMC and the perimetrium. If the mass is contiguous to these structures, this increases the suggestion of
an intraligamentous fibroid. The demonstration of a normal ovary on the affected side
is crucial to this diagnosis.[3] The presence of intrauterine fibroids also increases the
suggestion of this type of pathologic disorder.

Uterine Fluid Collections

Several different types of pathologic processes can lead to fluid accumulations in the uterus, cervix, and vagina. **Hydrometra** refers to fluid accumulation in the uterus; **hydrocolpos** refers to fluid in the vagina; **pyometra** is a superimposed infection in the uterine cavity; and **hematometra** is blood in the uterine cavity, usually as a result of menstruation. Hydrometra may also result from obstruction in one horn of a bicornuate uterus. In young patients, **hematocolpometra** may develop secondary to an imperforate hymen or vaginal atresia.[4] Typically, this condition becomes symptomatic at the usual age of the onset of menstruation. The patient complains of pelvic pain and cramping but experiences very little or no menstrual flow. In older patients, hydrometra, pyometra, or hematometra may stem from a cervical or endometrial carcinoma or from radiation-induced cervical stenosis. Another cause may be cervical stenosis caused by adhesions that have developed after surgery. The possible differential diagnosis regarding the type of fluid comes from the patient's clinical history, from the results of laboratory tests, and from a histologic evaluation.

The classic sonographic pattern is a cystic enlargement of the uterine and cervical and/or vaginal cavities (Fig. 13-8). The sonographer must try to determine the level and cause of the obstruction. Debris may suggest hematometra or pyometra, but a clinical history and the results of

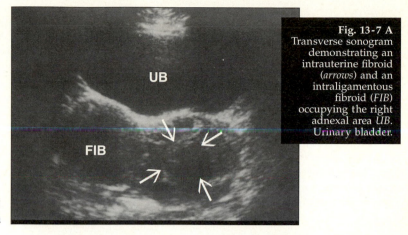

Fig. 13-7 A Transverse sonogram demonstrating an intrauterine fibroid (*arrows*) and an intraligamentous fibroid (*FIB*) occupying the right adnexal area *UB*, Urinary bladder.

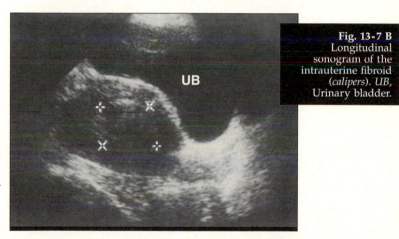

Fig. 13-7 B Longitudinal sonogram of the intrauterine fibroid (*calipers*). *UB*, Urinary bladder.

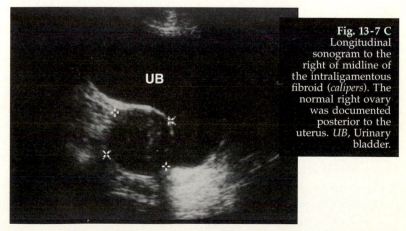

Fig. 13-7 C Longitudinal sonogram to the right of midline of the intraligamentous fibroid (*calipers*). The normal right ovary was documented posterior to the uterus. *UB*, Urinary bladder.

laboratory tests are usually needed to make a specific diagnosis.

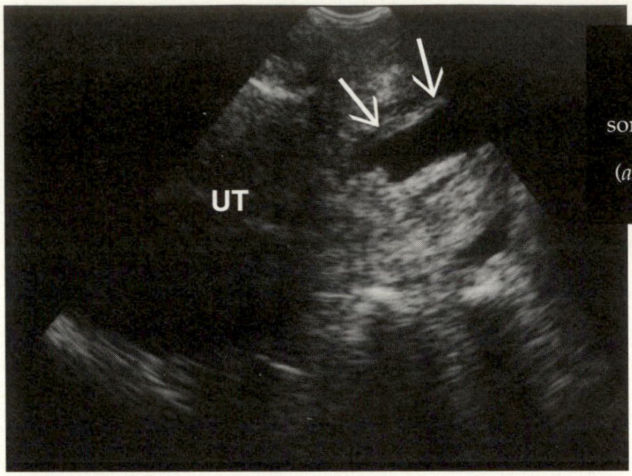

Carcinoma

Endometrial carcinoma accounts for 90% of malignancies of the uterine body and is the second most common cancer of the female reproductive system. The typical age ranges from 50 to 70 years, and the most common symptom is abnormal vaginal bleeding. Risk factors include nulliparity, obesity, and diabetes. The malignancy may obstruct the cervical cavity, resulting in hematometra or pyometra. In Stages I and II, endometrial carcinoma is limited to the uterus. In Stages III and IV the carcinoma has metastasized to distant sites.

In the early stages of the disease the sonographic pattern exhibits a prominent, often inhomogeneous EMC echo complex (Fig. 13-9). In the postmenopausal group the EMC should not measure more than 5 mm. With obstruction of the EMC, the sonographer may discover he-

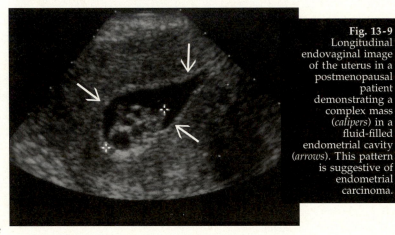

Fig. 13-8 Endovaginal longitudinal sonogram illustrating fluid in the cervix (*arrows*). *UT*, Uterine body.

Fig. 13-9 Longitudinal endovaginal image of the uterus in a postmenopausal patient demonstrating a complex mass (*calipers*) in a fluid-filled endometrial cavity (*arrows*). This pattern is suggestive of endometrial carcinoma.

matometra, which appears as a distended EMC containing fluid with debris. To more accurately stage the disease, the sonographer should scan the urinary bladder and the pelvic and retroperitoneal lymph nodes for evidence of distant metastasis.

Leiomyosarcoma accounts for only 3% of uterine tumors but is the most frequent uterine sarcoma. Arising from fibroids, the symptoms are often indistinguishable from myomas and include uterine bleeding and pelvic pain in the later stages of the disease. When confined to the uterus, the sonographic pattern is often indistinguishable from myomas. Suspicious patterns may include large areas of degeneration and atypical hyperechoic patterns. Local invasion indicated by a disruption of the perimetrium and evidence of lymphadenopathy allow leiomyosarcoma to be included in the differential diagnosis.

Endometrial Hyperplasia

Endometrial hyperplasia is a condition where the endometrium proliferates as a result of excessive hormonal stimulation. The typical symptom is irregular bleeding. Certain pathologic types of hyperplasia have an increased risk for the development of endometrial carcinoma. Determining the exact pathologic type requires a biopsy procedure.

The typical sonographic pattern for simple hyperplasia is a prominent EMC echo complex (Fig. 13-10). The pattern may appear inhomogeneous, and thus a differentiation from endometrial carcinoma may be difficult.

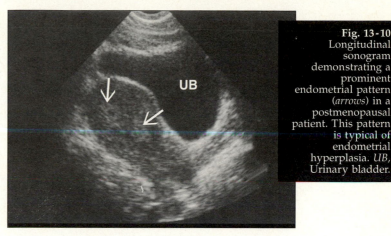

Fig. 13-10 Longitudinal sonogram demonstrating a prominent endometrial pattern (*arrows*) in a postmenopausal patient. This pattern is typical of endometrial hyperplasia. *UB*, Urinary bladder.

Adenomyosis

Adenomyosis, or internal endometriosis, occurs when the endometrial tissue diffusely invades the myometrium. A more rare form, adenomyoma, forms an encapsulated mass of endometrial tissue in the myometrium. Typically, the patient is between 40 and 50 years of age and complains of a gradual development of dysmenorrhea and menorrhagia. The pelvic examination usually reveals an enlarged uterus that is typically tender to palpation during the menstrual period. The diagnosis is usually confirmed only with pathologic evaluation of the uterus after a hysterectomy. The patient may also have external endometriosis.

The typical sonographic pattern is cystic areas in the myometrium, called the "swiss cheese" pattern.[2] Differentiation from fibroids may be difficult. The sonographer should look for signs of external endometriosis, such as the "chocolate cysts" of the ovaries.

PELVIC INFLAMMATORY DISEASE

Pelvic inflammatory disease (PID) results from an ascending infection that travels through the vagina into the EMC, the fallopian tubes, and the peritoneal cavity. Without prompt treatment, adhesions may develop, causing pelvic pain. If the adhesions obstruct a fallopian tube, the patient is at increased risk for ectopic pregnancy and infertility problems. The most common cause of PID is venereal disease, specifically gonorrhea. Another classification, termed pyogenic, can occur in the postpartum or postabortion patient and in patients wearing intrauterine contraceptive devices (IUCDs).[10] Patients typically have a fever, an elevated WBC count, a creamy vaginal discharge, and pelvic pain. On pelvic examination the cervix and adnexal areas are quite painful when manipulated. The disease may be either acute or chronic.

The sonographic patterns vary with the stage and severity of the infection. One of the first sonographic signs may be a prominent EMC as a result of endometritis. As the infection involves the fallopian tubes, it causes salpingitis that can evolve into a pyosalpinx, an enlarged tube filled with pus[1] (Fig. 13-11). Once the pus exsanguinates out of the fallopian tube, the exudate may layer in the posterior cul-de-sac (Fig. 13-12). If an ovary becomes involved, a tubo-ovarian abscess may develop, which classically presents as a tubular and circular cystic to complex mass in the adnexal area, superior to the cul-de-sac. This abscess rarely destroys the ovary. An abscess may develop in the cul-de-sac and may contain septations. The most serious stage is when general peritonitis develops. A detailed clinical history is crucial, since these sonographic patterns are also associated with endometriomas, ectopic pregnancy, and ovarian neoplasms. The sonographer must remember that if free fluid is seen in the pelvis, all potential peritoneal spaces should be evaluated for signs of further contamination.

INTRAUTERINE CONTRACEPTIVE DEVICES

Several years ago many IUCDs were removed from the market because of a rash of lawsuits. However, since several have re-appeared on the market, sonographers may encounter this type of patient. Usually sonography is used to determine if the IUCD is located in its proper position in the fundal portion of the EMC. The most common signs of an IUCD out of position include a "lost" string, symptoms of PID, a positive pregnancy test, or severe pelvic pain, which suggests the possibility of perforation. The most common complication associated with IUCD use is pregnancy, although the risk is small. However, the risk of spontaneous abortion of an intrauterine pregnancy with a coexisting IUCD is high. There is also a slight increased risk of ectopic pregnancy and a higher risk for the development of PID in certain types of patients.

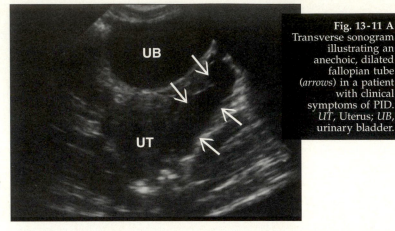

Fig. 13-11 A Transverse sonogram illustrating an anechoic, dilated fallopian tube (*arrows*) in a patient with clinical symptoms of PID. *UT*, Uterus; *UB*, urinary bladder.

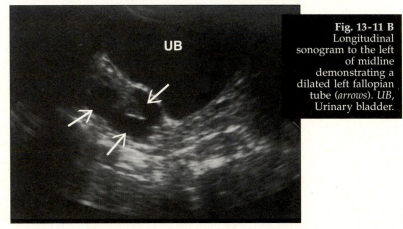

Fig. 13-11 B Longitudinal sonogram to the left of midline demonstrating a dilated left fallopian tube (*arrows*). *UB*, Urinary bladder.

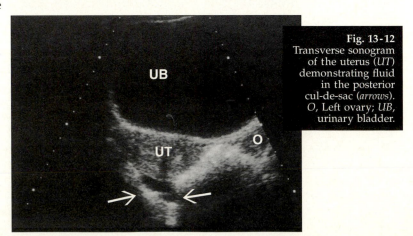

Fig. 13-12 Transverse sonogram of the uterus (*UT*) demonstrating fluid in the posterior cul-de-sac (*arrows*). *O*, Left ovary; *UB*, urinary bladder.

The sonographic patterns associated with a properly positioned IUCD include a hyperechoic structure in the fundal EMC that exhibits acoustic shadowing. The shadow is a very important sign, since a portion of the endometrium may appear to resemble an IUCD.[8] To display this pattern, the sonographer may need to use a 5.0 MHz transducer or perform an endovaginal examination. Several specific types of IUCDs can be identified by observing their shape on transverse and longitudinal scans. The Lippes Loop usually appears as a series of five interrupted hyperechoic lines on longitudinal scans, whereas tranverse images demonstrate longer segments of the loops (Fig. 13-13). As its name implies, the Copper-7 is shaped like a 7, with the short arm usually displaying as a hyperechoic line on transverse scans and the long arm being demonstrated on longitudinal scans. If an IUCD is not demonstrated in the EMC, the sonographer should carefully

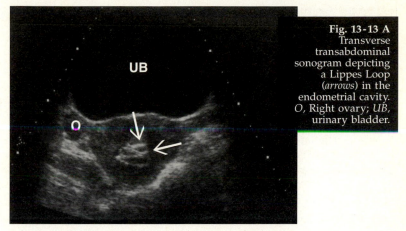

Fig. 13-13 A Transverse transabdominal sonogram depicting a Lippes Loop (*arrows*) in the endometrial cavity. *O*, Right ovary; *UB*, urinary bladder.

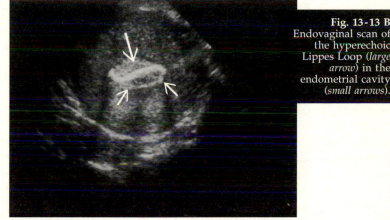

Fig. 13-13 B Endovaginal scan of the hyperechoic Lippes Loop (*large arrow*) in the endometrial cavity (*small arrows*).

examine the cul-de-sac and adnexal areas for a hyperechoic structure, but the surrounding bowel and fascia make this task difficult. In this situation the usual protocol is to obtain a radiograph of the pelvis, since the IUCDs are also radiopaque.

TECHNICAL PITFALLS

One of the most common pitfalls in the sonographic evaluation of the uterus is the improper use of the urinary bladder as an acoustic window for the entire uterus. Usually the transducer must be placed inferiorly at the symphysis and angled superiorly, forming an approximate 90-degree angle to the anterior and posterior borders of the uterus. The lateromedial angulation must also vary until all the uterine borders appear distinctly and the EMC appears in the midportion of the body and fundus. Slight pressure just before freezing the image will often allow better resolution and visualization of the superior border. Another common pitfall is not scanning superiorly to the urinary bladder, which could lead to missing a pedunculated fibroid or ovarian cyst. A ligamentous fibroid will initially present as an adnexal mass. The

TABLE 13-1 UTERINE PATHOLOGY–Correlation with Clinical Laboratory Tests	
CONDITION	LABORATORY TEST
CERVICAL CARCINOMA	+ PAP Smear
ENDOMETRIAL CARCINOMA	+ Biopsy
PELVIC INFLAMMATORY DISEASE	Increased White Blood Cell Count
INTRAUTERINE CONTRACEPTIVE DEVICE	Increased White Blood Cell Count with Infection + Pregnancy Test with Intrauterine Pregnancy

sonographer must ensure that the ovary on that side is demonstrated and that the uterus is examined carefully, since many patients will have additional fibroids, which allows a more narrow differential diagnosis. Inexperienced sonographers may misidentify the rounded fundus of a retroflexed uterus as a variety of fibroid. The sonographer should always demonstrate the continuity of the cervix and EMC, as well as the acoustic shadow that may occur at the bend of the lower uterine segment with the body and fundus. If in doubt, the sonographer should perform an endovaginal examination.

SUMMARY

There are many technical considerations and potential pitfalls that the sonographer must keep in mind when performing gynecologic sonography. The widespread use of the endovaginal examination has certainly improved the differential diagnosis by allowing better visualization of the retroflexed and retroverted uterus, as well as enhancing the demonstration of small masses. Although uterine pathologic conditions may be more limited than in other organs, the clinical history and the results of other diagnostic procedures still play a crucial role in improving the accuracy of this sonographic examination. Table 13-1 contains pertinent clinical laboratory test results for uterine pathologic disorders.

REFERENCES

1. Berland LL, Lawson T, et al: Ultrasound evaluation of pelvic infections, *Radiol Clin North Am* 20:367, 1982.
2. Bohlman M, Ensor R, Sanders R: Sonographic findings in adenomyosis of the uterus, *AJR* 148:765-766, 1987.
3. Dudiak CM, Turner DA, et al: Uterine leiomyomas in the infertile patient: preoperative localization with MR imaging versus US and hysterosapingography, *Radiology* 176:627-630, 1988.
4. Fleischer AC, Shawker TH: The role of sonography in pediatric gynecology, *Clin Obstet Gynecol* 30:735-746, 1987.
5. Fogel S, Slasky B: Sonography of nabothian cysts, *AJR* 138:927, 1982.
6. Gross BH, Siver TM, Jaffe MH: Sonographic features of uterine leiomyomas: analysis of 41 proven cases, *J Ultrasound Med* 2:401-406, 1983.
7. Malini S, Valdes C, Malinak R: Sonographic diagnosis and classification of anomalies of the female genital tract, *J Ultrasound Med* 3:397-404, 1984.
8. Najarian KE, Kurtz AB: New observations in the sonographic evaluation of intrauterine contraceptive devices, *J Ultrasound Med* 5:205-210, 1986.
9. Pennes DR, Bowerman RA, Silver TM: Congenital uterine anomalies and associated pregnancies, *J Ultrasound Med* 4:531-538, 1985.
10. Swayne L, Love M, Karasick S: Pelvic inflammatory disease: sonographic-pathologic correlation, *Radiology* 151:751-755, 1989.
11. Viscomi G, Gonzales R, Taylor K: Ultrasound detection of uterine anomalies after diethylstilbestrol (DES) exposure, *Radiology* 136:733, 1980.

ovarian pathology

INSTRUCTIONAL OBJECTIVES

At the completion of this chapter, the reader will be able to:

1. Describe the clinical problems that are typical reasons for the sonographic evaluation of the ovaries.
2. Describe the various causes of infertility, the types of treatment, and the sonographic procedure for monitoring follicular development.
3. Describe the clinical symptoms and pathologic and physiologic basis for functional ovarian cysts, Turner's syndrome, and Stein-Leventhal syndrome and identify the characteristic sonographic patterns of each.
4. Describe the clinical symptoms and pathologic basis for the disease processes of the ovaries, including ovarian torsion, cystadenomas and cystadenocarcinomas, benign and malignant teratomas, dysontogenetic neoplasms, external endometriosis, fibroma and Brenner tumors, primary ovarian malignancy, and metastasis to the ovary.
5. Identify on sectional sonograms the above-mentioned disease processes of the ovary, based on the sonographic appearance, the clinical history, and the results of other diagnostic procedures.
6. Describe several technical pitfalls associated with the identification of ovarian pathology.

THE CLINICAL PROBLEM

The clinical management of a patient who has an adnexal mass usually requires a pelvic sonogram. Again, the results of the bimanual pelvic examination may not provide a specific diagnosis regarding the consistency of a mass or the organ of origin. If the sonographic examination reveals a simple cyst, the referring physician may request a repeat examination in approximately one month to differentiate between a physiologic cyst and a neoplastic cyst. A complex cyst, particularly if it contains solid projections from the wall, suggests the possibility of malignancy, and surgery is usually indicated. The early detection of ovarian cancer remains a challenge. Recent research indicates that the use of endovaginal pulsed and color Doppler has some merit, but a reliable screening method remains elusive. Once again, the clinical history plays a crucial role in determining a sonographic differential diagnosis.

CLINICAL LABORATORY TESTS

Providing a specific diagnosis for ovarian tumors presents a challenge to the primary physician. Several clinical laboratory tests may provide additional information. Several tumor markers may prove useful for distinguishing ovarian tumors. **Carcinoembryonic antigen** (CEA) is produced by both normal and abnormal tissue. Malignancies linked to abnormally high production of CEA include primary tumors of the ovary, lung, colon, breast, urinary bladder, and prostate. Because of this broad range of malignancies, a positive CEA increases the possibility of a malignancy, but further diagnostic tests must narrow the organ of origin. Other pathologic conditions may produce an abnormal elevation of CEA, such as pancreatitis, bowel inflammation, chronic renal failure, and cirrhosis.[7]

Ca125 is another tumor marker that may provide a more restricted list of pathologic conditions. Abnormal elevations of Ca125 are associated with ovarian, cervical, fallopian tube, and pancreatic malignancies. However, benign gynecologic diseases can produce abnormally high levels.[7] Ovarian tumors that autonomously secrete female or male hormones may produce an abnormal serum elevation of the related hormone, such as testosterone, estrogen, or progesterone.

Vaginal cytologic smears, or the **Papanicolaou smear (Pap),** are used primarily for the early detection of cervical cancer and may provide additional information regarding a number of gynecologic conditions. The epithelial cells that line the vagina, cervix, and endometrial cavity (EMC) typically shed in reaction to malignancies of the genital tract. These cells also respond to normal and abnormal hormonal stimulation. In conjunction with an accurate menstrual history, the smear examination can diagnose hormonal-related conditions such as Stein-Leventhal syndrome and feminizing and masculinizing ovarian tumors.[7]

RELATED IMAGING PROCEDURES

Plain-film radiography usually provides little information on ovarian tumors. Large tumors may produce a mass effect in relation to the urinary bladder. This sign is more often seen with the performance of an intravenous pyelogram (IVP) examination. **Computed tomography** and **magnetic resonance imaging** allow the diagnosis of ovarian masses, as well as lymphatic involvement. These procedures also allow the detection of distant metastasis.

Hysterosalpingography is a radiographic procedure where a contrast medium is introduced into the uterine cavity. As part of the diagnostic work-up for infertility, this procedure allows the visualization of the fallopian tubes. If the tube is patent, the contrast material flows into the peritoneal cavity. However, a tubal spasm may lead to a false diagnosis of tubal obstruction. Chapter 13 contains a discussion of this procedure for the diagnosis of uterine abnormalities.

SCANNING PROTOCOLS AND TECHNIQUES

The scanning protocol and related techniques for the gynecologic sonographic examination are discussed in Chapter 12. Accurate identification of the ovaries poses a challenge to the inexperienced sonographer. The use of oblique patient positions and using the filled urinary bladder as an acoustic window enhances the visualization of the ovaries on the transabdominal examination. Evidence of follicles during the reproductive period also aids identification, although adjacent vessels can initially mimic the follicular pattern. The use of color flow can readily distinguish between these vascular structures and the follicles. If the ovaries are not optimally demonstrated on transabdominal images, the endovaginal examination often provides high-resolution images. However, a very superior or lateral ovary may be out of the maximum imaging depth of an endovaginal transducer.

BASIC SCANNING PROTOCOL

Transabdominal Examination

- ✔ **Longitudinal views of the midline uterus,** demonstrating the vagina, cervix, corpus, and fundus with EMC. Longitudinal and posteroanterior measurements should be obtained.
- ✔ **Longitudinal views to the right of midline,** demonstrating the lateral aspect of the uterus and the right ovary. Longitudinal measurement of the ovary should be obtained.
- ✔ **Longitudinal views to the left of midline,** demonstrating the lateral aspect of the uterus and the left ovary. Longitudinal measurement of the ovary should be obtained.
- ✔ **Transverse views from inferior to superior or from superior to inferior,** demonstrating the true transverse plane of the vagina, cervix, isthmus, and corpus with EMC.
- ✔ **Fundus with EMC,** obtaining transverse and posteroanterior measurements of the uterus and posteroanterior measurement through the thickest portion of the EMC.
- ✔ **Right ovary,** obtaining transverse and posteroanterior measurements.
- ✔ **Left ovary,** obtaining transverse and posteroanterior measurements. Dominant follicle(s) on ovary(ies) may also be measured.

Endovaginal Examination

- ✔ **Longitudinal view of the cervix,** including the posterior cul-de-sac.
- ✔ **Longitudinal view of the uterine body and fundus,** with the EMC. Longitudinal measurement should be obtained.
- ✔ **Longitudinal views of the right lateral aspect of the uterus.**

The scanning protocol for gynecologic sonography appears on the previous page and at right.

INFERTILITY

Coinciding with the trend of starting families later in life, problems related to infertility have increased during the last 10 years. Fertility usually declines during the fourth decade of life. This decrease in fertility appears to be related to the normal aging process of the oocytes and a decreased ability of the zygote to properly implant in the endometrium. A couple is usually diagnosed as infertile when they have failed to achieve a pregnancy in 12 months. A fertile couple usually has a 90% chance of achieving pregnancy during this same time interval.[6]

BASIC SCANNING PROTOCOL

Endovaginal Examination (continued)

- **Longitudinal views of the left lateral aspect of the uterus.**
- **Longitudinal views of the right and left ovaries,** obtaining longitudinal measurement. Dominant follicle(s) on the ovary(ies) may be measured.
- **Transverse view of the cervix,** including the posterior cul-de-sac.
- **Transverse views of the uterine body and fundus,** obtaining posteroanterior and transverse measurements of the fundus and posteroanterior measurement of the EMC.
- **Transverse views of both ovaries,** obtaining transverse and posteroanterior measurements. Dominant follicle on the ovary(ies) may be measured.

Causes

The causes of infertility are numerous and stem from both male and female conditions.

Male infertility factors include decreased or abnormal sperm production, obstruction of the efferent ducts, and ejaculation malfunction. Decreased sperm production may be caused by a varicocele, hormonal imbalances, a high testicular temperature, smoking, stress, or infections. Epididymitis may cause an obstruction of the efferent ducts. Retrograde ejaculation into the urinary bladder may be a result of an ejaculatory duct obstruction or a complication after prostatic surgery.[6]

Female infertility factors include tubal obstruction, ovulation failure, obstruction or other anomalies of the vagina, cervix or uterus; immunologic incompatibility; and nutritional and metabolic factors. Ovulation failure is the cause of infertility in 15% to 20% of women.[6] Usually this condition produces symptoms such as irregular menstrual cycles. In some cases ovulation does occur, but the ovum remains in the follicle. These patients may benefit from ovulation-inducing agents, such as Clomid or Pergonal. Tubal obstruction may occur anywhere along the fallopian tube. Causes for obstruction include tubal and pelvic infections, adhesions resulting from pelvic surgery, and endometriosis. Approximately 25% to 30% of patients are infertile as a result of tubal obstruction. Conditions of the vagina, cervix, and uterus associated with infertility include anomalies such as the T-shaped uterus associated with diethylstilbestrol (DES) exposure, cervical stenosis, and vaginitis or cervicitis. Examples of metabolic causes of infertility, comprising roughly 5% of infertility patients, include thyroid disorders, diabetes, and hyperprolactinemia.[6]

Assisted Reproductive Technology (ART) Procedures

In vitro fertilization (IVF) and embryo transfer (ET) are common infertility treatments when the condition is caused by a low sperm count or by female organic conditions that affect tubal patency, or when the cervical mucus is inadequate.[6] The patient is initially administered an ovulation-inducing agent, such as Clomid, and serial plasma estradiol levels are obtained. By the ninth day of the cycle, a patient with two ovaries should have a plasma estradiol level greater than 700 pg/ml or a level greater than 500 pg/ml if only one ovary is present. Hormonal and sonographic monitoring is crucial in order to prevent the development of **ovarian hyperstimulation syndrome.** This syndrome occurs with excessive administration of an ovulation-inducing agent, resulting in the formation of numerous, large ovarian cysts. These may rupture or leak, producing ascites and more severe symptoms.[5]

The follicle should measure greater than 16 mm before oocyte retrieval is attempted. If a mature follicle is present and the estradiol levels are adequate, an intramuscular injection of human chorionic gonadotropin (hCG) is given to produce the luteinizing hormone (LH) surge that stimulates the final maturation of the ovum and follicle rupture. Oocyte retrieval is usually scheduled approximately 36 hours after the hCG injection. Once the ova are retrieved, they are placed in special media, the sperm are introduced, and hopefully conception occurs. Typically, four embryos ranging from the 4- to 16-cell stage are transferred to the uterine cavity. After transfer, the patient receives injections of progesterone for the first 8 days. The β-hCG levels are monitored for evidence of implantation.

In **gamete intrafallopian transfer (GIFT)** the patient is again placed on an ovulation-induction regimen with hormonal and sonographic monitoring. After oocyte retrieval the ova and sperm are placed in the ampulla of the fallopian tube via a catheter. The success rate averages 25%.[6]

In **zygote intrafallopian transfer (ZIFT)** the ova are retrieved, and fertilization occurs in vitro. The resulting zygotes are placed in the fallopian tube.

The Role of Sonography in Infertility

Transabdominal and endovaginal sonography can identify some of the causes of infertility, such as pelvic masses and uterine anomalies. Further examination of the ovaries can reveal the presence and number of follicles, which is important information in determining the cause of infertility.[9]

The most common use of sonography in the infertile patient is the monitoring of follicular number and size during treatment. In a spontaneous cycle the sonographer usually performs a baseline scan on day 2 or day 3 of the menstrual cycle. This examination evaluates the patient for any adnexal masses or uterine pathology and documents the presence of any residual follicles from the previous ovulatory cycle. Another scan is performed on the day of the LH surge, which occurs approximately 36 hours before ovulation. The mature follicle ranges in size from 16 to 20 mm.[22] To confirm ovulation, a repeat examination is performed 2 to 3 days later, in which the decreased follicular size and evidence of an early corpus luteum are noted. The sonographic pattern of an early corpus luteum consists of a small area with irregular borders containing internal echoes. Some patients will have a small amount of fluid in the posterior cul-de-sac.[18]

For patients receiving ovulation-inducing agents, the sonographic protocol varies with the specific medication. Clomid is a synthetic drug that is given on day 5 through day 9 of the cycle. Sonographic examination begins on day 10 and is usually repeated every other day until ovulation occurs. The mature follicle ranges from 20 to 25 mm. With Pergonal, injections begin on day 2 or day 3 of the menstrual cycle. Usually daily sonograms and estradiol measure-

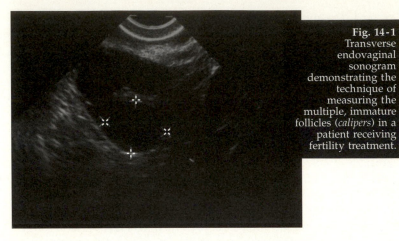

Fig. 14-1 Transverse endovaginal sonogram demonstrating the technique of measuring the multiple, immature follicles (*calipers*) in a patient receiving fertility treatment.

ments begin on day 8. The mature follicle ranges from 16 to 17 mm. The endovaginal examination is preferred, since the enhanced resolution allows more accurate identification and measurement of the follicles.

The sonographer measures all follicles in both the longitudinal and coronal planes (Fig. 14-1). After the initial examination, the sonographer should check the previous examination to verify the position of all measured follicles and ensure that the new measurements correlate. All measurements are recorded and presented to the interpreting physician. The referring physician is interested in whether the serial examination demonstrates interval growth and whether one or more follicles have attained mature size.[18] An additional sonographic sign that signals impending ovulation is the demonstration of the **cumulus oophorus.** This structure is made up of granulosa cells and surrounds the ova in the follicle. With the endovaginal technique, the cumulus oophorus sometimes appears as an echogenic, small structure in the fluid of the follicle.[22] The sonographer should also image the endometrium and obtain measurements. The endometrium measures from 2 to 4 mm in the preovulatory phase and 5 to 6 mm in the postovulatory phase.[13]

Ultrasound-guided aspiration of the follicles for oocyte retrieval is often used instead of laparoscopy. The transabdominal technique may be used with a periurethral or transvaginal aspiration procedure. The transvaginal technique may also be used. Ultrasound guidance is also used when performing the embryo transfer with IVF and ZIFT.[15]

CONGENITAL ANOMALIES

Turner's Syndrome

Turner's syndrome is a chromosomal anomaly in which there are 45 chromosomes, including a single X chromosome. This syndrome can produce various anomalies, including dwarfism, a webbed neck, and infantile sexual development. Various mosaic chromosomal patterns may produce variations of the full syndrome. The ovaries contain no primordial follicles and may consist of only fibrous connective tissue, termed the "fibrous streak." The uterus and vagina are usually present, but the lack of functional ovarian tissue causes an absence of female steroid hormone secretion. This absence produces an atrophic uterus and the characteristic infantile sexual development. Hormone supplementation can cause the development of secondary female sex characteristics and a further development of the uterus.

Turner's syndrome usually becomes clinically suggestive at an early age. The pelvic sonogram will typically reveal an atrophied uterus and no apparent ovaries, although normal ovaries in children under 5 years of age have a volume of less than 1 cc (1 × 1 × 0.5),[21] which can make their identification difficult.

Polycystic Ovary Syndrome

Polycystic ovary syndrome, also known as Stein-Leventhal syndrome, is characterized by a lack of ovulation caused by steady hormone levels, instead of the normal hormonal fluctuations during the monthly cycle. The partial suppression of follicle-stimulating hormone (FSH) results in a continuous stimulation of the ovarian follicles, which grow larger and persist through several cycles. This hormonal imbalance can lead to an increased production of ovarian androgens, such as testosterone. In classic Stein-Leventhal syndrome, this excess testosterone can lead to the development of male secondary sex characteristics, such as hirsutism. However, a number of patients will not develop these rather severe symptoms. The most common symptoms include irregular menstrual periods, obesity, and infertility problems. If the patient wants to become pregnant, the typical treatment includes Clomid administration. Otherwise the patient may be given progestin to achieve a more normal hormonal balance.[12]

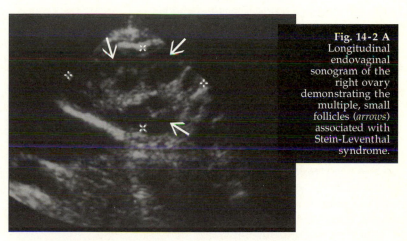

Fig. 14-2 A Longitudinal endovaginal sonogram of the right ovary demonstrating the multiple, small follicles (*arrows*) associated with Stein-Leventhal syndrome.

Typically sonography reveals bilaterally enlarged ovaries containing numerous small cysts (Fig. 14-2). With transabdominal examinations, poor resolution may not allow visualization of discrete cysts, demonstrating a more homogeneous, hypoechoic pattern of the ovaries. In these cases endovaginal examination will provide a more clear depiction of the status and severity of the disease.

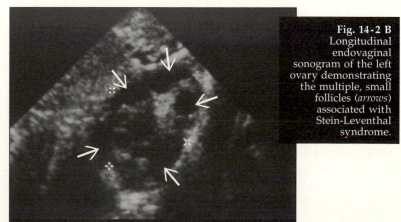

Fig. 14-2 B Longitudinal endovaginal sonogram of the left ovary demonstrating the multiple, small follicles (*arrows*) associated with Stein-Leventhal syndrome.

PATHOLOGIC PROCESSES OF THE OVARIES

Functional Ovarian Cysts

Functional, physiologic, or nonneoplastic ovarian cysts include follicle cysts, corpus luteum cysts, paraovarian cysts, and theca lutein cysts, as well as Stein-Leventhal syndrome. In all instances the cysts develop in response to hormonal stimulation or imbalance.

During the normal ovarian cycle, the immature follicle grows to an average size of 2 cm. **Follicular cysts** occur when the dominant follicle does not undergo ovulation but remains active. These cysts have thin walls, may be single or multiple, and contain a watery fluid. The size varies from 1 to 8 cm, although sonography cannot usually distinguish between a small follicular cyst and a normal dominant follicle on one examination. Therefore these cysts must measure 2.5 cm or larger before this possiblity should be recorded in the differential diagnosis. These cysts disappear spontaneously and therefore no treatment is required.[12] Follicular cysts generally meet the three sonographic criteria of a cyst: smooth thin walls, anechoic interior, and acoustic enhancement (Fig. 14-3). These cysts must reach a size of 2.5 cm before they can be differentiated from a dominant follicle. On transabdominal examinations the sonographer may need to use a 5.0 MHz transducer to improve resolution and depict the cyst's true sonographic characteristics. If the size of the patient prohibits the use of a higher frequency, an endovaginal examination may be necessary.

Corpus luteum cysts result from hemorrhage in a persistently mature corpus luteum and vary in size from 1 to 10 cm. These cysts can cause menstrual irregularities and pain, which can mimic ectopic pregnancy. During a normal pregnancy, the cyst measures less than 2 cm in diameter and often contains hypoechoic echoes. As the pregnancy advances, the cyst enlarges to an average size of 4 cm and remains active until approximately the twelfth week of pregnancy. Corpus luteum cysts may appear cystic or complex (Fig. 14-4). They tend to bleed, result-

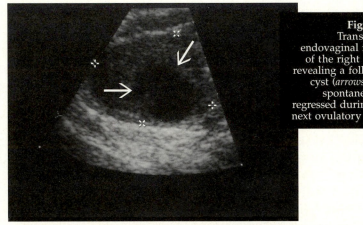

Fig. 14-3 Transverse, endovaginal image of the right ovary revealing a follicular cyst (*arrows*) that spontaneously regressed during the next ovulatory cycle.

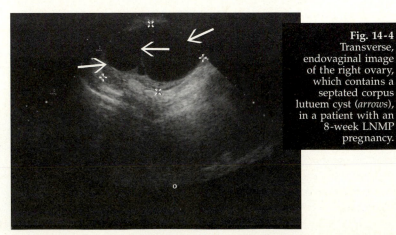

Fig. 14-4 Transverse, endovaginal image of the right ovary, which contains a septated corpus lutuem cyst (*arrows*), in a patient with an 8-week LNMP pregnancy.

ing in a complex pattern.[4] A more atypical pattern is a partially solid appearance. Color-flow Doppler often demonstrates a peripheral, higher resistance flow pattern.[8]

Paraovarian cysts arise from the remnants of the wolffian duct system, or Gartner's duct, which courses through the mesovarium. They typically measure 2 to 3 cm but may become larger. Usually Gartner's duct cysts have thin walls; they may contain a septum or become pedunculated. They are typically located adjacent to the uterus or vagina in the broad ligament.[1] Paraovarian, or Gartner's duct, cysts have thin walls, an anechoic interior, and distal acoustic enhancement. The sonographer must demonstrate that the cyst is not arising from the ovary in order for the interpreting physician to include this entity in the differential diagnosis.

Theca lutein cysts develop secondary to hyperstimulation of the ovary, which can occur with the hydatidiform mole, with ovulation induction therapy, and in multiple gestation.[19] These typically multiple bilateral cysts can attain a rather large size and may cause torsion of the ovary, or they can leak and produce fluid in the posterior cul-de-sac. Severe cases can produce very serious symptoms, including shock. Sonographically, theca lutein cysts usually display as bilateral, multiple cysts with thin to slightly thicker walls (Fig. 14-5). They may contain debris and may leak, resulting in free fluid in the posterior cul-de-sac. Since these cysts are most often associated with the hydatidiform mole, the sonographer should carefully evaluate the adnexal areas when the uterine pattern is suggestive of this pathology.

Neoplastic Ovarian Cysts

The **serous cystadenoma,** one of the most common benign epithelial tumors of the ovary, typically occurs between the ages of 30 and 50 years. Usually unilocular and unilateral, these cysts range in size from 5 to 15 cm and have thin, smooth walls containing a thin, straw-colored fluid. When small, these cysts may be clinically asymptomatic and may be first discovered during a routine pelvic examination. As the cyst attains a larger size, the patient may complain of urinary frequency as the mass applies pressure to the urinary bladder, and the patient may experience a recent, unexplained increase in abdominal size. Usually these cysts do not cause menstrual irregularities. The treatment of choice is surgical removal.

The serous cystadenoma typically appears as a rather large, unilocular cyst in the adnexal area (Fig. 14-6). The sonographer should use optimum resolution and check for any solid masses or papillomas projecting internally into the cyst or externally into the surrounding tissue. Multiple scanning angles should also be used, since some of the cysts are multilocular and the septa are angle dependent. The presence of solid masses in the cyst suggests the possibility of malignancy.[20] An endovaginal examination may be

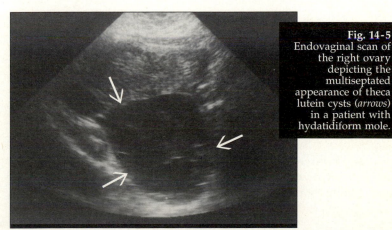

Fig. 14-5 Endovaginal scan of the right ovary depicting the multiseptated appearance of theca lutein cysts (*arrows*) in a patient with hydatidiform mole.

indicated to more accurately examine the mass for these signs. Since approximately 15% are bilateral, the sonographer should carefully evaluate the opposite adnexal area.

The **mucinous cystadenoma** is not quite as common as the serous cystadenoma and typically occurs between 30 and 50 years of age. This tumor is usually a unilateral, multilocular mass containing a more viscid fluid, which is similar to the secretions of the intestinal mucosa. These neoplasms can gain gigantic proportions, fill the entire abdominal-pelvic cavity, and weigh over 150 pounds. The mucinous variety may develop from a teratoma or from the epithelial layer of the ovary. Occasionally this neoplasm will rupture and allow the viscous material into the peritoneal cavity, which can stimulate the peritoneal mesothelium to secrete mucus. This condition is called **pseudomyxoma peritonei.** Although this condition is benign, it can cause symptoms similar to malignancy, such as the wasting of muscular tissue and malnutrition.[20] The primary clinical symptom is unexplained weight gain and increased abdominal size. The treatment of choice is surgical removal.

The sonographic pattern of the mucinous cystadenoma is a smooth-walled, lobulated, multiseptated adnexal mass, which may contain a hypoechoic pattern as a result of the higher viscosity of the fluid (Fig. 14-7). The sonographer should always

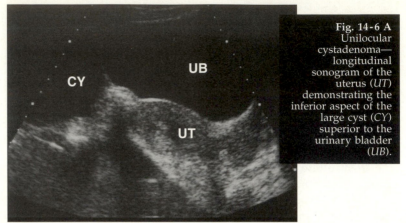

Fig. 14-6 A Unilocular cystadenoma—longitudinal sonogram of the uterus (*UT*) demonstrating the inferior aspect of the large cyst (*CY*) superior to the urinary bladder (*UB*).

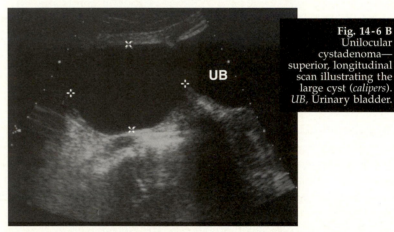

Fig. 14-6 B Unilocular cystadenoma—superior, longitudinal scan illustrating the large cyst (*calipers*). *UB,* Urinary bladder.

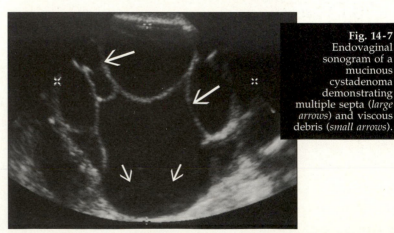

Fig. 14-7 Endovaginal sonogram of a mucinous cystadenoma demonstrating multiple septa (*large arrows*) and viscous debris (*small arrows*).

check for free fluid in the posterior cul-de-sac and in the other pelvic spaces for evidence of pseudomyxoma peritonei. Very large tumors will exceed the maximum image size of many current real-time systems, allowing only an approximation of the longitudinal and transverse dimensions. The use of a split screen or simultaneous dual imaging will allow a larger field of view and a better estimate of the tumor size.

The **serous cystadenocarcinoma,** the most common variety of malignant cystic neoplasm, is made up of serous epithelium and may attain a large size. This neoplasm usually contains septations, a clear, watery fluid, and solid external or internal papillary projections. The early clinical symptoms do not generally allow the differentiation from benign neoplasms, since the patient usually complains of unexplained weight gain and increasing abdominal girth.[20] The pelvic examination may reveal a fixated pelvic mass, which raises the suggestion of malignancy. The treatment of choice is surgical removal.

Sonographically, the serous cystadenocarinoma usually appears as a multilocular, complex mass in the adnexal area (Fig. 14-8). Because some of these neoplasms are bilateral, the sonographer should carefully scan the opposite adnexal area. However, many of these tumors totally fill the pelvic cavity, and the determination of whether

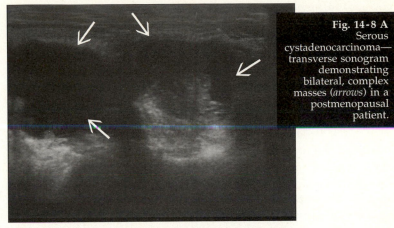

Fig. 14-8 A Serous cystadenocarcinoma—transverse sonogram demonstrating bilateral, complex masses (*arrows*) in a postmenopausal patient.

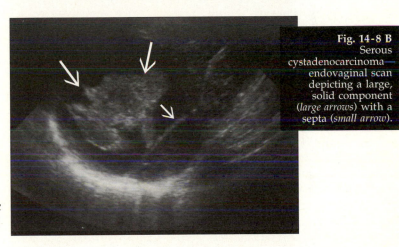

Fig. 14-8 B Serous cystadenocarcinoma—endovaginal scan depicting a large, solid component (*large arrows*) with a septa (*small arrow*).

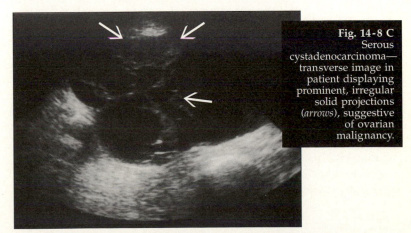

Fig. 14-8 C Serous cystadenocarcinoma—transverse image in patient displaying prominent, irregular solid projections (*arrows*), suggestive of ovarian malignancy.

they are unilateral or bilateral can be very difficult. The sonographer should check for malignant ascites in the peritoneal spaces.

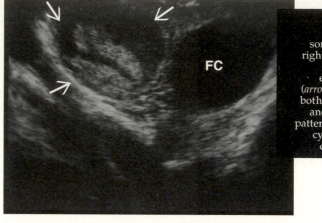

Fig. 14-9 Endovaginal sonogram of the right adnexal area depicting an endometrioma *(arrows)* exhibiting both a hypoechoic and hyperechoic pattern. A follicular cyst *(FC)* is also demonstrated.

The **mucinous cystadenocarcinoma** is typically unilateral and is not as common as the serous variety. It may be unilocular or multilocular, with localized solid projections. This neoplasm is also associated with pseudomyxoma peritonei. Again, the common presenting symptom is unexplained weight gain and increased abdominal girth. The treatment of choice is surgical removal.

Sonography typically reveals a multilocular, septated cyst with solid internal projections. The sonographer should check for the presence of pseudomyxoma peritonei and lymphadenopathy.

External Endometriosis

Endometriosis is the ectopic location of endometrial tissue. When it invades the myometrium of the uterus, the condition is called **internal endometriosis,** or **adenomyosis** (discussed in Chapter 13). In **external endometriosis** the endometrium invades the tissues and organs in the pelvic cavity, such as the fallopian tubes, suspensory ligaments, ovaries, and cul-de-sac. This type is more common than adenomyosis. More than half of the patients complain of unilateral or bilateral pelvic pain, which increases during menstruation. The endometrial nodules may obstruct the fallopian tubes, leading to infertility. Suggestive signs of endometriosis on the bimanual pelvic examination include the palpation of nodules on the uterosacral ligaments with a semifixated, retroverted uterus. However, laparoscopic examination is often required for a definitive diagnosis. According to surgical findings, endometriosis affects the following areas in decreasing order: one or both ovaries, the broad ligament, the posterior cul-de-sac, and the uterosacral ligaments.[16]

The endometrial deposits may form dense, hyperechoic nodules on the surfaces of the suspensory ligaments and other organs. These nodules are not routinely demonstrated on sonography. The endometrial deposits in an ovary may cause the development of **endometriomas,** or **chocolate cysts,** which appear as well-defined, slightly thick-walled cysts containing debris or a diffuse hypoechoic pattern. The latter has been termed the "ground glass" pattern (Fig. 14-9). Since these cysts contain blood, their pattern varies and may appear anechoic or contain hyperechoic areas. The sonographer should always carefully examine the adnexal areas, since these cysts can be unilateral or bilateral. Endometriomas may also leak, producing fluid in the posterior cul-de-sac. Once again, the clinical history is important, because these patterns can also occur with other ovarian neoplasms.

Teratoma

The **benign cystic teratoma,** or the dermoid cyst, is a very common germ-cell tumor that occurs during the reproductive years. This tumor contains areas of ectodermal tissue, hair balls, sebaceous material, and sometimes a tooth or bone fragment, and it ranges in size from 1 to 30 cm. Roughly 1% to 2% of these tumors are malignant, and 5% to 10% are bilateral. During a routine pelvic examination, these cysts often present as asymptomatic masses located anteriorly in the pelvis. Dermoids may become pedunculated and torse on their pedicle, causing minor to severe pelvic pain. The treatment of choice is surgical removal from the affected ovary.

The classic sonographic appearance of a cystic teratoma is a complex mass containing hyperechoic areas corresponding to hair or bone, which may exhibit acoustic shadowing that is referred to as the "tip of the iceberg" sign (Fig. 14-10). These masses are frequently located superior to the uterine fundus. However, teratomas have a wide range of patterns, including a rather homogeneous, hyperechoic pattern that often melds into the surrounding fascia.[20] The sonographer must look for signs of bladder indentation and ensure that the gain settings are not set too high to identify this type of pattern (Fig. 14-11). Another pattern includes the demonstration of a fat-fluid level, which relayers when the pa-

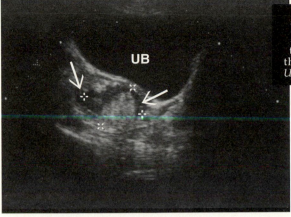

Fig. 14-10 A Longitudinal image of a solid, benign teratoma (*arrows*) in the left adnexal area. *UB,* Urinary bladder.

Fig. 14-10 B Transverse image of a solid, benign teratoma (*arrows*) in the left adnexal area. *UB,* Urinary bladder; *UT,* uterus.

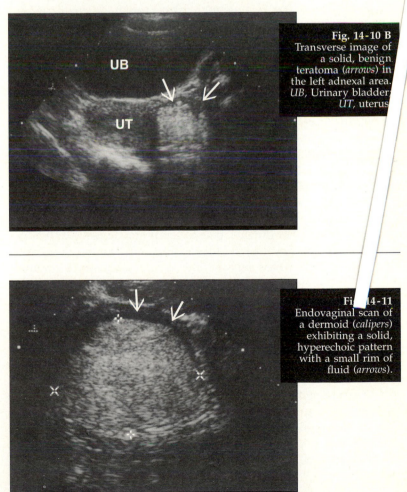

Fig. 14-11 Endovaginal scan of a dermoid (*calipers*) exhibiting a solid, hyperechoic pattern with a small rim of fluid (*arrows*).

tient's position is changed. The sonographer should always check the opposite adnexal area, since there is a risk for bilateral tumors.

The **malignant or immature teratoma** is typically unilateral and is usually seen in young children. These are fast-growing neoplasms and therefore tend to experience necrosis and hemorrhage. Sonographically they often appear to have more solid components than the benign variety, but histologic examination is necessary to confirm the diagnosis. The sonographer should look for signs of lymphadenopathy, which would increase the suggestion of malignancy.

Ovarian and Adnexal Torsion

Ovarian torsion most often occurs in children and young adults. Conditions that may cause torsion include an ovarian cyst, or neoplasm, and ovarian hyperstimulation syndrome. In these cases the growth of the mass displaces the ovary and twists the ovarian suspensory ligaments, which impede or occlude the vascular supply.[11] Adnexal torsion refers to the twisting of the fallopian tube and surrounding veins. The factors that can cause adnexal torsion include an excessively long tube, an enlarged tube, tortuosity of the tubal veins, a tubal ligation, or trauma. After normal labor and delivery, the prominent adnexal vasculature may cause an adnexal or ovarian torsion to occur. Bilateral torsion can occur, but it is rare. The clinical symptoms usually consist of severe pelvic pain, anorexia, and nausea and vomiting. The patient may have a palpable mass and leukocytosis. However, a partial torsion may produce less severe symptoms. This condition must be diagnosed as quickly as possible to save the ovary.

The most important sonographic criterion is the documentation of a decreased or absent flow to the ovary and adnexa with pulsed and color-flow Doppler.[8] Gray scale signs include an enlarged, hypoechoic ovary that may contain cystic areas. The sonographer should also scan the cul-de-sac, since the torsion can produce free fluid.

Ovarian Carcinoma

Each year, the cases of ovarian carcinoma exceed the total number of endometrial and cervical cancer cases combined. A woman has a chance of 1 in 70 to develop ovarian carcinoma during her lifetime. Because current diagnostic techniques do not allow for early diagnosis of this malignancy, the long-term prognosis at the time of diagnosis is poor, with a 37% 5-year survival rate. Adenocarcinoma is the most common pathologic type.[14] Clinical symptoms present late in the disease. By the time the neoplasm is palpable during a pelvic examination, there is usually evidence of distant metastasis. Often the symptoms are associated with the metastatic processes, such as liver metastasis or lymphadenopathy. Risk factors for ovarian carcinoma include a high fat diet, smoking, and alcohol consumption. Additional risk factors are women with two first-degree relatives who have had ovarian or breast cancer or women with a history of breast, colon, or endometrial cancer.

The International Federation of Gynecology and Obstetrics (FIGO) classifies ovarian cancer in four stages. Stage I exists when the neoplasm is limited to one or both ovaries. Stage II exists when pelvic extension of the malignancy has occurred. Stage III results when there are peritoneal implants beyond the pelvis and/or positive retroperitoneal or inguinal nodes. Stage IV exists when there is distant metastasis, such as liver metastasis, or when there is malignant pleural effusion.[14]

Typically the sonographic pattern for Stage I ovarian carcinomas present as primarily small solid ovarian masses with a hypoechoic pattern (Fig. 14-12). In the postmenopausal woman, a cystic area in an ovary requires further investigation, although this type of patient may still develop follicles and functional cysts.[10] The use of color-flow and pulsed Doppler to detect early ovarian carcinoma remains in the research stages. The theory underlying this technique relates to the development of abnormal vessels in malignant neoplasms. These vessels do not contain the normal arterial wall layers, specifically the elastic muscular layer that increases the resistance to flow in a normal artery. This decrease in elasticity allows more diastolic flow, which causes an abnormal systolic-to-diastolic flow ratio or a lower resistive index. Malignant tumors must reach a certain size threshold before they become vascular. Some research studies have indicated that a resistive index of less than 1 indicates malignancy,

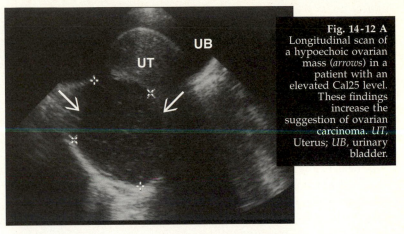

Fig. 14-12 A Longitudinal scan of a hypoechoic ovarian mass (*arrows*) in a patient with an elevated Cal25 level. These findings increase the suggestion of ovarian carcinoma. *UT*, Uterus; *UB*, urinary bladder.

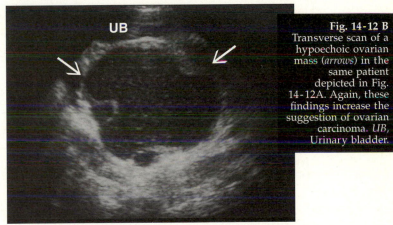

Fig. 14-12 B Transverse scan of a hypoechoic ovarian mass (*arrows*) in the same patient depicted in Fig. 14-12A. Again, these findings increase the suggestion of ovarian carcinoma. *UB*, Urinary bladder.

but this discriminatory zone has not been fully researched and correlated.[8] Other investigators believe that a resistive index of 0.5 or less is more discriminatory for malignancy. A pitfall in using this technique is the fact that low resistance flow also occurs with abscesses and chronic inflammatory conditions. After clinical correlation, these patients may proceed to a laparoscopic examination or exploratory surgery.[17]

Advanced-stage ovarian carcinoma may appear as a predominantly solid, rather large mass, with areas of necrosis and hemorrhage (Fig. 14-13). The sonographer should examine the inguinal and retroperitoneal nodes, the pelvic and abdominal peritoneal spaces for malignant ascites and peritoneal implants, and the liver for evidence of metastasis. This additional information will assist in accurately staging the disease.

Ovarian Metastasis

Several primary malignancies tend to invade the ovaries, although the ovaries rank rather low in the overall incidence of metastasis. Carcinoma of the breast ranks as the highest in ovarian metastatic involvement, occurring in approximately 6% to 10% of cases.[14] These metastatic deposits usually remain small and are typically discovered as incidental findings after oophorectomy is peformed for other clinical reasons. Primary tumors of the stomach or intestines may produce bilateral metastasis to the ovaries, which are called **Kruckenberg's tumors.** These tumors usually visualize as bilateral, solid to complex masses in the adnexal areas. Occasionally they present as a unilateral mass, usually affecting the right ovary. Endometrial carcinoma may also metastasize to the ovaries, but pathologic correlation is necessary to determine which location contained the primary tumor. Lymphoma may also metastasize to the ovary, usually producing a hyperechoic pattern. Metastasis from leukemia usually produces a cystic pattern. The sonographer must remember that a number of nonovarian types of pathology can produce solid adnexal masses, including a ligamentous

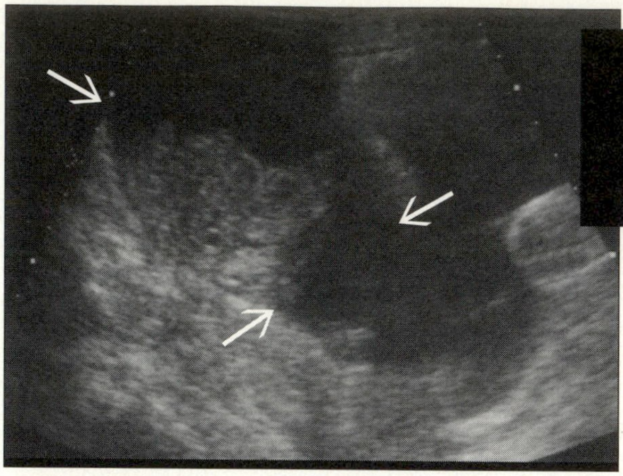

Fig. 14-13 A Longitudinal sonogram to the right of midline displaying a large, complex ovarian carcinoma (*arrows*).

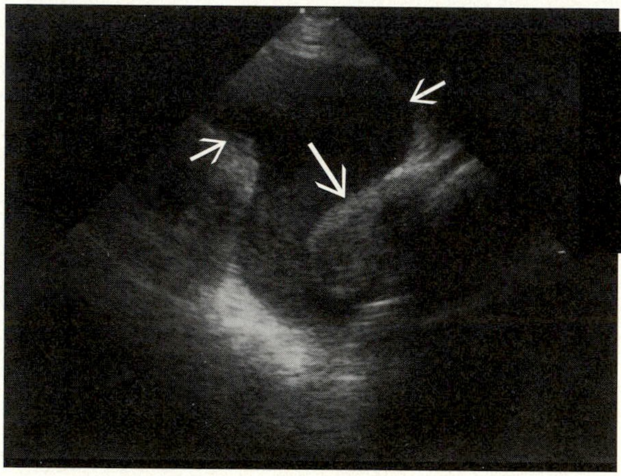

Fig. 14-13 B Longitudinal sonogram demonstrating malignant ascites (*small arrows*) and a peritoneal implant (*large arrow*).

broid, hematoma, thickened mesentery, and congealed omentum. A clinical history of previous pelvic surgery, which could have produced adhesions, or a history of infections or inflammatory pelvic masses may allow the interpreting physician to narrow the differential diagnosis.

Brenner Tumor and Fibroma

Brenner tumors consist of solid, epithelial tissue and are usually benign. Most of these tumors are unilateral, but bilateral tumors occur in approximately 7% to 13% of cases. Although the Brenner tumor may occur in any age group, about 50% appear in the postmenopausal patient. The typical clinical symptom is vaginal bleeding. These tumors are made up of fibrous connective tissue and range from less than 1 to 30 cm in size. **Meigs' syndrome,** which consists of ascites and right hydrothorax, can occur with the Brenner tumor.[3] Treatment requires the surgical removal of the affected ovary.

Sonographically, the Brenner tumor typically presents as a solid, echogenic tumor that may undergo cystic degeneration, producing several cystic areas. The malignant variety may appear larger than the benign tumor and may contain more cystic areas.[3] The sonographer should scan the opposite adnexal area to rule out bilateral involvement and check the pelvic and abdominal recesses and the pleural spaces to rule out Meigs' syndrome.

The **fibroma** tumor is relatively rare, typically occurs in menopausal or postmenopausal women, and is usually unilateral. **Meigs' syndrome** occurs in approximately 1% of cases, whereas ascites develops in about 15% of cases. **The basal cell nevus syndrome** is a hereditary condition that produces bilateral tumors along with basal cell carcinomas and keratocysts of the jaw.[2]

Typically the fibroma appears as a hypoechoic mass that produces acoustic shadowing. Again, the sonographer should check the opposite adnexal area to rule out bilateral masses and scan the pelvic and abdominal peritoneal spaces and the right pleural space to rule out Meigs' syndrome.

Granulosa Cell Tumor

The granulosa cell tumor, the most common hormonal neoplasm, typically occurs in postmenopausal women. These tumors often produce estrogen, which causes enhanced feminine characteristics, such as endometrial hyperplasia. Clinical symptoms include the discovery of a palpable mass during pelvic examination and vaginal bleeding. The grandulosa cell tumor usually exhibits low-grade malignant characteristics and may recur as long as 20 years after the initial diagnosis.[2] Ranging in size from 1 to 40 cm, these neoplasms metastasize through the lymphatic and circulatory systems.

When small, the granulosa cell tumor typically appears as a solid, rather homogeneous adnexal mass. Larger masses may contain cystic areas or appear septated. The sonographer should look for evidence of lymphadenopathy to assist the clinical staging of the disease.

Sertoli-Leydig Cell Tumor

The Sertoli-Leydig cell tumor, also known as the **arrhenoblastoma,** secretes male steroid hormones in 50% to 80% of cases, causing the development of male secondary sex characteristics. These tumors typically develop in patients 20 to 30 years of age, range in size from 3 to 5 cm, and are unilateral. Approximately 90% of these tumors are benign.[20] Clinical symptoms include the development of axillary and facial hair and menstrual irregularities or amenorrhea.

The Sertoli-Leydig cell tumor usually visualizes as a unilateral, solid ovarian mass. Although the sonographic pattern is not specific, correlation with the clinical symptoms, particularly if they include virilization, can allow a more specific differential diagnosis.

Dysgerminoma

The dysgerminoma, one of the most common types of germ cell neoplasms, usually occurs in the pediatric and adolescent patient. This neoplasm may measure only 3 to 5 cm, but it has a tendency to grow rapidly, producing the primary clinical symptom of pelvic pain. The dysgerminoma also invades the lymph nodes rather early in the disease. The tumor may rupture and cause intraperitoneal bleeding. Less than 10% of patients may have a positive serum β-hCG.[20] The dysgerminoma responds well to radiation and chemotherapy.

Sonographically, the dysgerminoma may appear as a solid ovarian mass when small, but large tumors may contain cystic areas secondary to necrosis and hemorrhage. The sonographer should scan the inguinal and retroperitoneal nodes for evidence of lymphadenopathy and the pelvic peritoneal spaces for signs of intraperitoneal bleeding.

Thecoma

The thecoma, a benign, unilateral stromal tumor that produces estrogen, usually appears in the postmenopausal woman but may occur from age 15 to 86 years. These neoplasms range in size from 1 to 30 cm. The common symptom in the typical age group is irregular vaginal bleeding. The luteinized thecoma, a subtype, occurs in younger patients during the reproductive years and secretes male steroid hormones, producing virilization in up to 50% of cases. The typical sonographic pattern is a hypoechoic mass, which usually produces acoustic shadowing distal to the entire neoplasm.[2]

TECHNICAL PITFALLS

One of the most common technical pitfalls in the sonographic evaluation of the ovaries is misidentifying a portion of the piriformis muscle or even a loop of the bowel for an ovary. The sonographer must use the anatomic landmarks and search all of the variable locations to confidently identify the ovaries. Another common pitfall is the misidentification of the sonographic characteristics of an ovarian mass on transabdominal sonography. Because of the degradation of resolution in the far field, cystic masses may appear solid, whereas solid masses may look cystic. Artifacts such as side lobe production, acoustic shadowing, and enhancement may also mask true sonographic patterns. An endovaginal examination will often allow a more accurate depiction of the sonographic characteristics, which could avoid unnecessary surgery for the patient.

SUMMARY

After reading this chapter, the sonographer should realize that the sonographic patterns for many ovarian tumors are quite similar and that obtaining a good clinical history may enable the interpreting physician to narrow the differential diagnosis. The sonographer must demonstrate that the mass is uterine, ovarian, extrauterine, or extraovarian in origin by changing the scanning window and the scanning angulation. The sonographer must use the posterior oblique positions and obtain color and pulsed Doppler information, which not only adds additional information for the interpreting physician but contributes to the ongoing research in the field and the quest to improve the diagnostic accuracy of gynecologic sonography. Table 14-1 contains pertinent clinical laboratory test results for ovarian pathology.

REFERENCES

1. Athey PA, Cooper NB: Sonographic features of paraovarian cysts, *AJR* 144:83-86, 1985.
2. Athey PA, Malone RS: Sonography of ovarian fibromas/thecomas, *J Ultrasound Med* 6:431-436, 1987.
3. Athey PA, Siegel MF: Sonographic features of Brenner tumor of the ovary, *J Ultrasound Med* 6:367-372, 1987.

TABLE 14-1 OVARIAN PATHOLOGY – Correlation with Clinical Laboratory Tests	
CONDITION	**LABORATORY TESTS**
TURNER'S SYNDROME	Decrease Estrogen and Progesterone
POLYCYSTIC OVARY SYNDROME	Partial Suppression of Follicle Stimulating Hormone Can Cause Increased Testosterone
OVARIAN CARCINONA	Increased Carcinoembryonic Antigen and Ca125
GRANULOSA CELL TUMOR	Increased Estrogen
SERTOLI-LEYDIG CELL TUMOR	Increased Testosterone
DYSGERMINOMA	Occasionally + β-hCG
LUTEINIZED THECOMA	Increased Testosterone

4. Baltarovich OH, Kurtz AB, et al: The spectrum of sonographic findings in hemorrhagenic ovarian cysts, *AJR* 148:901-905, 1987.
5. Blankenstein J, Shalev J, et al: Ovarian hyperstimulation syndrome: prediction by size and number of preovulatory ovarian follicles, *Fertil Steril* 47:597-602, 1987.
6. Dunnihoo DR: *Fundamentals of gynecology and obstetrics,* ed 2, Philadelphia, 1992, JB Lippincott, pp 635-647.
7. Fishbach F: *A manual of laboratory and diagnostic tests,* ed 4, Philadelphia, 1992, JB Lippincott, pp 700-706.
8. Fleischer AC: Transvaginal color Doppler sonography of ovarian masses with pathologic correlation, *Ultrasound Obstet Gynecol* 275(1):181-186.
9. Fleischer AC, Daniel JF, et al: Sonographic monitoring of ovarian follicular development, *J Clin Ultrasound* 9:275-280, 1981.
10. Goldstein SR, Subramanyam B, et al: The postmenopausal cystic adnexal mass: the potential role of ultrasound in conservative treatment, *Ostet Gynecol* 73:8-10, 1989.
11. Graif M, Itzchak Y: Sonographic evaluation of ovarian torsion in children and adolescence, *AJR* 150:647-649, 1988.
12. Hall DA: Sonographic appearance of the normal ovary, of polycystic disease, and of functional ovarian cysts, *Semin Ultrasound* 4:146, 1983.
13. Hann LE, Crivello M, et al: In vitro fertilization: sonographic perspective, *Radiology* 163:665-668, 1987.
14. Heintz APM, Hacker NF, Lagasse LD: Epidemiology and etiology of ovarian cancer: a review, *Obstet Gynecol* 66:127-135, 1985.
15. Jansen RPS, Anderson JC: Catheterization of fallopian tubes from the vagina, *Lancet* 10:309-310, 1987.
16. Kang H, Choi B, et al: Endometriosis: CT and sonographic findings, *AJR* 148:523-524, 1987.
17. Khan O, Cosgrove DO, et al: Ovarian carcinoma follow-up: US vs laparotomy, *Radiology* 159:111-113, 1986.
18. Mendelson EB, Friedman H, et al: The role of imaging in infertility management, *AJR* 144:415-420, 1985.
19. Montz FJ, Schlaert HB, Morrow LP: The natural history of theca lutein cysts, *Obstet Gynecol* 72:247-251, 1988.
20. Moyle JW, Rochester D, et al: Sonography of ovarian tumors: predictability of tumor type, *AJR* 241:985-991, 1983.
21. Munn CS, Kiser CC, et al: Ovary volume in young and premenopausal adults: US determination, *Radiology* 159:731-732, 1986.
22. Ritchie WG: Sonographic evaluation of normal and induced ovulation, *Radiology* 161:1-10, 1986.

15

clinical obstetrics

INSTRUCTIONAL OBJECTIVES

At the completion of this chapter, the reader will be able to:

1. Describe the procedures for the dating and clinical staging of pregnancy.
2. Define and describe the stages of labor and delivery.
3. List and discuss the clinical factors that place a pregnancy in a high-risk category.
4. Discuss the clinical and sonographic criteria for determining fetal presentation.
5. Describe the clinical laboratory tests for determining pregnancy, including serum and urine tests and their sensitivity and specificity.
6. Explain the physiology of amniotic fluid production and the clinical tests for determining fetal maturity, genetic screening, and other related applications.
7. Describe the role of sonography in chorionic villus sampling and amniocentesis.
8. Define the clinical role of the nonstress and contraction stress tests, describe the procedures, and discuss the clinical implications of the interpretation of each test.

THE CLINICAL PROBLEM

Determinating an accurate estimate of gestational age has always posed a problem to the obstetrician. The patient who has regular menstrual cycles and has kept track of the first day of the last menstrual period will allow a more accurate estimate of the expected due date than the patient who has irregular periods or has not kept track of the start of each menstrual cycle. Even with the former condition the date of conception is not usually known, since the day of ovulation can vary within the standard 28-day cycle. The clinical estimate of fundal height may also assist in determining gestational age, but accuracy decreases if the examination is initially performed in the second trimester or if the patient is obese. Under either circumstance a sonographic examination will often provide a more accurate estimate of gestational age.

The clinical determination of fetal presentation may also pose a dilemma in the obese patient or during the stages of labor. Sonography provides an easy remedy by visualizing the presenting part and thus allowing the obstetrician to determine if the patient can deliver vaginally or if a cesarean section is indicated.

During the past few years the development of more sensitive pregnancy tests has had an enormous impact on the clinical management of the obstetric patient. The use of the β-subunit hCG (human chorionic gonadotropin) test has allowed the early determination of intrauterine pregnancy, and it has improved the diagnosis of complications during the first trimester of pregnancy. The use of chorionic villus sampling during the first trimester has also assisted in the early determination of a genetically normal fetus. Amniocentesis and nonstress and contraction stress tests have allowed for more accurate monitoring of the second- and third-trimester fetus for signs of fetal distress and fetal maturity.

During the past 10 years, obstetric sonography has experienced a tremendous growth in sophistication. The sonographer plays a crucial role in the quality of the examination, as well as in the accuracy of the differential diagnosis. As in all sonographic specialties, the clinical history and the results of clinical laboratory tests and other diagnostic procedures play a critical role in the development of a refined differential diagnosis, which provides the necessary information to allow high-quality obstetric care.

OBTAINING THE CLINICAL HISTORY

As part of the standard clinical history, the patient's obstetric history in relation to the number of pregnancies, deliveries, abortions, and ectopic pregnancies is obtained by the sonographer before performing the examination. The term **gravida (G)** refers to the total number of conceptions, including normal pregnancies, elected and spontaneous abortions, hydatidiform moles, and ectopic pregnancies. This term is abbreviated as "G" with a subscript used for the number of conceptions, such as G_3, which indicates three pregnancies. **Parity (P)** refers to a patient who has given birth to at least one infant, alive or dead, that weighed more than 500 g. If the weight is unknown, an estimated gestational length of 20 or more weeks is used. A multiple birth is counted as one parous experience. Thus, for the patient who is currently pregnant and has a history of one full-term singleton pregnancy and one twin pregnancy (delivered at 36 weeks gestation), the history would be written as G_3 P_2. A woman who has not delivered an infant weighing 500 g or more or carried a pregnancy to at least 20 weeks is called a **nullipara. Primipara** is the term used to describe the patient who has delivered at least one infant. **Multipara** describes a patient who has given birth to more than one infant. An **abortion** is defined as a delivery that occurs before viability, which is usually set at 23 to 24 weeks. Abortions are classified as either elected or spontaneous and may be indicated in the history as A_e, with the appropriate number for elected abortions, or A_s, with the number for spontaneous abortions. The term **miscarriage** refers to a spontaneous abortion occurring before the middle of the second trimester, but patients often use this term to also describe fetal death later in the pregnancy.[8]

The obstetrician obtains an extensive history of the patient during the first office visit to determine if the pregnancy is at risk for the development of any abnormalities. A history of any of the following conditions classifies the pregnancy as high risk for complications[10]:

1. Hereditary abnormality, such as Down's syndrome, or previous infants with anomalies
2. Premature or small newborn infant (for gestational age) from most recent pregnancy
3. Genital tract anomaly, such as bicornate uterus or incompetent cervix
4. Preeclampsia or eclampsia
5. Severe social problem, such as teenage pregnancy, drug addiction, or alcoholism
6. Long-delayed or absent prenatal care
7. Age less than 18 years or greater than 35 years
8. Teratogenic viral illness or dangerous drug administration in first trimester
9. Fifth or subsequent pregnancy, particularly when over 35 years of age
10. Prolonged infertility or essential drug or hormone treatment
11. Heavy cigarette smoking
12. Pregnancy within 2 months of previous delivery

Or a diagnosis of any of the following during the pregnancy:

1. Little or no weight gain during first half of pregnancy
2. Obstetric complications, such as preeclampsia or hydramnios
3. Abnormal fetal presentation, such as breech or transverse
4. Fetal abnormal growth rate
5. Fetus at greater than 42 weeks gestation

For many of these conditions, sonography allows the definitive diagnosis of the suspected abnormality and the serial monitoring for further complications. The referring physician should provide the pertinent clinical history and the suspected abnormality. When obtaining the clinical history for the interpreting physician, the sonographer should ask the patient if she has any history of birth defects in the family, if she has diabetes or hypertension, if she smokes, and if her physician feels she is small or large for the gestational age of the fetus.

CLINICAL STAGING OF PREGNANCY

The primary clinical method for determining gestational age is based on the date of the last normal menstrual period (LNMP). Based on the first day of the LNMP, the normal gestation lasts 280 days, or 40 weeks, which equals 9 calendar months or 10 lunar months. Based on the premise that ovulation occurs on day 14 of a 28-day cycle, or 2 weeks after the last menstrual period, the gestational length is 38 weeks. This method correlates more with the actual development of the embryo and fetus, starting with the first developmental stages after conception. However, the sonographer should remember that the time of ovulation varies, and many patients cannot provide this type of information. The infertility patient is one major exception to this statement, since she is monitored chemically and with sonography to determine when ovulation will occur or when it has occurred. Other patients may record mittelschmerz (German for "middle pain"), a peritoneal irritation from the fluid of the ruptured follicle, which causes some pelvic pain or discomfort. Some patients keep track of the dates when they have sexual intercourse which can also provide a more accurate date of conception. Even with these exceptions, the sonographer should always obtain the menstrual history and calculate the current stage of pregnancy and the estimated date of confinement (EDC) on the basis of the first day of the last menstrual period. If the patient cannot remember the date of her LNMP, the sonographer should ask the patient what date her physician is currently using for the EDC. Using a gestational calculation wheel, the sonographer can determine the date the physician used for the LNMP. The tables used to sonographically determine fetal age are based on the LNMP, unless the tables specify otherwise.

Another method that the obstetrician uses to determine the stage of pregnancy is based on the clinical palpation of the uterine fundal height. On pelvic examination the uterus becomes flexible at the junction of the uterus and cervix during weeks 7 to 8 of the pregnancy and is referred to as **McDonald's sign.**[7] At this stage the uterine fundus is normally palpable at the level of the pubic symphysis. During the rest of the pregnancy the fundal height is determined by measuring the distance from the symphysis to the superior border of the fundus. By 15 weeks the fundus has reached the midpoint between the symphysis and the umbilicus and by 20 weeks the fundus has reached the umbilicus. The fundal height progresses superiorly during the remainder of the pregnancy, typically reaching its greatest height at 38 weeks, with a decrease through 40 weeks as a result of the engagement of the head in the lower pelvis in preparation for labor and delivery (Fig. 15-1). The accuracy of this clinical determination varies according to several factors, including the skill of the physician and the obesity of the patient. During a sonographic examination, the sonographer may note that the superior border of the fundus roughly correlates with the clinical determination of fundal height. In addition, a disparity between the gestational age (based on fundal height) and the menstrual history usually requires a sonographic examination to determine the cause of this discrepancy.[1]

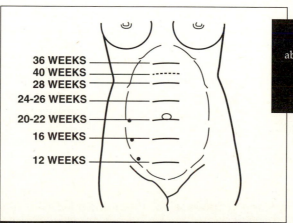

36 WEEKS
40 WEEKS
28 WEEKS
24-26 WEEKS
20-22 WEEKS
16 WEEKS
12 WEEKS

Fig. 15-1
The maternal abdomen correlating the fundal height with the approximate gestational age.

The obstetrician will also ask the patient to indicate when she first feels fetal movement, which is referred to as **quickening.** Usually the primigravida first feels movement at 18 weeks, whereas the multigravida, now familiar with the sensation, typically feels the first fetal movements at 17 weeks. However, some patients may dismiss these early sensations as being caused by other conditions. The physician uses this information only as an additional hallmark for pregnancy dating, as well as an early indication of fetal well being. Fetal heart tones may be heard with a fetoscope starting at 20 weeks, but a fetal heart rate may be documented earlier with the skilled use of a continuous-wave Doppler instrument. Again, patient obesity, as well as how early in the pregnancy the initial clinical examination is performed, affects the accuracy of the clinical staging of pregnancy.[1]

Stages of Labor and Delivery

Although assisting during labor and delivery does not fall within the normal responsibilities of the sonographer, many patients in labor arrive in the ultrasound department for sonographic evaluation. Consequently, the sonographer must be able to monitor the patient's condition and know when the patient requires further obstetric care. A patient in the later stages of labor should not come to the ultrasound department without a nurse or a member of the attending obstetric team. Often these examinations will be performed at bedside in the labor room. The sonographer may be asked to assist in a delivery when the patient is not accompanied by the proper personnel. In general, this occurs with a patient who is experiencing spontaneous abortion or with the patient who is rapidly advancing through the stages of labor.

False labor usually occurs late in pregnancy and consists of brief, irregular uterine contractions accompanied by less severe abdominal and/or back pain. False labor does not progress but remains inconsistent in strength and duration. There is no change or dilatation of the cervix, and the fetus does not descend. **True labor** occurs when there is a regular sequence of uterine contractions that become progressively stronger and closer together. The cervix experiences effacement and dilatation, and the fetus descends.[9]

Usually several events occur before the commencement of labor. Ranging from several days to several weeks before labor, the cervix softens and begins to dilate and often measures between 1 and 3 cm by the time labor starts. Just before labor the patient may pass a small amount of red-tinged mucus, referred to as the "cervical plug." The fetal membranes rupture, causing the external leakage of amniotic fluid, and 90% of patients will begin labor within 24 hours. If labor does not start within this time frame, the condition is referred to as prolonged premature rupture of membranes (PROM). This condition increases the risk of fetal infection and distress.[9]

Four major factors influence the progress and outcome of labor. Referred to as the four "Ps" of labor, they are the passage, powers, passenger, and placenta.[9] Passage refers to the condition of the bony and soft tissue areas of the maternal pelvis and includes such parameters as the size of the pelvic inlet. Powers refer to the strength and duration of the uterine contractions and whether the contractions are progressing satisfactorily. Passenger refers to the fetus and includes such criteria as the presenting part and the presence of any anomalies, which would contraindicate a vaginal delivery. The placenta is a very crucial factor, since the presence of placenta previa or abruptio placentae could lead to serious maternal bleeding with increased maternal and fetal morbidity and mortality. Many of these factors that are related to the four "Ps" require the use of sonography to determine the clinical management of the patient.

The **first stage of labor** commences with the onset of true labor and ends when the cervix fully dilates at 10 cm. Usually the longest stage of labor, the primipara usually spends 8 to 12 hours in this first stage, but the number of hours decreases to an average of 6 to 8 hours in subsequent pregnancies. The **second stage of labor** begins with the full dilatation of the cervix and ends with the birth of the baby, with the length varying from several minutes to several hours. The **third stage of labor** commences with the birth of the baby and ends with the delivery of the placenta, or afterbirth.[9] The obstetrician examines the afterbirth to ensure the complete delivery of the placenta and membranes. Sometimes a fourth stage is identified as the hour immediately following the third stage, since the risk of postpartum bleeding is still high.[2]

Fetal Presentation

Fetal presentation refers to the fetal part that is located over the pelvic inlet, and it consists of five broad categories: **vertex, breech, brow, face,** and **shoulder** (Fig. 15-2). Approximately 95% of patients will have a vertex, or cephalic, presentation, and 4% to 5% will have a breech presentation. The remaining categories (brow, face and shoulder) are rare presentations.[8] The normal vertex presentation occurs when the fetus's chin is tucked down, and the occipital region of the head is the lowest portion of the presenting part, referred to as the point of direction. In the typical breech presentation the sacrum is the point of direction. The **fetal lie** describes the position of the fetal longitudinal axis in relation to the maternal longitudinal axis. A **longitudinal lie,** the most common, occurs when the longitudinal axes of the fetus and mother are parallel. The **transverse lie** refers to the condition in which the fetal longitudinal axis is perpendicular to the maternal longitudinal axis. An **oblique lie,** technically a varia-

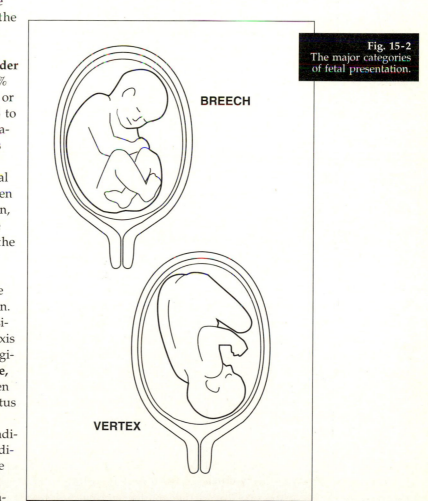

BREECH

VERTEX

Fig. 15-2
The major categories of fetal presentation.

tion of the transverse lie, refers to all other angles formed between the fetal and maternal longitudinal planes, although these angles must deviate substantially from the true transverse or longitudinal lies before this description is used[8] (Fig. 15-3). Typically the clinician uses physical palpation to determine the fetal lie and presentation. However, a number of factors, such as maternal obesity and the presence of polyhydramnios or multiple gestation, can interfere with an accurate determination; sonography can often alleviate this interference. Additionally, sonography allows the accurate determination of placental position and can diagnose placenta previa and umbilical cord prolapse.

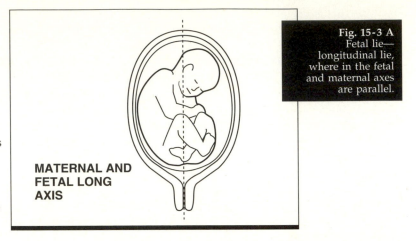

Fig. 15-3 A Fetal lie—longitudinal lie, where in the fetal and maternal axes are parallel.

MATERNAL AND FETAL LONG AXIS

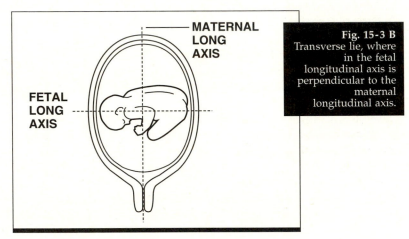

Fig. 15-3 B Transverse lie, where in the fetal longitudinal axis is perpendicular to the maternal longitudinal axis.

MATERNAL LONG AXIS

FETAL LONG AXIS

CLINICAL LABORATORY TESTS

Pregnancy Tests

The current clinical laboratory tests used to determine the status and duration of pregnancy are based on the evaluation of **human chorionic gonadotropin** (hCG), which is produced by the trophoblastic cells starting approximately 8 days after conception. Today's pregnancy tests are more sensitive and specific because they evaluate for a specific subchain of the hCG molecule, called the beta-subunit, or β-hCG. This evaluation decreases the false positive rate because the Alpha (α)–chain of the hCG molecule shares chemical similarities with the luteinizing hormone (LH) α–chain, whereas the beta (β)–chains are different.[3] The urine pregnancy test is the most common method of determining the existence of early pregnancy. The urine sample should be the first voiding in early morning, since the hCG level is typically higher, although later samples can provide clinically useful information. With normal renal function, urine pregnancy tests are typically positive 26 to 36 days after the first day of the last menstrual period or 8 to 10 days after conception. Current tests use monoclonal antibodies and a visible color change to indicate pregnancy. Typical sensitivity ranges from 25 to 50 milli-international units per milliliter (mIU/ml).[3] A quantitative analysis for β-hCG, often necessary for determining ectopic pregnancy, may require a 24- to 48-hour incubation time, but this analysis will provide enhanced sensitivity to the detection of a low hCG level. In a normal pregnancy the hCG level doubles approximately every 30 to 48 hours during the first month after conception. The hCG level peaks during the eighth week after conception, reaching an average level of 100,000 mIU/ml. The level rapidly decreases so that by approximately the sixteenth week after conception, the value has declined to 5000 mIU/ml, where it remains for the duration of the pregnancy. The hCG level returns to the normal nonpregnant range of less than 5 mIU/ml 10 to 14 days after delivery. The Second International Reference Standard (2nd IS) has a much greater sensitivity than the First International Reference Preparation (IRP), since the values are approximately 50% of the IRP values and, as a result, are more effective in the diagnosis of early intrauterine pregnancy and in the evaluation of ectopic pregnancy.[3] The exact values and their correlation with the sonographic findings are discussed in Chapter 17.

Amniocentesis

Amniocentesis is the removal of a small amount of amniotic fluid for laboratory analysis. Indications for performing this procedure include the following[7]:

1. Maternal age greater than 35 years
2. Previous child with chromosomal anomaly(ies)
3. Three or more spontaneous abortions
4. Patient or husband with chromosomal anomaly(ies)
5. Family history of chromosomal anomaly(ies)
6. Possible female carrier of X-linked disease
7. Metabolic disease link
8. Risk of neural tube defect

The evaluation of amniotic fluid can provide the diagnosis for over 100 metabolic diseases, as well as determine fetal sex and provide screening for chromosomal anomalies through the karyotype.[4]

Physiology. During the first half of pregnancy, the amniotic fluid probably originates from the transportation of maternal plasma across the membranes that cover the placenta and umbilical cord. At this stage of development the amniotic fluid is almost identical to plasma. In the second half of the pregnancy the fetal kidneys begin to function, creating a progressive mixture of fetal urine with a subsequent rise in the concentration of amniotic urinary metabolites. The amniotic fluid has a low specific gravity of 1.008 and a pH of 7.2. The amniotic fluid volume changes with the normal development of the fetus, ranging from approximately 30 ml at 10 weeks, to 350 ml at 20 weeks, to 800 ml at 38 weeks. After 38 weeks, the volume normally declines. In postmature pregnancies the volume may measure less than 500 ml, which is termed **oligohydramnios,** an abnormally low amniotic fluid volume. **Polyhydramnios,** or **hydramnios,** is usually defined as an abnormally high amniotic fluid volume of 2000 ml or greater.[7]

To maintain a stable amniotic fluid volume, the fetus must excrete approximately the same amount that it drinks. If a fetal disease or anomaly disrupts this balance, volume disturbances can occur, such as oligohydramnios with renal agenesis or polyhydramnios with duodenal atresia. During late pregnancy the amniotic fluid contains increasing quantities of particulate matter, such as desquamated cells, lanugo, scalp hairs, vernix caseosa, and a few leukocytes. By the late third trimester the fetus drinks approximately 400 to 500 ml of amniotic fluid per day, which is approximately the daily amount of milk a newborn will drink. Meconium is not normally excreted until after birth, and meconium in the amniotic fluid may be a sign of fetal stress or hypoxia.[7]

Technical Considerations. The prime time for performing a genetic amniocentesis is between 15 and 17 weeks, although it can be performed later. Some studies have shown that an amniocentesis before 15 weeks may be a good alternative to chorionic villus sampling.[5] **Chorionic villus sampling (cvs)** retrieves a chorionic villus sample from the decidua basalis during the first trimester, typically between 9 and 12 weeks. The sample can be obtained either transcervically or transabdominally, usually under ultrasound guidance. When performed by an expert, the risk of spontaneous abortion is approximately the same as in amniocentesis, roughly 2% to 5%.[12] Because of these statistics, chorionic villus sampling is usually performed only in large perinatal departments. This procedure allows for the diagnosis of genetic anomalies early in the pregnancy and makes a therapeutic abortion a safer procedure if the parents make that choice.

To perform amniocentesis, the physician inserts a 20- to 22-gauge needle through the maternal abdomen, advances it into the uterus, and usually removes 20 ml of amniotic fluid. To avoid excessive fluid removal, the maximum amount is limited to 1 ml per gestational week. For example, only 15 ml is removed if the gestational age is 15 weeks. The sonographer should have opaque tubes ready for the fluid samples or the room lights should be dimmed to avoid the breakdown of bilirubin. This is very important if Rh incompatibility is suspected.

The Role of Sonography. Before chorionic villus sampling, the sonographer should perform an examination and document:
1. Gestational age, number of fetuses, and fetal heart motion
2. Placental location
3. Presence of fetal anomalies
4. Presence of uterine and ovarian abnormalities
5. Identification of biopsy site.

The prime site for the biopsy is the portion of the placenta adjacent to the umbilical cord insertion, which is the thickest area of the placenta. The localization method is the same for both the transabdominal and endovaginal techniques. Using the transcervical method, a catheter is inserted through the vagina, advanced through the cervix, and introduced into the uterus. The course of the catheter is continuously monitored with sonography. The catheter is positioned next to the thickest portion of the placenta. At least one specimen is aspirated. With the transabdominal approach, the biopsy site is localized and a 20-gauge needle is introduced through the abdominal wall, advanced into the uterus, and positioned adjacent to the biopsy site. Again, the needle course is continuously monitored with sonography.

After the procedure the sonographer verifies fetal viability and checks for signs of hematoma development or other postbiopsy complications. A follow-up sonographic examination may be ordered up to a week later to rule out later complications.

Before amniocentesis, the sonographer should perform a routine sonographic examination and document:
1. Gestational age, number of fetuses, and fetal heart motion
2. Placental location
3. Adequacy of amniotic fluid (minimum of 2-cm pocket)
4. Presence of fetal anomalies

5. Presence of uterine or ovarian abnormalities

6. Identification of potential amniocentesis site

When identifying potential amniocentesis sites, the sonographer should follow the guidelines listed below:

1. Have patient void just before procedure to avoid accidental puncture.
2. Avoid needle trajectory that traverses placenta.
3. Avoid fetus, particularly the head and trunk.
4. Avoid umbilical cord.
5. Do not use a lateral needle entry site.
6. Provide a perpendicular needle entry path.
7. Document amniocentesis site.
8. Document fetal heart motion and rate after procedure.

The interpreting physician should verify that all the above guidelines have been followed. The physician performing the procedure may elect to advance the needle through an anterior placenta. For this approach the needle site should avoid the umbilical cord insertion and the central area of the placenta. If the patient has Rh incompatibility, the needle path should avoid the placenta. A number of fetal injuries during amniocentesis have been reported. Therefore the sonographer should always find a site away from the fetus. Using color Doppler will easily identify the position of the umbilical cord. The sonographer should localize a site on the anterior surface of the maternal abdomen. A lateral needle site may puncture the uterine arteries or veins, which are quite prominent.[6,13] The amniocentesis site should always be documented, using the calipers to measure the depth of the amniotic fluid pocket and, if possible, the needle path. Once the site has been selected, it should be marked and the area washed with an antiseptic solution. The procedure itself is performed using sterile techniques.

Laboratory Analysis. Normal amniotic fluid is clear to straw colored. A visual inspection of the color can provide some preliminary information. A yellow color may indicate the presence of bile pigment produced from red blood cell hemolysis caused by blood incompatibility. A red color indicates that blood contamination has occurred from either the mother or fetus; additional testing is necessary to determine the source. Meconium contamination produces a green fluid and indicates fetal distress, either one episode or a more serious case of fetal hypoxia.[7]

A genetic amniocentesis requires 1 to 2 weeks for laboratory analysis, since a culture of fetal cells must be grown to examine the karyotype for chromosomal anomalies. The laboratory can centrifuge fresh amniotic fluid, fix the cells on a slide, and stain them with Feulgen reagent to determine the presence or absence of sex chromatin. This procedure is indicated when one is looking for an X-linked congenital disorder.[4] The sonographer must check with the clinical laboratory regarding procedures, since these tests are often performed by an outside laboratory service.

Another common reason for amniocentesis is the determination of fetal maturity. Usually performed at 35 weeks gestational age or later, the **creatinine concentration** indicates mature renal function when the values reaches 1.8 mg/dl or greater. The exact values vary by individual laboratories. The **lecithin/sphingomyelin (l/s) ratio** is a routine test for the determination of fetal lung maturity. Produced by the lung tissue, these lipids prevent the collapse of the alveoli during expiration. By 30 to 32 weeks, the L/S ratio is approximately 1. By 35 weeks, the amount of lecithin begins to rapidly increase, whereas the sphingomyelin stays constant or decreases slightly. An L/S ratio of 2:1 or higher indicates lung maturity. One of the last lung surfactants to develop is **phosphatidylglycerol,** and its presence in the amniotic fluid is one of the most reliable indicators of fetal lung maturity. All values are less reliable in diabetic mothers, or if the amniotic fluid is contaminated by meconium, blood, maternal urine, or vaginal contents.[4]

The **bilirubin concentration** can assess the severity of an Rh+ fetus who is developing erythroblastosis. The severity of the anemia closely correlates with the bilirubin concentration. The more severe the disease, the higher the bilirubin concentration. Blood contamination in the fluid sample can make interpretation difficult.[4]

Nonstress and Contraction Stress Tests

The nonstress test is one of the most common methods for monitoring the fetus for signs of stress, and it is used to evaluate the function of the placenta. The foundation of the test relies on the fact that fetal movements during rapid eye movement (REM) sleep and periods of waking produce cardiac accelerations. Fetal movements decrease during periods of non–rapid eye movement (NREM) sleep, with certain central nervous system anomalies, alcohol consumption, and conditions that cause fetal hypoxia, as well as other abnormal conditions. The fetus is more active 1 to 2 hours after the mother eats, so this is the perfect time for the performance of this test. Using an external fetal monitor, the patient lies either supine or on her side, and the fetal heart rate is recorded. If a minimum of two cardiac accelerations occur in a 20-minute period (producing 15 beats above the baseline rate), and if these accelerations last for 15 seconds, the fetus is diagnosed as reactive, meaning that there is no evidence of fetal compromise. If less than two of these accelerations occur in a 45-minute period, the fetus is diagnosed as nonreactive, which may indicate fetal compromise and that further testing is necessary. A fetus in NREM sleep may have a nonreactive test, but the contraction stress test will usually differentiate this condition from fetal compromise.[11]

When the uterus contracts, the compression of the spiral arteries leading to the placenta causes a temporary decrease of oxygen and nutrients to the fetus. The normal fetus has enough reserves of oxygen and nutrients to prevent any deleterious effects. However, the compromised fetus does not often have a substantial reserve, and the stress produces cardiac deceleration. To perform the contraction stress procedure, an external fetal monitor is used, and the cardiac heart rate is monitored for 20 minutes. Uterine contractions are then stimulated either by having the mother stimulate her nipples or by administering oxytocin. The uterine stimulation is discontinued once three to five uterine contractions occur in a 10-minute period; the fetal heart rate is continuously monitored until all contractions stop. An absence of late decelerations indicates a negative study, whereas late decelerations occurring with each of the three contractions in a 10-minute period indicate a positive study.[11]

TECHNICAL PITFALLS

To keep legal liability at a minimum, the sonographer should always adhere to the guidelines for amniocentesis site localization and routinely document the findings and localization of the site. The interpreting physician should always be involved in these procedures and give the final approval for the needle site and path before the start of the procedure. If the sonographer finds contraindications or complications, such as oligohydramnios or an anterior placenta, the interpreting physician should be informed immediately.

SUMMARY

When an obstretric patient is referred for a sonographic examination, the importance of obtaining the clinical history cannot be overstressed. In many instances this duty initially involves the sonographer. Armed with this information, the sonographer can give more attention to certain anatomic areas and therefore help ensure a high-quality, diagnostic examination. Assisting physicians with invasive procedures, such as amniocentesis, carries additional legal responsibilities that the sonographer must be aware of to decrease legal risks.

REFERENCES

1. Dunnihoo DR: *Fundamentals of gynecology and obstetrics,* ed 2, Philadelphia, 1992, JB Lippincott, pp 63-66.
2. Dunnihoo DR: *Fundamentals of gynecology and obstetrics,* ed 2, Philadelphia, 1992, JB Lippincott, pp 369-370.
3. Fishbach F: *A manual of laboratory and diagnostic tests,* ed 4, Philadelphia, 1992, JB Lippincott, pp 219-221.
4. Fishbach F: *A manual of laboratory and diagnostic tests,* ed 4, Philadelphia, 1992, JB Lippincott, pp 938-939.
5. Hanson FW, Zorn EM, et al: Amniocentesis before 15 weeks gestation: outcome, risks, and technical problems, *Am J Obstet Gynecol* 156:1524, 1987.
6. Jeanty P, Rodesch F, et al: How to improve your amniocentesis technique, *Am J Obstet Gynecol* 146:593, 1983.
7. Pernoll ML, Benson RC, editors: *Current obstetric and gynecologic diagnosis and treatment,* ed 6, Norwalk, Conn, 1987, Appleton and Lange, pp 157-159.
8. Pernoll ML, Benson RC, editors: *Current obstetric and gynecologic diagnosis and treatment,* ed 6, Norwalk, Conn, Appleton and Lange, 1987, pp 178-180.
9. Pernoll ML, Benson RC, editors: *Current obstetric and gynecologic diagnosis and treatment,* ed 6, Norwalk, Conn, Appleton and Lange, 1987, pp 184-197.
10. Pernoll, ML, Benson RC, editors: *Current obstetric and gynecologic diagnosis and treatment,* ed 6, Norwalk, Conn, Appleton and Lange, 1987, pp 246-247.
11. Pernoll ML, Benson RC, editors: *Current obstetric and gynecologic diagnosis and treatment,* ed 6, Norwalk, Conn, 1987, Appleton and Lange, pp 285-289.
12. Rhoads GG, Jackson LG, et al: The safety and efficacy of chorionic villus sampling for early prenatal diagnosis of cytogenic abnormalities, *N Engl J Med* 320:609-617, 1989.
13. Romero R, Jeanty P, et al: Sonographically monitored amniocentesis to decrease intraoperative complications, *Obstet Gynecol* 65:426, 1985.

16

normal first-trimester pregnancy

INSTRUCTIONAL OBJECTIVES

At the completion of this chapter, the reader will be able to:

1. Describe the events that occur in the early stages of embryologic development, including fertilization, the formation of blastomeres, the morula and blastocyst stages, implantation, and the development of the primary germ layers.
2. Name the three layers of the decidua of pregnancy, and describe their development during the first trimester.
3. Describe the development of the major organ systems.
4. Discuss the development of the membranes and cavities during the first trimester.
5. Identify on both transabdominal and endovaginal sectional sonograms a normal first-trimester pregnancy.
6. Describe the basic scanning protocol for both transabdominal and endovaginal examinations of the first-trimester pregnancy, including the calculation of the size of the gestational sac and the crown-rump length.
7. List several technical pitfalls associated with the sonographic evaluation of the first-trimester pregnancy.

THE CLINICAL PROBLEM

The advent of endovaginal sonography has transformed the management of the patient during the first trimester of pregnancy. The clinician can now verify an intrauterine pregnancy as early as 4 weeks after the last normal menstrual period (LNMP) and, as a result, can rule out a number of other conditions. However, the clinical expectations in relation to endovaginal sonography are occasionally too high, and the use of follow-up examinations are still necessary to make a definitive diagnosis. Because of the enhanced resolution of endovaginal transducers, the sonographer can depict detailed anatomy of the embryo and its related structures, which was previously impossible with most transabdominal systems. Therefore the sonographer must understand detailed embryology and the related sonographic patterns in order to perform a high-quality examination.

CLINICAL LABORATORY TESTS

The primary pregnancy test for accurately determining an early first-trimester gestation is the human chorionic gonadotropin (β-hCG) serum test. Clinical laboratories may use either the First International Reference Preparation (IRP) or the Second International Reference Standard. To compare the two standards, 2.2 mIU/mL using the second standard equals 1 mIU/ml using the first standard. The **discriminatory zone** is the β-hCG level at which the normal gestation is visible with sonography. This level will vary with the individual clinical laboratory and the type of equipment used in the ultrasound department. During the fourth week from the LNMP, the level varies from 400 to 800 mIU/ml (using IRP).[11] Performing a series of normal examinations using optimum resolution, noting the β-hCG level, and correlating this information with the menstrual history will allow each sonography department to establish its own discriminatory zone.[8]

EMBRYOLOGY

In embryology, developmental events are referenced to conception. That is, day 1 of embryologic development coincides with fertilization. In clinical sonography the duration of the pregnancy is calculated from the first day of the LNMP. Therefore the reader must remember that fertilization occurs approximately 2 weeks *after* the LNMP, using the standard 28-day menstrual cycle. In the embryology sections of this chapter the timing of developmental events is keyed to fertilization, whereas the normal sonographic patterns section uses the LNMP with the embryologic dates in parentheses.

Fertilization and Early Embryologic Development

Fertilization typically occurs in the distal fallopian tube when one sperm penetrates the ovum. Both the sperm and ovum normally carry a haploid complement of 23 chromosomes, which unite at the time of fertilization to form a full set of 46 chromosomes. The term **zygote** refers to the united ovum and sperm. This single cell experiences its first mitotic division approximately 30 hours after fertilization, forming two smaller duplicates, which are the first in a series of divisions called **cleavage.** During cleavage the individual cells become smaller, and the overall size of the cell mass does not increase. The cells that are formed during cleavage are called **blastomeres.** By the third day after fertilization, the blastomeres form a berrylike solid

mass of cells called the **morula.**
All of these early developments
occur in the fallopian tube (Fig.
16-1). The morula reaches the
endometrial cavity (EMC) 3 to 4
days after fertilization. As the
cells continue to divide, they
form a hollow, fluid-filled mass
called the **blastocyst.** The blastocyst floats freely in the EMC for
several days. During this time
the cells of the blastocyst differentiate into an outer layer, called
the **trophoblast,** and an inner
cluster of cells, called the **inner**

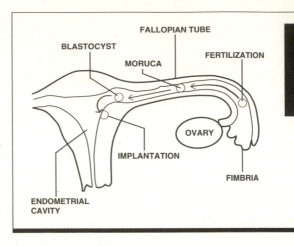

Fig. 16-1
Coronal illustration
depicting the initial
embryologic stages
that occur during
migration through
the fallopian tube.

cell mass. The inner cell mass divides into two fluid-filled cavities, the **amniotic cavity**
and the **primitive yolk sac.** The trophoblast contains two layers, the outer **syncytiotro-**
phoblast and the inner **cytotrophoblast.** The syncytiotrophoblast grows and projects
into the endometrial lining of the uterine cavity and secretes proteolytic enzymes,
which allow it to sink into the endometrium. This layer is the fetal component of the
placenta. By day 7 the blastocyst has implanted into the endometrium, and implantation is complete by approximately day 10. Implantation normally occurs in the upper
third of the uterus and gives rise to the endometrial divisions of pregnancy, referred to
as **decidua,** which means "to shed." The decidua is made up of three parts: (1) the
decidua basalis, the portion of endometrium on which the implanted embryo rests; (2)
the decidua capsularis, the endometrium covering the gestational sac; and (3) the
decidua parietalis, the remaining endometrial lining, exclusive of the area surrounding
the gestational sac[2] (Fig. 16-2).

Development of Extraembryonic Membranes and Cavities

The extraembryonic membranes are the chorion, amnion, allantois, and secondary
yolk sac. The two predominant cavities formed during early pregnancy are the
amniotic and chorionic cavities. The **chorionic villi** first appear at the end of the
second week and continue to proliferate, totally covering the blastocyst by the third
week. As the blastocyst continues to grow, the villi adjacent to the decidua capsularis
become compressed and begin to degenerate, producing a bare area, termed the
chorionic laeve, which will later become the **chorion.** At approximately day 12 a new
cavity begins to develop, called the **extraembryonic coelom.** At the same time the
primary yolk sac shrinks in size, and the **secondary yolk sac** begins to develop. This
sac arises from the cells of the hypoblast from the embryonic disk and is located in the
primary yolk sac. By the third week the extraembryonic coelom has become the
chorionic cavity, within which a connecting stalk suspends the embryonic disk,
amnion, and yolk sac (Fig. 16-3). By the end of the third week the chorionic cavity is
well developed and, at this stage, the amniotic cavity is much smaller than the
chorionic cavity. The edges of the amniotic cavity have fused with the embryonic disk.
During the fourth week the flat embryonic disk folds both longitudinally and

transversely. As it folds the posterior curvature of the embryo
bows into the amniotic sac, and
its attachment to the amnion is
then located on its anterior aspect. Concurrently, a portion of
the yolk sac is used to form the
midgut, and the remainder of
the yolk sac is attached to the
midgut by the yolk stalk. The
umbilical cord starts to form,
and the size of the amniotic cavity begins to increase. After the
folding process is complete, the
embryo then lies in the amniotic
cavity. The **allantois** begins to
form during the third week and
is derived from the digestive
tract of the embryo. It initially
aids in the excretion of wastes,
but later it becomes incorporated
into the fetal urinary system. By
the end of the first trimester the
embryo fills the entire EMC.
This growth causes the **decidua
capsularis** to come into contact
with the **decidua parietalis,** both
of which eventually fuse. Consequently, the decidua capsularis
degenerates and disappears, and
the chorion becomes fused to the
decidua parietalis. At approximately the same time the amniotic cavity grows to the extent
that the amnion is in contact
with the chorion. These two extraembryonic membranes fuse
and form the amniochorionic
membrane.[3]

The Placenta

As previously mentioned, the
chorionic villi begin to proliferate
during the second week. The
chorion frondosum, the fetal
component of the placenta, de-

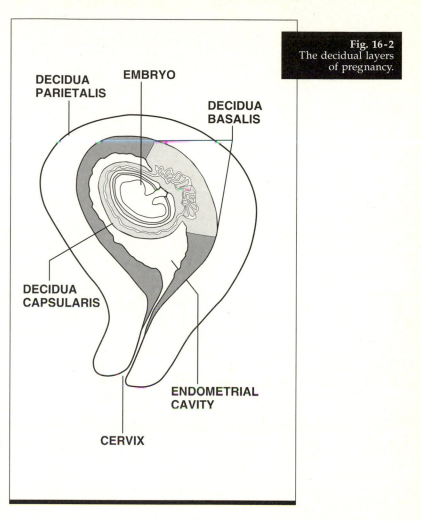

Fig. 16-2
The decidual layers
of pregnancy.

DECIDUA
PARIETALIS

EMBRYO

DECIDUA
BASALIS

DECIDUA
CAPSULARIS

ENDOMETRIAL
CAVITY

CERVIX

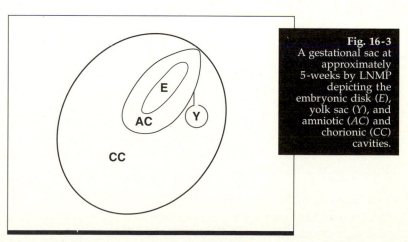

Fig. 16-3
A gestational sac at
approximately
5-weeks by LNMP
depicting the
embryonic disk (*E*),
yolk sac (*Y*), and
amniotic (*AC*) and
chorionic (*CC*)
cavities.

E

Y

AC

CC

velops adjacent to the imbedded portion of the blastocyst by the inner cell mass. The chorionic villi rapidly grow in this area. The maternal component of the placenta is the **decidua basalis.** By the fourth week the physiologic exchange of oxygen, nutrients, and waste products begins. The chorionic membrane is attached to the placenta. The villi in the mature placenta allow the diffusion of oxygen, nutrients, and waste products between the mother and fetus. There is no direct mingling of the maternal and fetal circulations. By the middle of the first trimester the umbilical cord is fully functional, containing one vein that transports oxygen and nutrients to the fetus and two arteries that convey waste products from the fetus to the placenta.[6]

Development of Primary Germ Layers

Approximately 2 weeks after fertilization the blastocyst has become a hollow ball of cells that surround two cavities, which are separated by a double-layered plate of cells, called the **embryonic disk.** With this development the conceptus is now called an **embryo,** and this term is used until the end of the eighth week after conception, when the rudimentary structures of all major systems have been formed. The two early cavities are the initial development of the **amniotic cavity,** which will later surround the embryo and the secondary yolk sac. Initially the embryonic disk differentiates into the **epiblast** and **hypoblast.** At the start of the third week the midline portion of the epiblast layer begins to thicken, forming the **primitive streak,** which produces mesenchymal cells that form the **mesoderm.** At this point the epiblast is called the **ectoderm,** and the hypoblast is termed the **entoderm.** Thus the **three primary germ layers** are formed: the inner layer (entoderm), the middle layer (mesoderm), and the outer layer (ectoderm). These three layers will further differentiate into the following structures[3]:

ECTODERM—from which are developed the central and peripheral nervous systems; epidermis, hair, and nails; the mammary, subcutaneous, and pituitary glands; and teeth enamel.

MESODERM—from which are developed the serous linings of the peritoneal, thoracic, and pericardial cavities; cartilage, connective tissue, bone, and muscle; heart, blood vessels and cells, and lymph vessels and cells; and kidneys, ovaries, testes, adrenal cortex, and spleen.

ENTODERM—from which are developed the parenchyma of the liver, pancreas, thymus, thyroid glands, epithelial linings of the urinary bladder, and a majority of the urethra, respiratory, and gastrointestinal tracts.

As one can appreciate from this list, many organ systems have elements from more than one germ layer. Cells migrate, form groups, and experience further differentiation according to the blueprint encoded in the chromosomes. By the time a woman has missed the first menstrual period, organogenesis is well underway. During this period of rapid growth and accelerated mitotic activity, the embryo is highly susceptible to the actions of **teratogens,** which are substances that cause abnormal development and include viral infections (such as measles), toxic agents such as alcohol, and exposure to ionizing radiation.

Development of Major Organ Systems

The Central Nervous System. During the third week the ectoderm thickens at the midline, forming the **neural plate.** The lateral edges of the plate thicken to form the

neural folds, which fuse along the midline to form the **neural tube.** As further differentiation occurs during the next several weeks, the walls of the neural tube will form the spinal cord and brain, and the lumen will evolve into the spinal canal and the cerebral ventricular system. During the fourth week the three primitive divisions of the brain appear. The **forebrain** differentiates into the cerebral hemispheres. The **midbrain** gives rise to several structures, including the cerebral peduncles. The **hindbrain** will eventually differentiate into the medulla oblongata, the pons, and the cerebellum.[4]

The Gastrointestinal System. During the fourth week the primitive gut forms and divides into the foregut, midgut, and hindgut. The **foregut** gives rise to the esophagus and stomach, the first and some of the second portions of the duodenum, the liver and pancreas, the gallbladder and bile ducts, the pharynx, and the lower portion of the respiratory system. The celiac artery provides circulation to a number of these structures. The **midgut** produces the small bowel, cecum, and appendix, the ascending colon, and a portion of the transverse colon. The superior mesenteric artery supplies most of these structures. At the beginning of the sixth week (eighth week by LNMP), the midgut herniates into the base of the umbilical cord, producing a **normal physiologic herniation,** which is necessary for the further development of the midgut. During the tenth week (twelfth week by LNMP), the midgut *moves back into the abdominal cavity.* The **hindgut** differentiates into the descending colon, part of the transverse colon, the sigmoid colon, the rectum, the superior anal canal, and the epithelium of a majority of the urethra and the urinary bladder.[4]

The Urinary System. The kidneys derive from the mesoderm and go through three developmental stages. During the fourth week the **pronephroi** form, made up of a small cluster of cells with primitive ducts. Later in the fourth week the **mesonephroi** develop and include rudimentary tubules and glomeruli. By the fifth week the **metanephroi** begin to form and will become the permanent kidneys. The kidneys first produce urine between 11 and 13 weeks (13 to 15 weeks by LNMP).[5] The kidneys begin their development in the pelvic cavity, anterior to the sacrum, with the hilums pointing anteriorly. As the fetal abdomen continues to grow, the kidneys migrate to their typical location in the renal fossae lateral to the spine. The kidneys reach their normal position during the ninth week. Fetal kidneys appear lobulated and do not attain their normal smooth contours until later in infancy.

As the rudimentary **urinary bladder** begins to form, it is continuous with the allantois, one of the early extraembryonic membranes. This portion of the allantois constricts and forms the **urachus,** which becomes the medial umbilical ligament in the adult. The bladder enlarges, and the ascent of the kidneys causes the ureteral orifices to migrate to their typical position in relation to the trigone.[4]

The Reproductive System. During the fifth week an area of mesodermal tissue on the medial aspect of the mesonephros thickens and develops primary sex cords, referred to as the **indifferent gonads.** Although the sex is determined at the time of fertilization, the gonads of the male and female remain identical until the seventh week. By the twelfth week, the development of the external genitalia in both sexes allows identification. In the male the testes develop in the abdominal cavity and typically begin their migration toward the scrotal sac during the twenty-eighth week. By the thirty-second week the testes have usually entered the scrotum, and the inguinal canal has closed around the spermatic cord.[4]

The Cardiovascular System. This is the first system to function in the embryo. Development starts with the formation of the **cardiogenic cords** during the third week. These cords develop lumens, called **endocardial heart tubes,** which fuse to form a single heart tube, called the **primitive heart.** The primitive heart begins to beat at the end of the third week (end of the fifth week by LNMP). During the fourth through the seventh weeks, the four heart chambers form. This crucial period of development can give rise to a number of cardiac congenital anomalies, such as septal defects. Because the lungs do not function in utero, and since the fetus receives its oxygen and nutrient supply from the placenta, there are several unique connections in the fetal heart. The **patent ductus arteriosis** allows blood to flow between the pulmonary arteries and the aorta. The **ductus venosus** allows blood to flow from the fetal portal system directly into the inferior vena cava. The **foramen ovale** allows blood to course from the right atrium into the left atrium.[4]

The Skeletal System. The skeletal system, derived from the mesoderm, initially begins as collections of mesoderm cells that later differentiate into osteoblasts, chondroblasts, and fibroblasts. During the fourth week these mesenchyme cells form three primary centers of activity: the areas of the vertebral bodies, the vertebral arches, and the thoracic ribs. During the sixth week these areas develop cartilage tissue, and ossification of the vertebral arches can be seen by the eighth week. However, the **clavicles** begin to ossify before any other bone in the body. Early ossification also occurs in the maxillae and mandible. The **limb buds** can be seen by the fourth week, and by the fifth week they have differentiated into the upper and lower legs and arms, with hands and feet. By the eighth week the **long bones** first begin to ossify in the shafts.[4]

SCANNING PROTOCOLS AND TECHNIQUES

Transabdominal Sonography

The scanning protocol for a gynecologic examination is the basic protocol for the first-trimester pregnancy (see Chapter 12). Sequential survey longitudinal and transverse images of the uterus and adnexal areas allow the identification of the gestational sac, any uterine pathology (such as myomas), a corpus luteum cyst, or other adnexal pathology. The patient must have a full urinary bladder. The normal-size patient requires the use of a 3.5 MHz transducer with the focal zone coinciding with the areas of interest. The sonographer may use a 5.0 MHz on thin patients, and obese patients may need a 2.25 MHz transducer. If the sonographer visualizes an early gestational sac but not the embryo, the primary measurement is the mean sac diameter (MSD). The sonographer should localize the true longitudinal axis of the gestational sac through its largest dimension, and place the calipers at the decidua-fluid interface. A true transverse image should be obtained through the largest sac diameter, placing the calipers at the decidua-fluid interface and measuring the posteroanterior and transverse diameters of the sac (Fig. 16-4). Although many ultrasound units will automatically calculate the MSD and the corresponding gestational age, the formula is:

$$MSD = \frac{\text{length} + \text{width} + \text{height}}{3}$$

If an embryo is demonstrated, the sonographer should verify fetal heart motion and obtain the crown-rump length (CRL) measurement, the most accurate gestational age determinant. The sonographer should localize the longitudinal axis of the embryo. If possible, the spine should be used for this localization procedure. If feasible, an image with the fetus in full extension should be obtained. The sonographer can exert pressure on the maternal abdomen to demonstrate **Moro's reflex,** which consists of the fetus fully extending and moving anterior in the amniotic fluid and then relaxing and returning to the dependent portion of the gestational sac. This will increase the accuracy of the CRL. The calipers should be placed from the superior aspect of the head to the tip of the buttocks

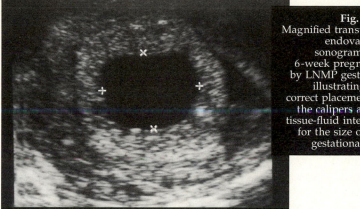

Fig. 16-4 Magnified transverse endovaginal sonogram of a 6-week pregnancy by LNMP gestation illustrating the correct placement of the calipers at the tissue-fluid interface for the size of the gestational sac.

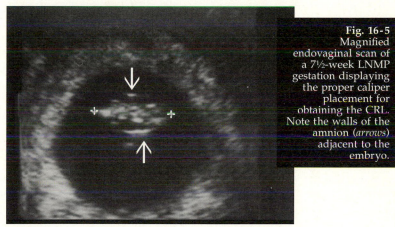

Fig. 16-5 Magnified endovaginal scan of a 7½-week LNMP gestation displaying the proper caliper placement for obtaining the CRL. Note the walls of the amnion (*arrows*) adjacent to the embryo.

(Fig. 16-5). Several measurements are obtained, with the longest measurement typically used for the gestational age calculation. Some obstetric calculation packages use an average value from a series of CRL measurements.

In summary the first-trimester sonographic examination should accomplish the following:

1. Verify an intrauterine pregnancy, and calculate the gestational age. If at all possible, the CRL should be used, since it is more accurate than the gestational sac size.
2. Verify the number of gestational sacs, and check for fetal viability.
3. Examine the uterus for any abnormalities, such as myomas.
4. Examine the adnexal areas, documenting the presence of a corpus luteum cyst or other types of adnexal pathology.
5. Check the posterior cul-de-sac for evidence of fluid.

If the scan is performed later in the first trimester, a limited fetal anatomy survey can be performed to rule out gross abnormalities.

The scanning protocol is similar to the standard gynecologic examination, discussed in Chapters 12 through 14. The protocol is summarized in the box at right.

Endovaginal Examination

The scanning protocol for an endovaginal examination of the first-trimester pregnancy should follow the transabdominal protocol previously listed. The high-resolution capabilities of the endovaginal technique allows an earlier identification of the gestational sac and CRL than does the transabdominal examination, and it allows earlier documentation of the heart motion.[1] Again, the entire uterus and adnexal areas should be scanned sequentially. If transabdominal sonography reveals an abnormal sac or a gestational sac in a retroverted uterus, the endovaginal examination will often improve the reso-

---

BASIC SCANNING PROTOCOL

- ✔ **Longitudinal midline uterus,** demonstrating the vagina, cervix, corpus, and fundus with the gestational sac. The longitudinal measurement of gestational sac should be obtained and, when feasible, the crown-rump length.
- ✔ **Longitudinal views to the right and left of midline,** demonstrating the lateral aspect of the uterus and gestational sac and the ovaries. The longitudinal measurement of the ovaries should be obtained.
- ✔ **Transverse views from inferior to superior or from superior to inferior,** demonstrating the true transverse plane of the vagina, cervix, isthmus, corpus, fundus, and ovaries. The transverse and posteroanterior measurements of the gestational sac should be obtained if the crown-rump length is not feasible.

---

lution to the extent that a definitive diagnosis can be made. The motto in obstetric sonography is to "give the fetus the benefit of the doubt." That is, the sonographer should request a follow-up scan or refer the patient to a high-risk ultrasound laboratory if the current examination does not allow a confident diagnosis of normality or abnormality.

NORMAL SONOGRAPHIC PATTERNS

This section will discuss the normal sonographic appearance of the first-trimester pregnancy on both endovaginal and transabdominal examinations by week, based on the age from the LNMP, with the age from conception indicated in parentheses.

Fourth Week (Second Week)

On endovaginal examination the blastocyst can be visualized when its size reaches 2 to 3 mm, corresponding to the optimum lateral and axial resolution of the transducer frequency used. This size is typically correlated to an LNMP ranging from 4 weeks and 1 day through 4 weeks and 5 days.[1] Since the gestational sac grows approximately 1 to 2 mm per day at this stage of the pregnancy, repeating the scan several days later can allow visualization. No internal contents can be demonstrated; consequently, a definitive diagnosis of a viable intrauterine pregnancy cannot be made at this early stage. The gestational sac appears as a small, fluid-filled circular structure in the hyperechoic endometrium (Fig. 16-6).

On transabdominal examination a 4-week pregnancy can occasionally be demonstrated with optimum resolution. With the failure to visualize an intrauterine pregnancy, the patient should undergo an endovaginal examination or receive a repeat transabdominal scan a week to 10 days later, if the clinical symptoms do not contraindicate this delay.

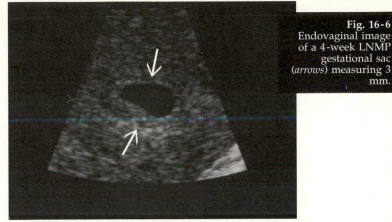

Fig. 16-6 Endovaginal image of a 4-week LNMP gestational sac (*arrows*) measuring 3 mm.

Fifth Week (Third Week)

By the fifth week the gestational sac has reached at least 5 mm, and the endovaginal examination can easily document the pregnancy as a hyperechoic, circular structure with an anechoic interior (Fig. 16-7). The early corpus luteum cyst may be demonstrated. By the end of the fifth week the sac has approached 10 mm in size, which can allow the early visualization of the embryo and the first identification of the heart motion.[9]

A transabdominal examination can visualize a gestational sac in the 0.5 to 1 cm range. However, overdistension of the urinary bladder can easily compress the small sac so that it fails to be demonstrated.[13] The patient who is obese or has a retroflexed uterus will often not allow adequate resolution for proper identification.

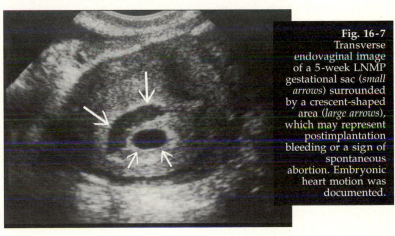

Fig. 16-7 Transverse endovaginal image of a 5-week LNMP gestational sac (*small arrows*) surrounded by a crescent-shaped area (*large arrows*), which may represent postimplantation bleeding or a sign of spontaneous abortion. Embryonic heart motion was documented.

Sixth Week (Fourth Week)

By the sixth week the gestational sac ranges from approximately 15 to 20 mm, allowing a reliable identification of intrasac structures. With endovaginal sonography the first structures identified are the yolk sac and the amniotic sac[7] (Fig. 16-8). The primitive embryonic disk demonstrates as a linear group of echoes between the secondary yolk sac and the amniotic cavity, allowing a more confident documentation of the primitive heart motion. During this period the first CRL can be obtained, with values ranging around 5 mm. Image magnification is required to correctly position the calipers. The primitive limb buds may be seen. The decidual layers can now be seen. The decidua basalis, located deep to the embryo in relation to the surrounding endometrium, appears as a slightly thickened, hyperechoic rim. The decidua capsularis surrounds the rest of the gestational sac and is often separated from the decidua parietalis by the hypoechoic to anechoic appearance of the empty portion of the uterine cavity. This pattern is called the "crescent" sign, or the double-decidua sign[13] (Fig. 16-9). Because of normal postimplantation bleeding, this area may appear more prominent and may contain debris. The corpus luteum cyst may contain debris and often appears as a cystic structure measuring between 2 and 4 cm (Fig. 16-10).

A transabdominal examination should reliably reveal a 6-week intrauterine pregnancy (Fig. 16-11), since the gestational sac has reached 2 cm, and since proper magnification techniques will often allow the documentation of the yolk sac and embryo. Fetal heart motion and a CRL may be obtained under optimum conditions.

Seventh Week (Fifth Week)

During the seventh week the gestational sac has reached approximately 3 cm in size, and the CRL is in the 1 cm range. The head has increased greatly in size, and the limb buds are formed. Endovaginal sonography can easily demonstrate the embryo with heart motion, the amniotic and chorionic cavities, and the yolk sac[10] (Fig. 16-12). Transabdominal sonography should routinely visualize the gestational sac. With optimum resolution and image magnification, the heart motion can be seen and the CRL obtained.

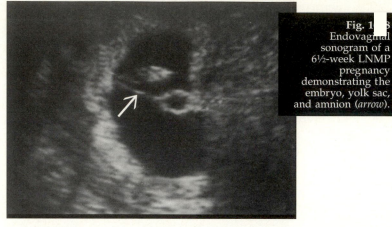

Fig. 16-8 Endovaginal sonogram of a 6½-week LNMP pregnancy demonstrating the embryo, yolk sac, and amnion (*arrow*).

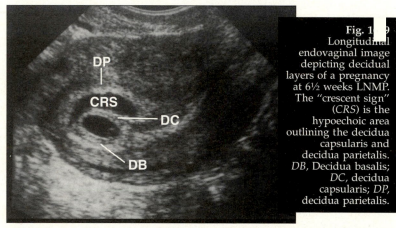

Fig. 16-9 Longitudinal endovaginal image depicting decidual layers of a pregnancy at 6½ weeks LNMP. The "crescent sign" (*CRS*) is the hypoechoic area outlining the decidua capsularis and decidua parietalis. *DB*, Decidua basalis; *DC*, decidua capsularis; *DP*, decidua parietalis.

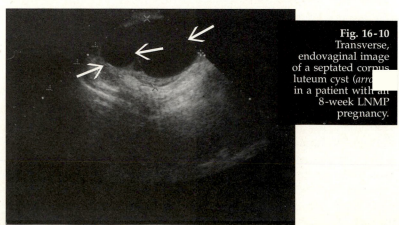

Fig. 16-10 Transverse, endovaginal image of a septated corpus luteum cyst (*arrow*) in a patient with an 8-week LNMP pregnancy.

Eighth Week (Sixth Week)

The head has become dominant in size, the embryo curvature has diminished, and the heart is formed. The midgut loop has herniated into the base of the umbilical cord. The CRL has approached 2 cm. Endovaginal sonography can reveal the physiologic herniation of the midgut[10] (Fig. 16-13). Using the transabdominal technique the sonographer should be able to obtain the CRL. The location of the placenta is more readily identifiable.

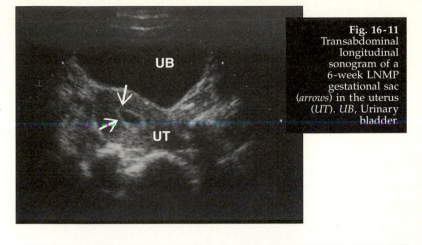

Fig. 16-11 Transabdominal longitudinal sonogram of a 6-week LNMP gestational sac (*arrows*) in the uterus (*UT*). *UB*, Urinary bladder.

Ninth Week (Seventh Week)

The CRL has approached 3 cm, the yolk sac may still be seen, and the size of the amniotic cavity has increased (Fig. 16-14). Early ossification may be seen in the clavicles, ribs, spine, maxillae, and portions of the calvaria.

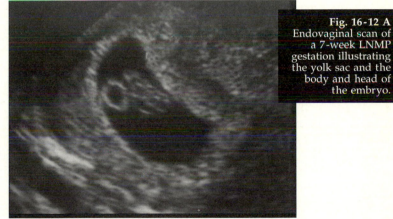

Fig. 16-12 A Endovaginal scan of a 7-week LNMP gestation illustrating the yolk sac and the body and head of the embryo.

Tenth Week (Eighth Week)

The CRL has now approached 4 cm, and typically fetal muscular movement has begun. On endovaginal examination amniotic fluid may be seen in the stomach (Fig. 16-15). The midgut has started to return into the abdominal cavity. The scan may demonstrate the hyperechoic choroid plexus in the lateral ventricles (Fig. 16-16). The rhombencephalon, the primitive fourth ventricle, may appear as a cystic area in the posterior fossa of the skull.[10] With endovaginal scans with optimum resolution, the sonographer may obtain a biparietal diameter (BPD) and the femur length. However, many ges-

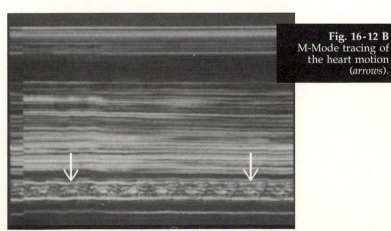

Fig. 16-12 B M-Mode tracing of the heart motion (*arrows*).

tational calculation charts are not extrapolated to this early age.

Twelfth Week (Tenth Week)

The CRL has reached the 7 cm range, but some charts may not extrapolate to this age range. However, many BPD and femur length charts cover this age range. The midgut has returned into the abdominal cavity, which rules out an omphalocele. The amnion is now close to the chorion, which will usually fuse by the fifteenth or sixteenth week.[10] Typically the yolk sac is no longer identifiable.

Fourteenth Week (Twelfth Week)

The sonographer should now obtain BPD and femur lengths. The fetal kidneys have begun to produce urine, allowing the early identification of the fetal bladder (Fig. 16-17). The spine and long bones display a hyperechoic pattern but have not experienced enough ossification to cast an acoustic shadow. On both endovaginal and transabdominal sonography, a fetal anatomy survey can be performed under optimum conditions.

TECHNICAL PITFALLS

One of the common technical pitfalls associated with transabdominal sonography relates to bladder distention. An underfilled bladder may allow visualization of the gestational sac, but its position in the uterine cavity and the inspection of the adnexal areas will be less than adequate. On the other hand, an overly distended bladder may

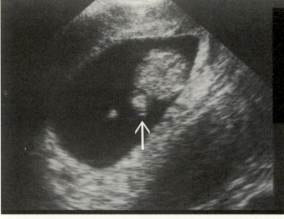

Fig. 16-13
Endovaginal scan depicting the physiologic herniation of the midgut into the base of the umbilical cord (*arrow*) in a 10-week LNMP pregnancy.

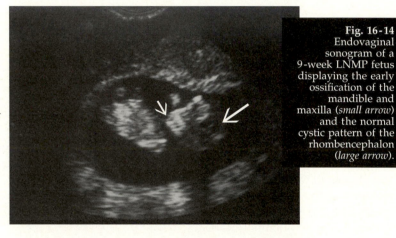

Fig. 16-14
Endovaginal sonogram of a 9-week LNMP fetus displaying the early ossification of the mandible and maxilla (*small arrow*) and the normal cystic pattern of the rhombencephalon (*large arrow*).

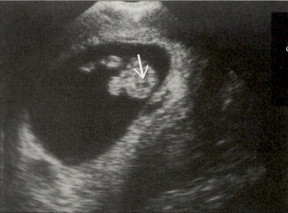

Fig. 16-15
Endovaginal image of a 10-week LNMP gestation demonstrating the stomach (*arrow*) in the fetal abdomen.

compress the gestational sac, leading to its nonvisualization or the distortion of its shape, so that it appears abnormal or empty. The sonographer must always recognize the resolution limitations of transabdominal sonography in the far field. A gestational sac may appear totally abnormal on a transabdominal scan, but an endovaginal examination may reveal a normal sac with a viable embryo (Fig. 16-18).

The most common mistake in relation to the CRL is overestimating the measurement by including the adjacent yolk sac. Early in pregnancy the fetal head and the yolk sac may look similar to the novice, but an examination of these structures transversely often provides differentiation. An oblique scan through the uterine myometrium can project this tissue into the gestational sac, and the sonographer can mistake this area for the embryo. Again, scanning in the opposite plane will usually prevent this pitfall. Identifying the early fetal heart motion can also present a challenge. The sonographer must magnify the image so that the embryo fills the viewing screen. It should be remembered that the fetal heart rate is in the 120- to 160-bpm range, whereas the maternal heartbeat is approximately one half of that rate. Monitoring the maternal pulse while observing the area of motion can clarify if the heartbeat represents the fetal or maternal circulation.

The endovaginal examination is not without its pitfalls.

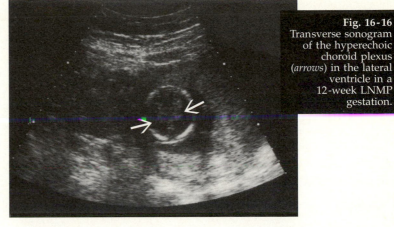

Fig. 16-16 Transverse sonogram of the hyperechoic choroid plexus (*arrows*) in the lateral ventricle in a 12-week LNMP gestation.

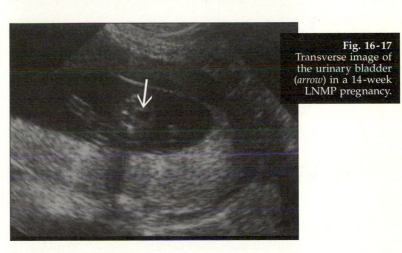

Fig. 16-17 Transverse image of the urinary bladder (*arrow*) in a 14-week LNMP pregnancy.

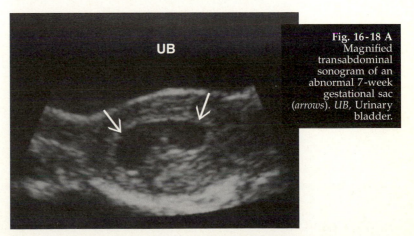

Fig. 16-18 A Magnified transabdominal sonogram of an abnormal 7-week gestational sac (*arrows*). *UB*, Urinary bladder.

The sonographer must increase the magnification to take advantage of the improved resolution and to identify the early gestational sac and its contents. Because of its limited scanning depth, a fundal pregnancy in an enlarged uterus may not appear on an endovaginal scan. Likewise, large adnexal masses may not be evident on an endovaginal examination.

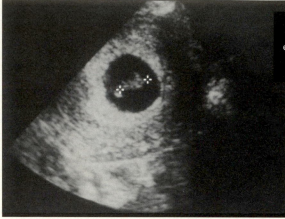

Fig. 16-18 B
The endovaginal examination revealed a viable 7.2-week embryo (*calipers*).

SUMMARY

The advent of endovaginal sonography has had an enormous impact on the diagnosis and management of the clinical complications of the first-trimester pregnancy. Enhanced resolution has required that the sonographer understand more about embryologic development than the sonographer entering the field in the early 1980s. The use of the β-hCG pregnancy test has allowed an earlier diagnosis of intrauterine pregnancy, as well as abnormal conditions. Table 16-1 provides a summary of normal β-hCG levels with the corresponding gestational age. The sonographer should remember that these are approximate values and that they will vary with the individual clinical laboratory ranges. Additionally, the visualization of the gestational sac and intrasac structures depends on the transducer characteristics and the body habitus of the patient.

TABLE 16-1 SONOGRAPHIC CRITERIA AND β-hCG CORRELATION – First Trimester			
GESTATIONAL AGE	ENDOVAGINAL	TRANSABOMINAL	β-hCG LEVELS
FOURTH WEEK LNMP	2 to 3 mm mean sac diameter*	Not usually seen	400 to 800[†]
FIFTH WEEK LNMP	6 mm mean sac diameter at 5.1 weeks; cardiac activity may be seen at 5.5 weeks; yolk sac may be seen	10 mm mean sac diameter at 5.7 weeks[†]	Decreased
SIXTH WEEK LNMP	15 mm at 6 weeks; crown-rump length = 3 mm; cardiac activity should be present if β-hCG is >5000	Should obtain mean sac diameter; may see cardiac motion; may obtain crown-rump length; may see corpus luteum	>3500
SEVENTH WEEK LNMP	24 to 30 mm mean sac diameter; crown-rump length	Should obtain crown-rump; may see yolk sac; document cardiac motion	>6000
EIGHTH WEEK LNMP	31 to 38 mm mean sac diameter	Crown-rump length = 13 to 20 mm	

*The consistency of sonographic visualization varies according to transducer resolution and the body habitus of the patient.

[†]These values are based on the Second International Preparation and serve only as examples. Actual normal ranges vary between clinical laboratories. The sonographer should always obtain the laboratory's normal ranges according to gestational age.

REFERENCES

1. Goldstein SR, Snyder JR, et al: Very early pregnancy detection with endovaginal ultrasound, *Obstet Gynecol* 72:204, 1988.
2. Moore KL: *The developing human: clinically related embryology,* ed 4, Philadelphia, 1988, WB Saunders, pp 28-35.
3. Moore KL: *The developing human: clinically related embryology,* ed 4, Philadelphia, 1988, WB Saunders, pp 38-42.
4. Moore KL: *The developing human: clinically related embryology,* ed 4, Philadelphia, 1988, WB Saunders, pp 65-85.
5. Moore KL: *The developing human: clinically related embryology,* ed 4, Philadelphia, 1988, WB Saunders, pp. 88-91.
6. Moore KL: *The developing human: clinically related embryology,* ed 4, Philadelphia, 1988, WB Saunders, pp 104-113.
7. Nyberg DA, Malk LA, et al: Value of the yolk sac in evaluating early pregnancies, *J Ultrasound Med* 7:129-135, 1988.
8. Peisner DB, Timor-Tritsch IE: The discriminatory zone of β-hCG for vaginal probes, *J Clin Ultrasound* 18:280-285, 1990.
9. Shenker L, Astle C, et al: Embryonic heartbeat before the seventh week, *J Reprod Med* 31:333-335, 1986.
10. Timor-Tritsch IE, Peisner DR, Raju S: Sonoembryology: an organ-oriented approach using a high frequency vaginal probe, *J Clin Ultrasound* 18:286-298, 1990.
11. Timor-Tritsch IE, Rottey S, editors: *Transvaginal sonography,* ed 2. New York, 1991, Elsevier, pp 233-235.
12. Yen H, Rabinowitz J: Amniotic sac development: ultrasound features of early pregnancy—the double sac sign, *Radiology* 166:97-103, 1988.
13. Zemlyn S: The effect of the urinary bladder in obstetric sonography, *Radiology* 128:169, 1978.

17

complications of the first-trimester pregnancy

INSTRUCTIONAL OBJECTIVES

At the completion of this chapter, the reader will be able to:

1. Describe the clinical problems that are typical reasons for the sonographic evaluation of the first-trimester pregnancy.
2. Describe the use of the β-human chorionic gonadotropin (hCG) pregnancy test during the first trimester of pregnancy, including the normal ranges and the values associated with pathologic conditions.
3. Describe the clinical symptoms and pathologic basis for complications of the first-trimester pregnancy, including spontaneous abortion and the other clinical categories of abortion, blighted ovum, ectopic pregnancy, trophoblastic disease, and pseudocyesis.
4. Discuss the conditions that can cause maternal pelvic masses or complications during pregnancy, including uterine anomalies, uterine myomas, corpus luteum cysts, and ovarian neoplasms.
5. Identify on sectional sonograms the above-mentioned pathologic or anomalous conditions of the first-trimester pregnancy, based on the sonographic appearance, the clinical history, and the results of other diagnostic procedures.
6. Describe several technical pitfalls associated with the sonographic examination of the first-trimester pregnancy.

THE CLINICAL PROBLEM

As previously mentioned, the use of endovaginal sonography combined with the interpretation of the quantitative β-hCG pregnancy test has enhanced the management of complications in the first-trimester pregnancy. During this period, the most common reasons for a sonographic examination include threatened abortion, size and date discrepancy, suspected ectopic pregnancy, and the evaluation of maternal pelvic masses. The most common clinical symptom that develops during the first trimester is vaginal bleeding, and it can occur with normal postimplantation changes, blighted ovum, ectopic pregnancy, and spontaneous abortion. Consequently, the clinician initially faces a broad differential diagnosis. Sonography can often narrow the diagnosis early in the first trimester, which allows the clinician a broader choice in interventional techniques, particularly in ectopic pregnancy. However, the accuracy of sonography often depends on a correlation with a single, and sometimes serial, β-hCG test. The interpreting physician must communicate with the clinicians, reinforcing the importance of routinely ordering this test when any of the pathologic conditions associated with the first trimester of pregnancy are suspected.

CLINICAL LABORATORY TESTS

The primary clinical laboratory test used for diagnosing and differentiating the abnormal conditions of the first-trimester pregnancy is the β-hCG radioimmunoassay test. In spontaneous abortion the death of the embryo causes an initial decline in serum hCG levels compared with the normal range for the gestational age according to the menstrual history. In ectopic pregnancy the embryo typically implants in the fallopian tube. This condition causes an increase in serum hCG, but the levels do not increase by the same amount as with an intrauterine pregnancy. With an intrauterine pregnancy, the hCG levels normally double every 2 to 3 days during the first 8 weeks of gestation. This abnormal **subdoubling** helps the clinician to differentiate between an ectopic pregnancy and other complications of the first trimester. However, if the patient's menstrual history is unreliable, interpretation of the hCG levels is more difficult. In these cases sonography can assist in more accurately dating an intrauterine pregnancy and in identifying an ectopic gestation. But in a number of patients, sonography cannot confidently diagnose an early ectopic pregnancy. Serial β-hCG tests can demonstrate that the hCG levels continue to fall below the normal range for the given menstrual age. Approximately 1 week later a repeat sonogram may then demonstrate evidence of an ectopic pregnancy.

SCANNING PROTOCOLS AND TECHNIQUES

The scanning protocols and techniques for the first-trimester sonographic examination are explained in Chapter 16. With the common use of endovaginal sonography, patients are referred for examinations early in pregnancy, typically 4 to 6 weeks from the last normal menstrual period (LNMP). Most department protocols still require a transabdominal examination to demonstrate any pathologic process in the superior portion of the pelvis, such as uterine fibroids and large adnexal masses. However, endovaginal images are often necessary to identify both normal intrauterine and ectopic pregnancies during this time frame. The scanning protocol for both the transabdominal and endovaginal examinations is presented in the box on the following page.

PATHOLOGIC PROCESSES OF THE FIRST TRIMESTER

Blighted Ovum

A blighted ovum, or anembryonic pregnancy, occurs when the zygote develops into a blastocyst, but the inner cell mass fails to develop. This condition occurs from approximately 2 weeks after conception until the end of the seventh or eighth week. Initially the patient exhibits all the symptoms of a normal pregnancy, such as a positive pregnancy test. But as the pregnancy advances, the patient frequently complains of vaginal spotting, and a repeat pregnancy test may display a weakly positive level or a negative value.

A major sonographic sign of a blighted ovum is a mean sac diameter (MSD) greater than 20 mm, which approximately corresponds to a 6½-week gestation LNMP, that does not contain a yolk sac. Another sonographic sign is an MSD greater than 25 mm, which approximately corresponds to an early 7-week gestation LNMP, that does not contain an embryo.[7] The gestational sac usually appears distorted in shape, and the decidual layers may look irregular (Fig. 17-1). Other sonographic signs include a fluid level in the sac as a result of intrasac bleeding and a gestational sac that occupies a disproportionately large area of the uterus (Fig. 17-2). If a repeat scan is performed approximately 1 week later, an increase in the MSD of less than 75% suggests a blighted ovum.[10] However, the sonographic differential diagnosis often includes early spontane-

---

BASIC SCANNING PROTOCOL

✔ **Longitudinal midline uterus,** demonstrating the vagina, cervix, corpus, and fundus with EMC and gestational sac. Images of the posterior cul-de-sac should be included. If demonstrated, the longitudinal measurement of the gestational sac should be obtained and, when feasible, the CRL measurement.

✔ **Longitudinal views to the right and left of midline,** demonstrating the lateral aspect of the uterus and gestational sac and the ovaries and adnexal areas. Longitudinal measurements of the ovaries should be obtained.

✔ **Transverse views from inferior to superior or superior to inferior,** demonstrating the true transverse plane of the vagina, cul-de-sac, cervix, isthmus, corpus, fundus, and ovaries. If demonstrated, transverse and posteroanterior measurements of the gestational sac should be obtained and, when feasible, the CRL measurement.

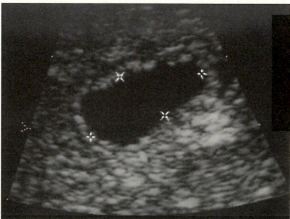

Fig. 17-1
Endovaginal image of a 6-week LNMP gestational sac (*calipers*) containing no evidence of an embryo, which is a typical pattern of a blighted ovum.

ous abortion, since the sonographic patterns of these two
anomalies can appear similar.

Threatened Abortion

The term threatened abortion
refers to the clinical situation of
a patient early in the first trimester who is experiencing vaginal
spotting or bleeding, as well as
some cramping, but has a cervix
that remains closed. These
symptoms occur in approximately 25% of clinically diagnosed pregnancies, and approximately one half of these
pregnancies end in spontaneous
abortion. With the death of the
embryo the chorionic tissue may
still function, producing a positive pregnancy test. However,
falling hCG levels on serial tests
is a reliable sign of pregnancy
failure. But since this pattern
may occur with ectopic pregnancy, sonographic correlation
often provides a definitive diagnosis. The primary role of sonography is to verify the viability or
nonviability of the pregnancy for
patients with the clinical diagnosis of threatened abortion. If a

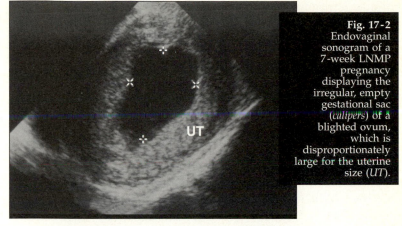

Fig. 17-2
Endovaginal
sonogram of a
7-week LNMP
pregnancy
displaying the
irregular, empty
gestational sac
(*calipers*) of a
blighted ovum,
which is
disproportionately
large for the uterine
size (*UT*).

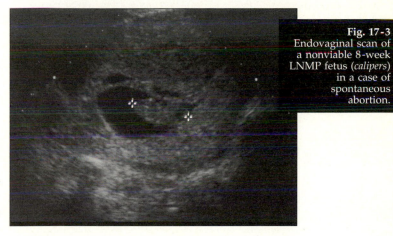

Fig. 17-3
Endovaginal scan of
a nonviable 8-week
LNMP fetus (*calipers*)
in a case of
spontaneous
abortion.

viable embryo is seen, 90% to 97% of these pregnancies will continue to develop
normally.[3,10]

The sonographic features of a normal first-trimester pregnancy are discussed in
Chapter 16. The sonographer should document the heart motion with M-mode or have
the interpreting physician verify the heart motion. Before pronouncing an embryo
nonviable, the sonographer should watch for heart motion over several minutes and
use color Doppler if heart motion is not demonstrated. The interpreting physician
should verify the diagnosis of a spontaneous abortion. The sonographic gray-scale
pattern of spontaneous abortion ranges from a normal depiction of an embryo with no
evidence of heart motion to a misshapen, inhomogeneous echo pattern (Fig. 17-3) with
debris in the sac and irregular sac walls.

Other Abortion Classifications

There are five additional abortion categories that are based on clinical symptoms and
findings: inevitable, incomplete, complete, missed, and habitual abortion. In **inevi-**

table, or **impending, abortion**
the patient experiences bleeding
and cramping, and the cervix is
open. **Incomplete abortion** occurs when some of the products
of conception have been expelled
from the uterus. Again, the patient complains of bleeding and
usually experiences cramping. In
many cases the embryo or fetus
is expelled first, since the placenta and membranes are attached to the uterine wall. In
complete abortion all the products of conception have been ex-

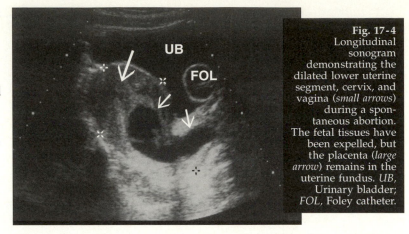

Fig. 17-4
Longitudinal
sonogram
demonstrating the
dilated lower uterine
segment, cervix, and
vagina (*small arrows*)
during a spon-
taneous abortion.
The fetal tissues have
been expelled, but
the placenta (*large
arrow*) remains in the
uterine fundus. *UB,*
Urinary bladder;
FOL, Foley catheter.

pelled from the uterus. The clinician has the tissue examined to accurately confirm that
all tissue from the fetus and placenta has been expelled. In **missed abortion,** which
typically occurs early in the second trimester, the nonviable fetus is retained in the
uterus for at least 8 weeks. The typical clinical signs include a decline in the normal
symptoms of pregnancy, a decrease in uterine size, no passage of fetal tissues, and a
cervix that remains closed. In **habitual abortion** the patient has experienced three
consecutive spontaneous abortions before 20 weeks LNMP. Risk factors include a
maternal age greater than 33 years and a history of a previous abortion, a stillbirth, or
a newborn with congenital anomalies.[12]

Once again, the results of the β-hCG test may be negative or display a weakly
positive level. Serial samples may be necessary to confirm the diagnosis and differentiate from other pathologic processes.

As in threatened abortion, the primary role of sonography is to document the
viability or nonviability of the fetus. Depending on the amount of elapsed time from
fetal demise, the fetal echo pattern ranges from a rather normal appearance to an
ill-defined, inhomogeneous mass.[10] Since the fetus is usually expelled first, the
sonographer should note the position of the fetus in relation to the internal cervical os
and determine whether the cervical canal appears dilated (Fig. 17-4). If the fetus is in
the lower uterine segment or in the cervical or vaginal canal, delivery may be
imminent and the sonographer should notify the obstetric staff immediately. In
incomplete abortion the typical sonographic pattern consists of retained products,
usually the placenta, in the uterine cavity (Fig. 17-5). Complete abortion is likely if the
endometrial echo complex appears fairly homogeneous and measures less than 7 mm.[8]
Missed abortion is actually a diagnosis based on clinical findings and does not exhibit
a unique sonographic pattern when compared with other classifications of abortion.
Usually sonography reveals a nonviable fetus, which may appear small for the
expected gestational age as a result of resorption.

Ectopic Pregnancy

Ectopic pregnancy, the implantation of the blastocyst in an abnormal site, occurs in
approximately 0.5% to 1% of all pregnancies. Predisposing factors include a history of

pelvic inflammatory disease, infertility, and therapeutic abortions, previous tubal reconstructive surgery, and the use of intrauterine contraceptive devices. Over 95% of ectopic pregnancies occur in the fallopian tube, with the ampullary portion being the most common tubal location. The remaining ectopic gestations occur in rare sites, such as the ovaries, abdomen, cervix, or retroperitoneal space. **Abdominal pregnancy** can be one of two types, primary or

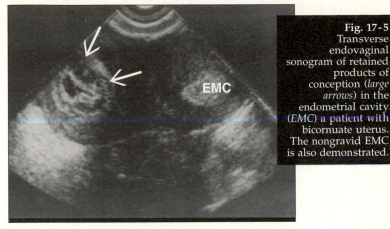

EMC

Fig. 17-5 Transverse endovaginal sonogram of retained products of conception (*large arrows*) in the endometrial cavity (*EMC*) a patient with bicornuate uterus. The nongravid EMC is also demonstrated.

secondary. In primary abdominal pregnancy the conceptus implants on the peritoneal surface, and the tubes and ovaries are normal. In secondary abdominal pregnancy, the most common, the embryo or fetus leaves the tube through a rupture of the fimbria and reimplants on maternal structures, such as the omentum or bowel. The clinician should become suspicious of abdominal pregnancy if the patient complains of unique gastrointestinal symptoms, has symptoms suggestive of spontaneous abortion or tubal ectopic, and experiences painful fetal movements or easily palpable movements. In **interstitial pregnancy,** implantation of the blastocyst occurs in the medial segment of the fallopian tube. Because this portion is surrounded by myometrial tissue or by the uterine vessels, this location presents a higher risk of serious hemorrhage when it ruptures. These ectopic gestations can survive to the end of the first trimester, which also increases the complication rate. Although still rare, the incidence of **heterotopic pregnancy,** or coexisting intrauterine and ectopic pregnancy, has increased. Clinical symptoms include a history of persistent pain after a spontaneous or therapeutic abortion or symptoms of ectopic pregnancy accompanied by uterine enlargement and other signs of intrauterine pregnancy.[11]

The most frequent clinical symptom of ectopic pregnancy is pelvic or lower abdominal pain that usually develops 1 to 8 weeks after the first missed menstrual period. Pain radiating to the shoulder or scapula area may indicate irritation from the leakage or rupture of the ectopic pregnancy. An increase in the severity of the pain is also indicative of a leak or rupture. Approximately 75% of patients will experience abnormal vaginal bleeding caused by the sloughing of the decidual casts in the uterine cavity. A pelvic examination usually reveals adnexal tenderness, and an adnexal mass is present in approximately one half of patients. Current treatment includes laparoscopic verification, if necessary, followed by surgical removal. In the case of an unruptured ectopic pregnancy the surgeon will attempt to save the fallopian tube and repair any other damage to increase the patient's chances for a subsequent intrauterine pregnancy.[14]

Over 80% of patients with an ectopic pregnancy will have a positive pregnancy test. The use of a β-hCG pregnancy test allows a highly sensitive quantification of maternal serum hCG, since ectopic gestations typically produce less hCG than a normal intrauterine pregnancy at the same gestational age. With endovaginal techniques, the discriminatory zone has been reported as 1025 mIU/ml (2nd IS), which corresponds to approximately a 5-mm to 6-mm gestational sac.[8,11] This gestational sac size is still fairly small, and maternal conditions such as uterine fibroids may impede visualization. In ectopic pregnancy, serial β-hCG tests usually reveal abnormal **subdoubling** when compared with an intrauterine pregnancy in which the hCG levels double every 2 to 3 days during the first 8 weeks.[13] With only transabdominal sonography, the discriminatory zone is approximately 1800 mIU/ml (2nd IS), since resolution parameters limit the ability to document a gestational sac of less than 1 cm.[8] Because of the high ligation rate involving ectopic pregnancies, the interpreting physician should request correlation of the sonographic findings with the β-hCG levels and request a repeat sonographic examination or additional clinical correlation if the sonographic findings are inconclusive.

The diagnostic sonographic signs for an ectopic pregnancy include documenting the lack of an intrauterine gestational sac and the visualization of an ectopic gestational sac containing a viable embryo (Fig. 17-6). The decidual reaction in the uterine cavity has been called the "pseudosac sign," since it can appear similar to an intrauterine gestational sac on transabdominal scans, and because it was a prime cause of misdiagnosis before the early 1980s.[9] On endovaginal sonography these sonographic signs may be seen from the beginning of the sixth week LNMP, but transabdominal techniques will not reliably visualize this pattern until 7 to 8 weeks LNMP. This time factor is crucial, since the risk of rupture increases by the seventh to eighth week. Suggestive signs for ectopic pregnancy include nonvisualization of an intrauterine pregnancy and a solid to complex extrauterine and extraovarian mass.[5] However, a corpus luteum cyst can form with an ectopic pregnancy, and it may visualize as a complex pattern. A leaking or ruptured ectopic pregnancy causes the development of free fluid or a hemoperitoneum in the posterior cul-de-sac (Fig.

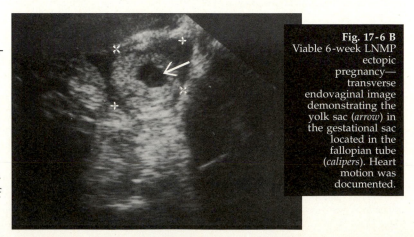

Fig. 17-6 A
Viable 6-week LNMP ectopic pregnancy—endovaginal scan demonstrating the left fallopian tube (*small arrows*) containing the hyperechoic "ring sign" (*large arrow*) suggestive of ectopic pregnancy.

Fig. 17-6 B
Viable 6-week LNMP ectopic pregnancy—transverse endovaginal image demonstrating the yolk sac (*arrow*) in the gestational sac located in the fallopian tube (*calipers*). Heart motion was documented.

17-7). The sonographer should examine the superior peritoneal spaces for evidence of further contamination (Fig. 17-8). Color-flow Doppler may provide additional information in locating the site of the ectopic pregnancy by demonstrating the increased vascularity at the implantation site and the lack of this pattern in the endometrial cavity (EMC).[4]

The sonographic verification of an abdominal pregnancy can be difficult. Suspicious signs include failure to visualize the uterine wall between the fetus and the urinary bladder, fetal parts adjacent to the maternal abdominal wall, and an abnormal fetal position in the maternal abdomen (Fig. 17-9). The definitive sonographic sign is the documentation of the uterus as a separate structure from the fetus.[15] This can be difficult, particularly later in the pregnancy. The placenta may appear in an unusual location, or it may lack its normal, regular borders (Fig. 17-10). An interstitial pregnancy can be difficult to differentiate. It may initially appear as if it is intrauterine, but closer evaluation can reveal that the myometrial mantle surrounding the sac is thinner than normal and that the sac has an abnormal location compared with the EMC. In heterotopic pregnancy both an intrauterine and ectopic pregnancy are visualized (Fig. 17-11). The sonographer must always perform a complete evaluation of the adnexal and cul-de-sac areas when an intrauterine pregnancy is seen.

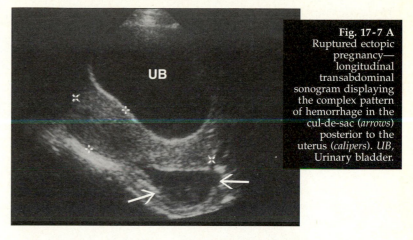

Fig. 17-7 A Ruptured ectopic pregnancy—longitudinal transabdominal sonogram displaying the complex pattern of hemorrhage in the cul-de-sac (*arrows*) posterior to the uterus (*calipers*). *UB*, Urinary bladder.

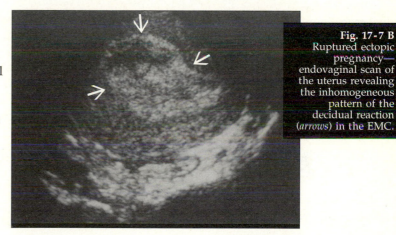

Fig. 17-7 B Ruptured ectopic pregnancy—endovaginal scan of the uterus revealing the inhomogeneous pattern of the decidual reaction (*arrows*) in the EMC.

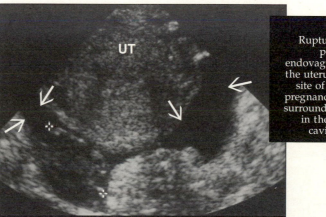

Fig. 17-7 C Ruptured ectopic pregnancy—endovaginal scan of the uterus (*UT*), the site of the ectopic pregnancy (*calipers*), surrounded by fluid in the peritoneal cavity (*arrows*).

Trophoblastic Disease

Trophoblastic disease consists of three categories: the hydatidiform mole, the invasive mole, and choriocarcinoma. All three derive from the fetal trophoblast. The benign hydatidiform mole, also called a complete or transitional mole, is the most common type with an incidence of 1:1500 pregnancies in the United States. This condition usually derives from a blighted ovum, but portions of the placenta may experience molar transformation during the second and third trimesters of pregnancy. One of the pathologic hallmarks of the hydatidiform mole is the marked edema and enlargement of the chorionic villi, producing the classic grapelike cluster of vesicles in the EMC. In invasive mole the molar tissue invades the myometrium or other adjacent structures and can produce distant metastasis. This neoplasm may cause hemorrhage if it disrupts the outer myometrium. Choriocarcinoma can develop during and after any pregnancy category, such as abortion or blighted ovum. Although capable of distant metastasis to the lungs and other organs, it is very responsive to chemotherapy.[1] Rarely, a fetus may coexist with a mole, but the fetus is usually triploidic with multiple congenital anomalies.[2]

The clinical symptoms for molar gestation include hyperemesis, the onset of hypertension before 20 weeks gestational age, vaginal bleeding or the passage of vesicular tissue, and a

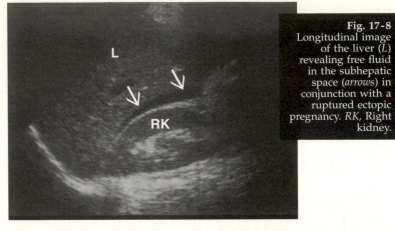

Fig. 17-8 Longitudinal image of the liver (*L*) revealing free fluid in the subhepatic space (*arrows*) in conjunction with a ruptured ectopic pregnancy. *RK*, Right kidney.

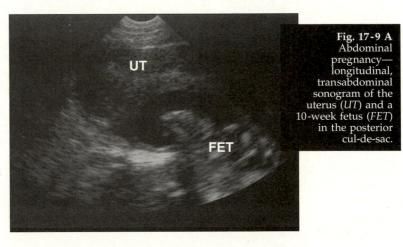

Fig. 17-9 A Abdominal pregnancy—longitudinal, transabdominal sonogram of the uterus (*UT*) and a 10-week fetus (*FET*) in the posterior cul-de-sac.

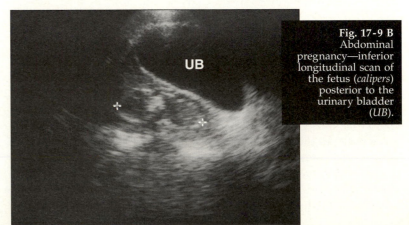

Fig. 17-9 B Abdominal pregnancy—inferior longitudinal scan of the fetus (*calipers*) posterior to the urinary bladder (*UB*).

large uterus for gestational age. Because of the autonomous secretion of hCG by the molar tissue, the hCG levels are abnormally high. This hypersecretion can produce ovarian theca lutein cysts, with a reported incidence ranging from 20% to 50% of patients.[1]

The classic sonographic pattern for the hydatidiform mole is a moderately hyperechoic soft tissue mass filling the EMC, which contains cystic vesicles of varying size[6] (Fig. 17-12). Although this pattern typically becomes apparent in the second trimester, the pattern may appear similar to a blighted ovum or an incomplete abortion during the first trimester. Correlation with β-hCG levels will allow a definitive diagnosis. Color Doppler may indicate increased vascularity in the molar tissue.[16] The sonographer should examine the adnexal areas for the presence of theca lutein cysts, which usually occur bilaterally and are often septated (Fig. 17-13). Differentiating the invasive mole is difficult. Suggestive signs include a loss of the myometrial mantle around the molar tissue and free-fluid or hemorrhagic areas adjacent to the uterus.[6] The uterine pattern of choriocarcinoma is usually the same as that demonstrated with the benign mole. The sonographer may examine the liver and lymph nodes for evidence of distant metastasis. The exact etiology is determined by the pathologic examination of the molar tissue after evacuation.

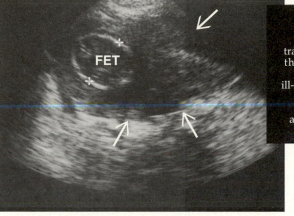

Fig. 17-9 C Abdominal pregnancy—transverse image of the fetal head (*FET, calipers*) and the ill-defined "uterine" walls (*arrows*) surrounding the amniotic fluid and fetus.

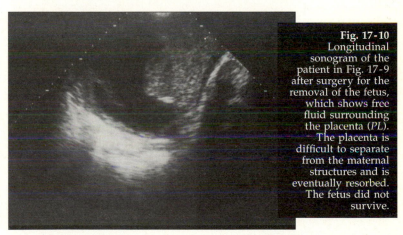

Fig. 17-10 Longitudinal sonogram of the patient in Fig. 17-9 after surgery for the removal of the fetus, which shows free fluid surrounding the placenta (*PL*). The placenta is difficult to separate from the maternal structures and is eventually resorbed. The fetus did not survive.

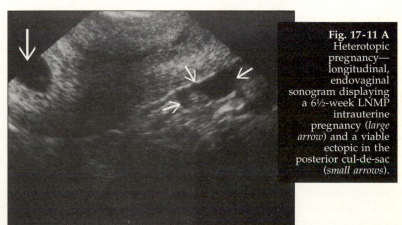

Fig. 17-11 A Heterotopic pregnancy—longitudinal, endovaginal sonogram displaying a 6½-week LNMP intrauterine pregnancy (*large arrow*) and a viable ectopic in the posterior cul-de-sac (*small arrows*).

Pseudocyesis

Pseudocyesis, or false pregnancy, is a psychologic condition wherein the patient exhibits many of the physical symptoms of pregnancy, including morning sickness and a distended abdomen, but is not pregnant. The typical patient either wants to become pregnant, but suffers from infertility, or is abnormally fearful of pregnancy. Some patients need intensive psychiatric treatment. The clinician may need to request a sonographic examination to rule out intrauterine or extrauterine pregnancy and may need to convince the patient that she is not pregnant.[12]

Uterine Anomalies

The clinician may experience difficulty in detecting uterine anomalies during pregnancy. However, diagnosing uterine anomalies is important, since they can lead to a higher incidence of spontaneous abortion, premature labor, and an increased perinatal morbidity and mortality.[12] In both uterus didelphys and the bicornate uterus, there are two EMC echo complexes, and sonography during the first trimester of pregnancy typically reveals a gestational sac in one cavity and a decidual reaction in the nongravid EMC (Fig. 17-14), which may be mistaken for a solid pelvic mass. In uterus septus or subseptus the amniotic fluid can allow the visualization of the septa as a moderately hyperechoic tissue band of varying thickness (Fig. 17-15). The sonographer must carefully follow the septa, noting

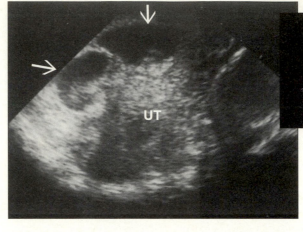

Fig. 17-11 B Heterotopic pregnancy—an endovaginal examination revealing an intrauterine twin gestation (*arrows*). *UT*, Uterus.

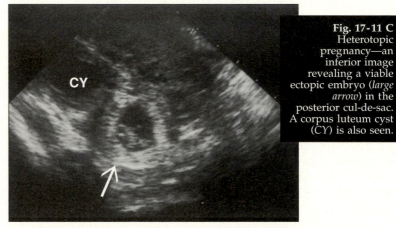

Fig. 17-11 C Heterotopic pregnancy—an inferior image revealing a viable ectopic embryo (*large arrow*) in the posterior cul-de-sac. A corpus luteum cyst (*CY*) is also seen.

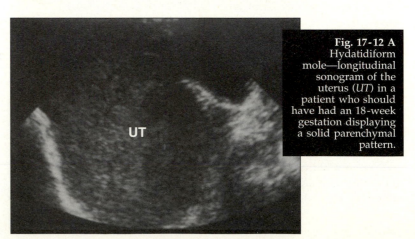

Fig. 17-12 A Hydatidiform mole—longitudinal sonogram of the uterus (*UT*) in a patient who should have had an 18-week gestation displaying a solid parenchymal pattern.

the position of the fetal structures and placenta, to determine where it terminates in relation to the lower uterine segment and the internal os.

Maternal Pelvic Masses

The clinician should to take a conservative approach in the management of a pelvic mass during pregnancy. Usually an obstetrician will simply monitor a pelvic mass during pregnancy if it appears to be benign, measures less than 6 cm, does not enlarge during the pregnancy, and does not threaten the normal development of the fetus or impede a normal vaginal delivery. The clinician will consider surgery for a mass that measures larger than 6 cm, enlarges during the pregnancy, or threatens the fetus. Surgeons prefer to perform surgery during the second trimester, since the effects of anesthesia on the fetus are more predictable, and surgery during the third trimester is more difficult as a result of the size of the fetus.[12]

Clinical symptoms of a pelvic mass during pregnancy include a palpable mass and pain. The consistency of the mass and its location are important, since some masses have a high risk of rupture during normal labor and delivery. The clinician will also determine if the mass is fixed or movable, which also influences the decision regarding a vaginal delivery or a cesarean section. The use of prevoid and postvoid images and the decubitus or Trendelenburg position can assess the movability of the

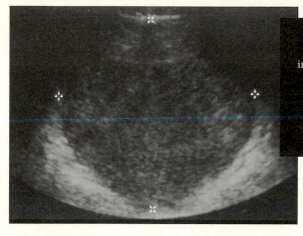

Fig. 17-12 B Hydfatidiform mole—transverse image of the uterus (*calipers*) with the characteristic soft tissue pattern of a molar pregnancy. The β-hCG levels were abnormally high.

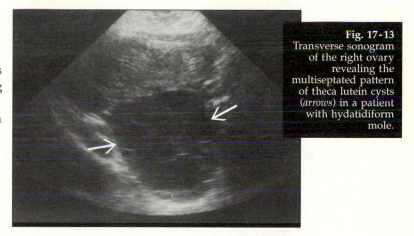

Fig. 17-13 Transverse sonogram of the right ovary revealing the multiseptated pattern of theca lutein cysts (*arrows*) in a patient with hydatidiform mole.

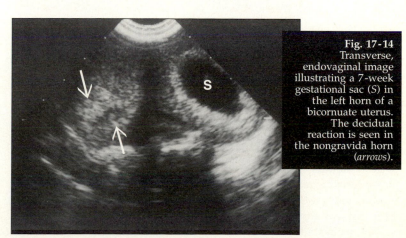

Fig. 17-14 Transverse, endovaginal image illustrating a 7-week gestational sac (*S*) in the left horn of a bicornuate uterus. The decidual reaction is seen in the nongravida horn (*arrows*).

mass. If the urinary bladder displaces the mass, it is probably movable. If the mass displaces the urinary bladder, it is probably fixed.

Uterine fibroids, one of the most common pelvic masses, may enlarge during pregnancy as a result of hormonal stimulation. The sonographic pattern ranges from hypoechoic to hyperechoic, with areas of calcification (Fig. 17-16), and may contain cystic areas of degeneration, which can occur if they grow quickly during the pregnancy. **Corpus luteum cysts,** a normal finding during early pregnancy, usually regress and are reabsorbed by 12 to 15 weeks LNMP. Occasionally they persist into the second trimester and may attain a size of 10 cm. These cysts have a tendency to bleed, leading to a complex pattern. As they resolve, they may appear as a solid mass. Serial scans will often reveal the continuing evolution of the cyst with a corresponding pattern change. A corpus luteum cyst and a cystic neoplasm are included in the differential diagnosis when an adnexal cyst is first discovered during the second trimester. Serial scans may again narrow the diagnosis if the cyst disappears later. **Dermoid cysts** may initially become symptomatic during pregnancy. Their sonographic pattern ranges from cystic to complex, with areas of acoustic shadowing, to a solid pattern. **Serous cystadenoma** may present as a unilocular or multilocular cystic adnexal mass, which may attain a large size. **Mucinous cystadenoma** typically

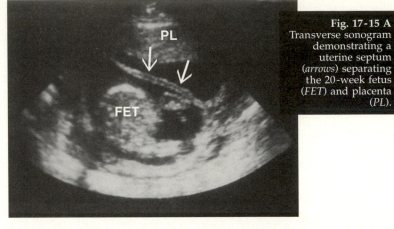

Fig. 17-15 A Transverse sonogram demonstrating a uterine septum (*arrows*) separating the 20-week fetus (*FET*) and placenta (*PL*).

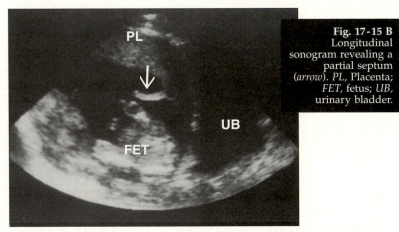

Fig. 17-15 B Longitudinal sonogram revealing a partial septum (*arrow*). *PL*, Placenta; *FET*, fetus; *UB*, urinary bladder.

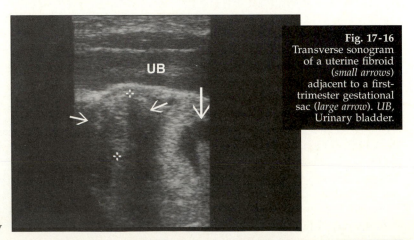

Fig. 17-16 Transverse sonogram of a uterine fibroid (*small arrows*) adjacent to a first-trimester gestational sac (*large arrow*). *UB*, Urinary bladder.

contains septations and a gelatinous material. For both of these masses the sonographer should look for ascites, which may indicate malignancy, and the presence of pseudomyxoma peritonei with mucinous cystadenoma. Other causes of ascites during pregnancy include toxemia of pregnancy and hepatic cirrhosis. **Theca lutein cysts** are the result of excessive hormonal stimulation and are typically associated with a molar pregnancy. However, they may also develop in a multiple pregnancy or in conjunction with fetal hydrops. They typically present as multilocular, bilateral cystic masses and usually regress after the pregnancy. **Pelvic inflammatory disease (PID)** and **intraabdominal abscess,** which rarely occur during pregnancy, may appear as cystic, complex, or solid adnexal or abdominal masses. With PID the sonographer may find an enlarged fallopian tube, a tubo-ovarian abscess, or an abscess in the posterior cul-de-sac. If not treated early, these infections can lead to increased maternal and fetal morbidity and mortality.

Ectopic organs, such as a pelvic kidney, can present as an adnexal mass and may interfere with a vaginal delivery. The sonographic pattern consists of a reniform solid mass with the hyperechoic central renal sinus. The sonographer should examine the distal ureter for signs of dilatation and the contralateral kidney for evidence of obstruction. The nongravid horn of a bicornate uterus may be mistaken for a solid adnexal mass, but the depiction of the hyperechoic EMC will allow proper identification. The sonographer should remember to scan the kidneys, since renal anomalies are associated with uterine anomalies. The patient may develop **hydronephrosis** during the latter half of the pregnancy. Because of the course of the right ureter, fetal pressure will more likely cause the development of right hydronephrosis. Although bilateral hydronephrosis is not common, the sonographer should examine both kidneys if the patient complains of flank or back pain. Other maternal complications include cholelithiasis, pancreatitis, vascular aneurysms, and bowel obstructions.

TECHNICAL PITFALLS

As mentioned previously, an overdistended urinary bladder can make an early normal pregnancy appear abnormal. Because of a lack of resolution, normal gestational sacs may appear abnormal on transabdominal examinations, but endovaginal scans will reveal a normal, viable pregnancy. The converse is also true. An early pregnancy can appear normal on transabdominal images, but endovaginal scans will reveal an abnormal gestation.

The sonographer should remember that ectopic pregnancies can lie superior to the uterine fundus and that this area must always be evaluated. If a transabdominal scan appears normal during the early part of the first trimester and the patient has a history that includes the possibility of an ectopic pregnancy, the patient should receive an endovaginal examination.

SUMMARY

Sonography plays a crucial role in the management of complications of the first trimester. The value of the β-hCG test cannot be overstressed. In many instances the correlation of the hCG levels with the sonographic examination is necessary to make a more confident diagnosis. Endovaginal sonography provides the necessary resolution to determine the findings earlier in the pregnancy than can be demonstrated with the transabdominal technique. Table 17-1 provides a summary of the related clinical laboratory test findings with the specific types of abnormal conditions during the first trimester.

TABLE 17-1   THE ABNORMAL FIRST-TRIMESTER PREGNANCY–Correlation with Clinical Laboratory Tests

	Gestational Age	*β-hCG*	*OTHER*
BLIGHTED OVUM	2 to 7 weeks*	Weakly positive to negative[†]	
THREATENED ABORTION	6 to 8 weeks	Positive to weakly positive	Positive or negative heart motion
INEVITABLE ABORTION	Varies	Weakly positive to negative	Negative heart motion
INCOMPLETE ABORTION	Varies	Weakly positive to negative	Retained products
COMPLETE ABORTION	Varies	Weakly positive to negative	Endometrial cavity < 7 mm
MISSED ABORTION	Varies	Weakly positive to negative	
ECTOPIC PREGNANCY	4 to 8 weeks	Weakly positive	No intrauterine pregnancy for corresponding LNMP
HYDATIDIFORM MOLE	Varies	High	
PSEUDOCYESIS	Varies	Negative	

*Based on last normal menstrual period (LNMP).
[†]Weakly positive values based on normal values according to LNMP and/or serial evaluations.

REFERENCES

1. Atrash HK, Hogne JR, Grimes DA: Epidemiology of hydatidiform mole during early gestation, *Am J Obstet Gynecol* 154:906-909, 1986.
2. Bree RL, Silver TM, et al: Trophoblastic disease with coexistent fetus: a sonographic and clinical perspective, *J Clin Ultrasound* 6:310-314, 1978.
3. Cashner KA, Christopher CR, Dysert GA: Spontaneous fetal loss after documentation of a live fetus in the first trimester, *Obstet Gynecol* 70:827-830, 1987.
4. Dillon EH, Taylor KJW: *Doppler ultrasound in the female pelvis and first trimester of pregnancy.* In Clinics in diagnostic ultrasound, Vol 26, New York, 1990, Churchill Livingstone, pp 106-109.
5. Filly RA: Ectopic pregnancy: the role of sonography, *Radiology* 162:661-668, 1987.
6. Munyer TP, Callen PW, et al: Further observations on the sonographic spectrum of gestational trophoblastic disease, *J Clin Ultrasound* 91:349-358, 1981.
7. Nyberg DA, Filly RA, et al: Abnormal pregnancy: early diagnosis by US and serum chorionic gonadotropin, *Radiology* 158:393-396, 1986.
8. Nyberg DA, Filly RA, et al: Ectopic pregnancy diagnosis by sonography correlated with quantitative β-hCG levels, *J Clin Ultrasound* 6:145-150, 1987.
9. Nyberg DA, Laing FC, et al: Ultrasonic differentiation of the gestational sac of early pregnancy from the pseudogestational sac of ectopic pregnancy, *Radiology* 146:755-759, 1978.
10. Nyberg DA, Laing FC, Filly RA: Threatened abortion: sonographic distinction of normal and abnormal gestation sacs, *Radiology* 158:397-400, 1986.
11. Nyberg DA, Mack LA, et al: Endovaginal sonographic evaluation of ectopic pregnancy: a prospective study, *AJR* 149:1181-1186, 1987.
12. Pernoll ML, Benson RC, editors: *Current obstetric and gynecologic diagnosis and treatment*, ed 6, Norwalk, Conn, 1987, Appleton and Lange, pp 255-270.
13. Pittway D: β-hCG dynamics in ectopic pregnancy, *Clin Obstet Gynecol* 30:130-132, 1987.
14. Russell JB: The etiology of ectopic pregnancy, *Clin Obstet Gynecol* 30:183-184, 1987.
15. Stanley JH, Horgen EO III, et al: Sonographic findings in abdominal pregnancy, *AJR* 147:1043-1046, 1986.
16. Taylor KJW, Schwartz PE, Koharn EI: Gestational trophoblastic neoplasia: diagnosis with Doppler ultrasound, *Radiology* 165:445-448, 1987.

normal second- and third-trimester pregnancy

INSTRUCTIONAL OBJECTIVES

At the completion of this chapter, the reader will be able to:

1. Describe the clinical problems that are typical reasons for the sonographic evaluation of the second- and third-trimester pregnancy.
2. Describe the basic scanning protocol for the sonographic examination of the second- and third-trimester pregnancy as recommended by professional organizations, including calculations for gestational dating and growth determinations.
3. Determine the fetal lie while performing a sonographic examination.
4. Identify on sectional sonograms the major anatomic structures of the fetus, including the spine, stomach, kidneys, urinary bladder, cord insert, heart, and intracranial structures, such as the ventricular system.
5. Describe the basic anatomic landmarks used for obtaining the biparietal diameter, occipitofrontal diameter, head circumference, cephalic index, femur length, and abdominal circumference.
6. Identify other measurement techniques, and describe the conditions that warrant their use.
7. Describe several technical pitfalls associated with the sonographic examination of the second- and third-trimester pregnancy.

THE CLINICAL PROBLEM

The patient who has a history of irregular menstrual periods or who is uncertain about the date of her last menstrual period will often require a sonographic examination for determining the gestational age. Also, it is more difficult to determine an accurate gestational age by physical examination in the patient who is obese or who did not receive obstetric care during the first trimester. Other reasons for sonography during the second and third trimesters include vaginal bleeding, small or large for gestational age, risk factors for congenital anomalies, maternal complications such as preeclampsia or diabetes, and suspected multiple gestation. These latter reasons are discussed in later chapters. This chapter discusses the basic scanning protocol, the normal fetal anatomy, and the determination of gestational age and growth calculations.

OBTAINING THE CLINICAL HISTORY

The sonographer should obtain the patient's pertinent clinical history, including the number of previous pregnancies, deliveries, and abortions (miscarriages), as well as the last normal menstrual period. To keep her anxiety to a minimum, the sonographer should always tell the patient that these are routine questions that are asked of every patient. The answers should provide any history of birth defects in previous pregnancies or in related family members, any occurrence of vaginal bleeding, and other maternal factors, such as hypertension or diabetes. Maternal smoking during pregnancy can cause intrauterine growth retardation and a lower birth weight in babies. If the patient smokes, she should be asked to estimate the number of cigarettes smoked per day. Another good question that the sonographer should ask every patient is if her physician informed her of the reason for the examination. This answer can provide correlation with the information provided by the referring physician at the time the examination was ordered. It may also allow the sonographer to determine the concerns of the physician, if no reason for the examination had been previously given.

CLINICAL LABORATORY TESTS

The primary screening clinical laboratory test is performed to determine the levels of the maternal serum **alpha-fetoprotein (AFP).** These levels become elevated with a number of fetal anomalies and other abnormalities. The most suspicious anomaly group is open neural tube defects, such as spina bifida and anencephaly. Other conditions associated with elevated AFP levels include gastrointestinal obstructions, omphalocele, fetal distress, fetal death, and severe Rh immunization. A normal multiple gestation can also produce elevated AFP levels, since the levels may be based on the normal ranges for a singleton pregnancy. A thorough sonographic evaluation is necessary to determine the cause for elevated AFP levels. Chapter 21 discusses the sonographic patterns for many of the fetal anomalies associated with abnormal AFP values.

SCANNING PROTOCOLS AND TECHNIQUES

Several professional organizations, including the American Institute of Ultrasound in Medicine (AIUM), the American College of Radiology (ACR), and the American College of Obstetricians and Gynecologists (ACOG), have published guidelines for the performance of obstetric sonographic examinations. These guidelines contain similar criteria, but the AIUM guidelines include the following major criteria.[1] For the second and third trimester, the routine examination should document the fetal number and presentation, as well as the fetal heart motion. The amount of amniotic fluid should be evaluated in comparison with the normal amount or to determine if oligohydramnios or polyhydramnios is present. The sonographer should document the position of the placenta, note the grade or abnormalities, and verify placental position in relation to the internal cervical os. The primary calculations for gestational age assessment are the biparietal diameter (BPD), head circumference, and the femur length. For fetal growth and weight estimates, the sonographer must also obtain the abdominal circumference. Each examination should also include an evaluation of the uterus and adnexal areas for the presence of maternal pathology. Every study should also include a survey of fetal anatomy to assess fetal physiologic functions and to exclude a number of anomalies. At a minimum the protocol during the second and third trimesters should survey the following:

Fetal Age and Growth
1. BPD
2. Head circumference or cephalic index
3. Abdominal circumference
4. Femur length
5. Estimation of fetal weight

Fetal Anatomy
1. Cerebral ventricles to rule out hydrocephaly
2. Four-chamber heart and heart position within the thoracic cavity
3. Spine to rule out spina bifida
4. Stomach to assess function and rule out anomalies
5. Kidneys to rule out anomalies and obstruction
6. Urinary bladder to assess renal function and rule out obstruction
7. Umbilical cord insertion to rule out abnormalities of the anterior abdominal wall
8. Three-vessel cord
9. Fetal lie in relation to maternal longitudinal axis

Placenta and Maternal Anatomy
1. Anatomic location and grade
2. Position of placenta in relation to internal cervical os
3. Amount of amniotic fluid
4. Uterus for fibroids and other abnormalities
5. Adnexal areas to rule out masses

Some ultrasound departments may include a more extensive survey as part of the routine examination. A patient who is at risk for congenital anomalies or other complications of pregnancy or has an anomaly that is discovered during a routine examination warrants a more extensive examination. An expanded protocol may include examining the nuchal skin fold on the posterior aspect of the neck, evaluating all extremities for normal growth and ossification, and including a detailed evaluation of the heart. Some ultrasound departments may not feel qualified to perform this type of advanced examination. Everyone involved in sonography must evaluate individual skills and limitations and determine when to refer a patient to a regional center that specializes in high-risk obstetrics. A department increases its legal risks if it attempts to manage a patient who has pathology that exceeds its level of expertise.

Determining the fetal position in relation to the maternal anatomy often poses a challenge to the inexperienced sonographer. The clinical categories of presentation are discussed in Chapter 15. During the sonographic examination the sonographer should document the presenting fetal part in relation to the internal cervical os. In the **vertex presentation,** the head of the fetus is adjacent to the internal cervical os, and the long axis of the fetus is parallel to the maternal long axis. In the **breech presentation** the fetal rump or lower extremities are adjacent to the internal cervical os, but the long axis of the fetus remains parallel to the maternal long axis. In the **transverse presentation** the long axis of the fetus is perpendicular to the maternal long axis, and there is no definitive presenting part. **Oblique presentations** are clinical variations of the transverse position, but the sonographer can often identify the head or the rump as the fetal part closest to the internal cervical os and obtain an oblique longitudinal scan that indicates the fetal lie in relation to the maternal long axis. The sonographer should remember that fetal position varies during pregnancy, but major changes of fetal presentation late in the third trimester are not as common as changes during the second trimester.

The sonographer must also identify the fetal left and right to determine the normal position of fetal structures, such as the stomach and heart. Scanning through the transverse axis of the fetus allows immediate identification of the fetal spine, but many sonographers prefer localizing the fetal spine on survey longitudinal images. In the **vertex** presentation the fetus is lying on its **right side** if the fetal spine is on the **maternal right** (Fig. 18-1). If the fetal spine is on the **maternal left,** the fetus is lying on its **left side.** In the **breech** presentation the fetus is lying on its **left side** if the fetal spine is on the **maternal right** (Fig. 18-2). If the fetal spine is on the **maternal left,** the fetus is lying on its **right side.** If this is difficult to conceptualize, the sonographer should use a doll, place it in the various types of presentation in relation to his or her abdomen, and then identify the fetal right and left.

NORMAL SONOGRAPHIC PATTERNS

The sonographer must recognize numerous maternal and fetal anatomic structures. This section describes the sonographic patterns for those structures, which are included in the minimum scanning guidelines. Examination of additional fetal organs and structures may allow differentiation of suspected fetal anomalies and, as a result, are used for advanced sonographic protocols. All scanning planes are in reference to the fetus; that

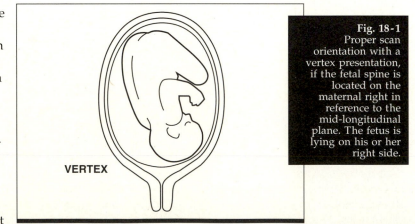

VERTEX

Fig. 18-1
Proper scan orientation with a vertex presentation, if the fetal spine is located on the maternal right in reference to the mid-longitudinal plane. The fetus is lying on his or her right side.

is, longitudinal refers to the long axis of the fetus.

The **fetal spine** has three ossification centers, which appear as hyperechoic, rounded structures arranged in the shape of a V on transverse images (Fig. 18-3). The bilateral back muscles should appear symmetrical, and the skin line should course as a continuous hyperechoic line. The entire spine should be scanned transversely, and several representative images can be preserved on hard copy, particularly the sacrolumbar area, which is the most common site for spina bifida. Longitudinal views of the spine depict the two posterior ossification centers coursing parallel with each other superiorly, tapering inferiorly, and merging in the region of the coccyx (Fig. 18-4). The cervical spine normally widens as it reaches the occipital area (Fig. 18-5). This view also depicts the soft tissue and posterior skin line, which can help in the identification of a meningocele. The sonographer should remember that a minimum of two scanning planes are necessary to adequately examine any fetal structure. The coronal view images the fetal body in the posteroanterior dimension and allows identification of more subtle spinal widening.[10] The normal coronal image of the sacrolumbar region should demonstrate a normal tapering of the ossification centers between the iliac wings (Fig. 18-6).

In the **fetal neck** the sonographer may identify the carotid arteries, thyroid, esophagus, and tongue. These structures have

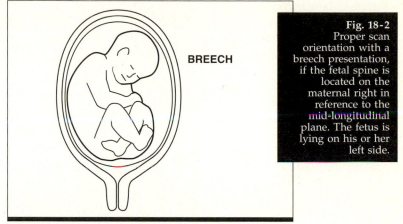

Fig. 18-2
Proper scan orientation with a breech presentation, if the fetal spine is located on the maternal right in reference to the mid-longitudinal plane. The fetus is lying on his or her left side.

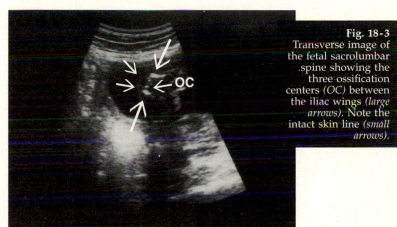

Fig. 18-3
Transverse image of the fetal sacrolumbar spine showing the three ossification centers *(OC)* between the iliac wings *(large arrows)*. Note the intact skin line *(small arrows)*.

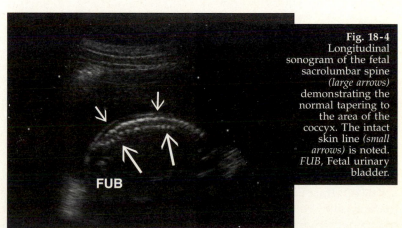

Fig. 18-4
Longitudinal sonogram of the fetal sacrolumbar spine *(large arrows)* demonstrating the normal tapering to the area of the coccyx. The intact skin line *(small arrows)* is noted. *FUB,* Fetal urinary bladder.

the same anatomic relationships as in the adult (see Chapter 9) and are not routinely evaluated. However, there have been reported cases of thyroid enlargement, or goiter,[2] and the esophagus must be imaged in suspected cases of esophageal atresia. The use of color-flow Doppler can identify the movement of amniotic fluid through the fetal mouth.

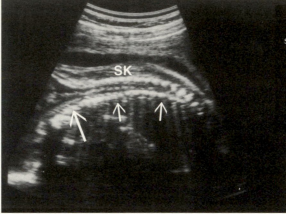

Fig. 18-5
Longitudinal sonogram of the fetal cervical spine (*small arrows*) displaying the normal widening in the occipital region (*large arrow*). Note the intact skin line (*SK*).

The sonographer can identify numerous structures in the **fetal brain.** In the transverse plane and beginning inferiorly at the level of the occiput, the petrous ridges and sphenoid wings form a hyperechoic X in the central portion of the calvaria. This is the location of the fourth ventricle and the **posterior fossa,** which is the prime location for a Dandy-Walker cyst and other anomalies. Scanning more superiorly in the fetal head, the **cerebellum,** a butterfly-shaped structure, is seen in the posterior portion of the skull, slightly inferior to the thalamus[14] (Fig. 18-7). Cerebellar measurements can be used as an additional gestational age estimate during the second trimester.[20] Moving slightly superior, the standard plane for the BPD comes into view. The **falx cerebri** connects the two cerebral hemispheres and appears as a hyperechoic line coursing through the midline from anterior to posterior (Fig. 18-8). The **thalami** are hypoechoic, diamond- or heart-shaped structures, which lie on either side of the falx in the central portion of the brain. The slitlike **third ventricle** lies between the thalami

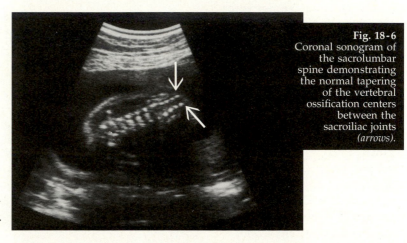

Fig. 18-6
Coronal sonogram of the sacrolumbar spine demonstrating the normal tapering of the vertebral ossification centers between the sacroiliac joints (*arrows*).

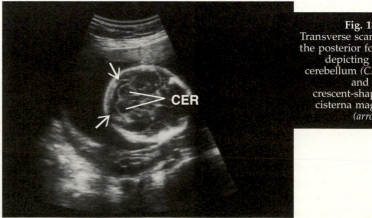

Fig. 18-7
Transverse scan of the posterior fossa depicting the cerebellum (*CER*) and the crescent-shaped cisterna magna (*arrow*).

and normally measures less than 3 mm.[4] Anterior to the thalami, the **cavum septum pellucidum** appears as a boxlike, hypoechoic to anechoic structure or may appear as a parallel, hyperechoic line on either side of the falx. Scanning superiorly, the bodies of the **lateral ventricles** appear adjacent to the falx (Fig. 18-9). The medial walls are close to the falx, and axial resolution limitations may not allow their discrete visualization. During the first trimester and early second trimester the ventricular diameter is normally larger in relation to the cerebral hemispheres, but this must not be mistaken for ventriculomegaly. Also, the choroid plexus is still prominent and must not be misidentified as a solid mass.

Scanning the **fetal chest,** rib ossification begins early and appears as hyperechoic areas, which produce acoustic shadowing. The scapula appears on a longitudinal or coronal scan of the fetus as a hyperechoic, linear structure seen posteriorly in the upper chest on either side of the vertebral column. The lungs, which contain no air, display a homogeneous echogenic pattern that is usually slightly hypoechoic when compared with the normal liver parenchymal pattern. The diaphragm appears as a hypoechoic, curved, linear area between the lungs and the liver (Fig. 18-10). During the third trimester the lungs may appear hyperechoic compared with the normal liver pattern.

The **heart** begins to beat at the end of the fifth week LNMP.

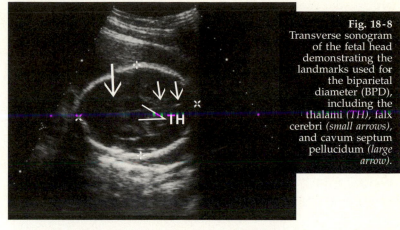

Fig. 18-8 Transverse sonogram of the fetal head demonstrating the landmarks used for the biparietal diameter (BPD), including the thalami *(TH)*, falx cerebri *(small arrows),* and cavum septum pellucidum *(large arrow).*

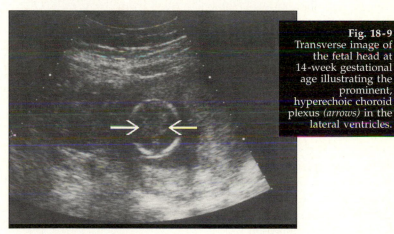

Fig. 18-9 Transverse image of the fetal head at 14-week gestational age illustrating the prominent, hyperechoic choroid plexus *(arrows)* in the lateral ventricles.

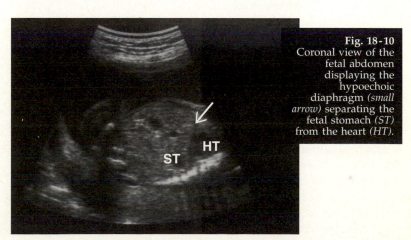

Fig. 18-10 Coronal view of the fetal abdomen displaying the hypoechoic diaphragm *(small arrow)* separating the fetal stomach *(ST)* from the heart *(HT).*

Cardiac valve motion and the movement of the foramen ovale are usually apparent by 16 weeks LNMP, and endovaginal techniques may allow earlier visualization. The fetal circulation has several unique pathways compared with the adult circulatory system (Fig. 18-11). Oxygenated blood leaves the placenta via the **umbilical vein,** enters the fetus through the umbilicus, and travels superiorly to the fetal liver where it connects with the portal system. In the adult the remnants of the fetal umbilical vein form the ligamentum teres. Some of this blood feeds the fetal liver cells and eventually leaves the liver through the hepatic veins into the inferior vena cava (IVC), entering into the right atrium of the heart. Most of the oxygenated blood reaches the right atrium through the **ductus venosus,** a small vessel that connects the portal system to the IVC. In the adult the remnants of the ductus venosus form the ligamentum venosum. Most of the blood that enters the **right atrium** passes into the left atrium via the **foramen ovale,** through the **mitral valve** into the left ventricle, and then into the ascending aorta through the **aortic valve.** The small amount of blood remaining in the right atrium passes through the **tricuspid valve** into the right ventricle and into the pulmonary artery via the **pulmonary valve.** Only a small amount of this oxygen-rich blood travels to the lungs, since it provides oxygen only to lung tissue. Therefore most of the blood courses from the pulmo-

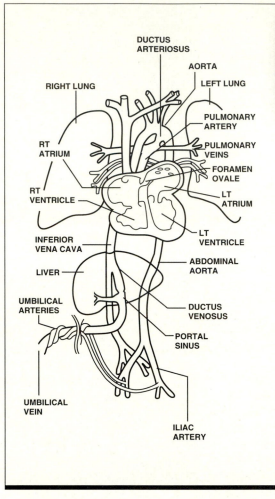

Fig. 18-11
Fetal circulatory system. Note the unique connections, including the ductus venosus, foramen ovale, and ductus arteriosus.

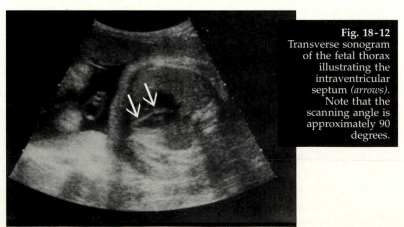

Fig. 18-12
Transverse sonogram of the fetal thorax illustrating the intraventricular septum *(arrows).* Note that the scanning angle is approximately 90 degrees.

nary artery into the aorta through the **ductus arteriosus.** The aorta then distributes the blood to all fetal tissue through its many tributaries. Approximately one half of this blood remains in the descending aorta and leaves the fetal circulation through the **umbilical arteries** and then on to the placenta for reoxygenation.

The fetal heart occupies approximately one third of the fetal thoracic cavity and lies with the apex, or inferior aspect, pointing to the left of midline. The right ventricle lies closest to the anterior chest wall, and the left atrium is usually the most posterior chamber. The two atrial chambers are approximately equal in size, and the foramen ovale will appear sonographically as a hyperechoic linear structure moving in the left atrium. The two ventricular chambers are usually equal in size, or the right ventricle may appear slightly larger than the left. The left ventricle will enlarge after birth as a result of increased demand. The **ventricular septum** divides the two ventricles and should appear as a continuous, echogenic border between them. To ensure that no septal defect is present, the ventricular septum must be scanned at a 90-degree angle to the transducer (Fig. 18-12), in order to use axial resolution and to properly image a specular reflector.[6]

The standard four-chamber view of the fetal heart is obtained on a transverse scan of the fetal thorax[5] (Fig. 18-13). This view allows an evaluation of chamber size and the position of the heart in the chest. The proper scanning window will allow a perpendicular angulation to evaluate the atrial septum, which should only demonstrate the small opening of the foramen ovale. The transverse plane may also allow for the evaluation of the ventricular septum, but an apical view may provide a better delineation of the septum, as well as the four heart chambers. For the apical view the transducer is placed inferior to the fetal heart and angled superiorly.

In the fetal abdomen the **liver** occupies the entire posteroanterior dimension of the right upper quadrant. The left lobe is more prominent in the fetus than it is in the adult. The liver parenchyma should display a homogeneous sonographic pattern that is slightly hyperechoic when compared with the normal lung pattern in the second-trimester fetus. The **gallbladder** often appears as an anechoic, ovoid-shaped structure located lateral to the umbilical vein (Fig. 18-14). It can be mistaken for the umbilical vein when obtaining the image for the abdominal circumference measurement. The **stomach** appears as a cystic structure in the left upper quadrant (Fig. 18-15), anterior to the left adrenal gland. Normally the left kidney lies inferior to the stomach. During the second trimester the **fetal bowel** usually appears as echogenic loops in the mid and lower abdomen because of the presence of normal meconium. Particularly in the third trimester, several fluid-filled loops of the bowel may be seen. Normal small bowel loops should measure less than 7 mm.[15] Meconium is not normally passed until after birth, but a normal fluid-

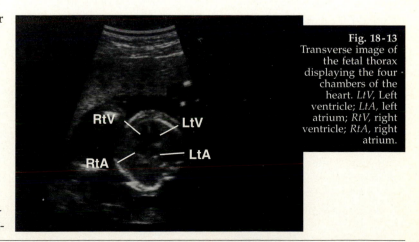

Fig. 18-13
Transverse image of the fetal thorax displaying the four chambers of the heart. *LtV,* Left ventricle; *LtA,* left atrium; *RtV,* right ventricle; *RtA,* right atrium.

filled colon (1 cm or less) and rectum may be seen, particularly during the mid to late third trimester.[18] The pancreas may be identified by the same vascular landmarks that are used in the adult. It is slightly hyperechoic to the liver, although a pancreas examination is rarely indicated.

The fetal **adrenal glands** are prominent structures that have a similar shape and sonographic pattern as the fetal kidneys. The adrenal glands are most consistently seen in the latter half of the third trimester. By the third trimester the medulla may appear as a hyperechoic central area surrounded by the hypoechoic cortex (Fig. 18-16). Early in the second trimester the fetal **kidneys** display as hypoechoic structures adjacent to the spine. Later in the second trimester and in the third trimester the sonographer can identify the renal sinus, renal pyramids, and perirenal fat[3] (Fig. 18-17). With normal function, the renal pelvis may appear as a cystic area at the medial aspect of the kidney and should not measure more than 5 mm in the posteroanterior dimension.[11,13] The **urinary bladder** displays as a rounded cystic structure in the fetal pelvis, bordered by the hyperechoic iliac wings (Fig. 18-18). It fills or partially empties in approximately 1 hour. The sonographer can identify the **external genitalia** as early as 14 weeks LNMP and consistently after 18 weeks.[8] On a transverse scan of the inferior fetal pelvis, the scrotum and penis typically appear as hyper-

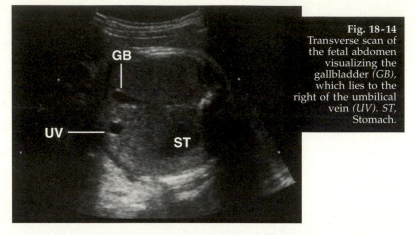

Fig. 18-14
Transverse scan of the fetal abdomen visualizing the gallbladder *(GB)*, which lies to the right of the umbilical vein *(UV)*. *ST*, Stomach.

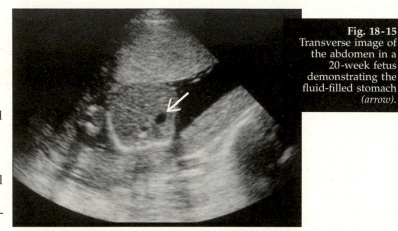

Fig. 18-15
Transverse image of the abdomen in a 20-week fetus demonstrating the fluid-filled stomach *(arrow)*.

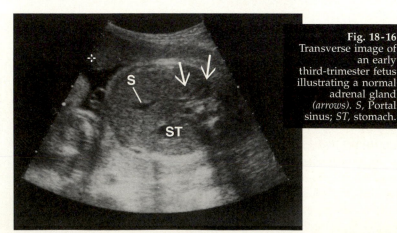

Fig. 18-16
Transverse image of an early third-trimester fetus illustrating a normal adrenal gland *(arrows)*. *S*, Portal sinus; *ST*, stomach.

echoic rounded masses (Fig. 18-19). Changing the scanning plane can allow the identification of the elongated penis surrounded by the scrotal sac. Since loops of umbilical cord can be mistaken for the scrotum, identification of the penis will allow a more confident identification of the sex. In the female fetus a transverse view of the inferior pelvis at the level of the buttocks allows visualization of the **labia,** which appear as two hyperechoic linear echoes (Fig. 18-20).

In a transverse plane slightly superior to the urinary bladder, the **umbilical cord insertion** should appear as one or more cord vessels bordered by the hyperechoic cord walls entering at the midline, with intact abdominal wall musculature, and with skin displayed as a moderately hyperechoic linear echo group (Fig. 18-21). The normal skin thickness is 2 to 3 mm. If the fetus remains in the prone position, the umbilical cord insertion cannot be optimally imaged.

The **umbilical cord** contains three vessels—the larger single umbilical vein and two smaller umbilical arteries, which are surrounded by the echogenic **wharton's jelly** (Fig. 18-22). The two arteries normally coil around the umbilical vein.

During the second and third trimesters the **fetal extremities** are readily identifiable as a result of bone ossification. However, identifying the extremities and performing a complete evaluation are difficult during the latter portion of the third trimester

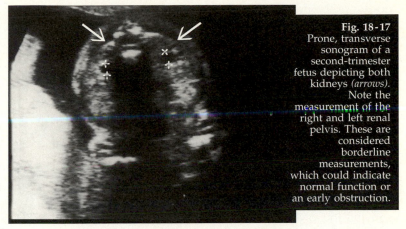

Fig. 18-17
Prone, transverse sonogram of a second-trimester fetus depicting both kidneys *(arrows)*. Note the measurement of the right and left renal pelvis. These are considered borderline measurements, which could indicate normal function or an early obstruction.

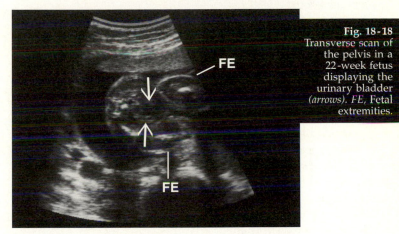

Fig. 18-18
Transverse scan of the pelvis in a 22-week fetus displaying the urinary bladder *(arrows)*. *FE,* Fetal extremities.

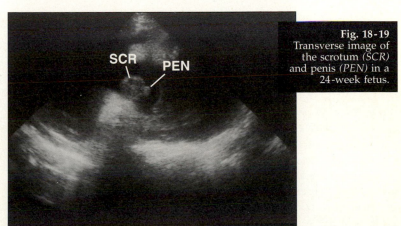

Fig. 18-19
Transverse image of the scrotum *(SCR)* and penis *(PEN)* in a 24-week fetus.

because of the tight fetal position and the normal decline in the amniotic fluid volume. During the second trimester, identification is easier and includes differentiation of the fingers and toes. The sonographer can identify the superior and inferior portions of each extremity by the number of bones. The upper arm contains the humerus, and the lower arm contains the ulna and radius. The upper leg contains the femur, and the lower leg consists of the tibia and fibula (Fig. 18-23). Some departments include documentation of the fetal extremities in its routine scanning protocol.

SONOGRAPHIC MEASUREMENTS FOR GESTATIONAL AGE

Biparietal Diameter

The biparietal diameter (BPD) is the most accurate measurement for predicting gestational age when obtained between 14 and 24 weeks; yet its accuracy declines during the third trimester. Usually the maximum rate of growth occurs between 14 and 20 weeks, averaging 3 to 4 mm per week. At approximately 30 weeks the growth rate slows to an average of 2 mm per week. The plane of section for the BPD is a transverse scan at the level of the thalamus and cavum septum pellucidum.[12] The scanning plane must be perpendicular to the lateral skull walls to display the falx cerebri as a midline structure. This angulation is referred to as the **angle of asynclitism** and varies according to fetal position. For example, if the fetus is in the vertex presentation

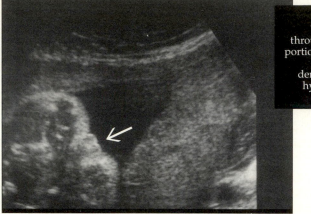

Fig. 18-20 Transverse scan through the inferior portion of the female fetal pelvis demonstrating the hyperechoic labia *(arrow)*.

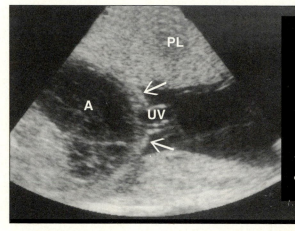

Fig. 18-21 Transverse scan of the fetal abdomen demonstrating the umbilical vein *(UV)* at the level of the cord insertion with intact skin to the right and left of midline *(small arrows)*. This fetus also has ascites *(A)*, which displays a complex pattern. *PL*, Placenta.

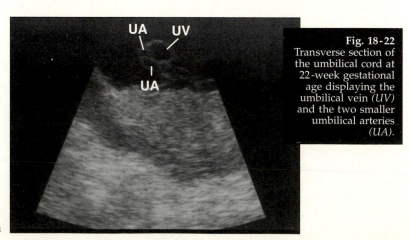

Fig. 18-22 Transverse section of the umbilical cord at 22-week gestational age displaying the umbilical vein *(UV)* and the two smaller umbilical arteries *(UA)*.

with the chin tucked toward the chest, the sonographer must scan in the transverse plane of the fetal head and angle superiorly. Additionally, the scanning plane must be obliqued to obtain a true transverse section. For example, if the orbits appear in the anterior portion of the image, the scanning obliquity is too steep, and the transducer should be pivoted to demonstrate the frontal bone superior to the orbits. If the occipital bone appears at the posterior aspect of the BPD plane, the transducer must be pivoted to demonstrate the smooth calvaria superior to the occiput. The proper BPD image should display the anatomic landmarks in the midline of the brain, and the calvarial outline should be smooth around the entire circumference (Fig. 18-24). Calipers should be placed from the outer surface of the near-field skull to the inner surface of the far-field bone table, positioned through the widest dimension on the image, usually slightly posterior to the thalami. The line connecting the two cali-

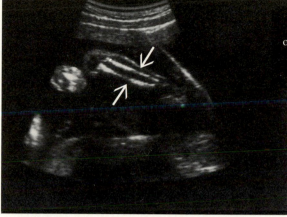

Fig. 18-23
Longitudinal image of the fetal lower leg demonstrating the shafts of the tibia and fibula *(arrows)*.

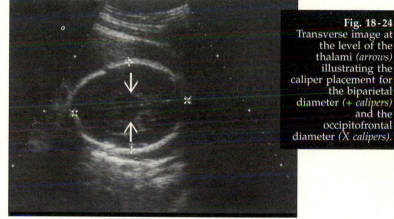

Fig. 18-24
Transverse image at the level of the thalami *(arrows)* illustrating the caliper placement for the biparietal diameter *(+ calipers)* and the occipitofrontal diameter *(X calipers)*.

per positions should form a 90-degree angle to the falx and other midline structures. This caliper placement uses the best axial resolution characteristics and, as a result, improves the accuracy of the calculation. Gain settings are adjusted so that the calvarial walls are not excessively hyperechoic and artifactually thickened, which could lead to an erroneous measurement.

There are several technical errors associated with the BPD measurement. A direct face-up or face-down presentation does not allow accurate identification of the landmarks; and landmarks that are identified are located in the same scanning depth of the sound field, which uses lateral resolution that results in image degradation. The use of an oblique patient position, a narrow aperture sector transducer, and a lateral scanning window may produce a satisfactory BPD image. When the fetal head is located deep in the maternal pelvis, the sonographer may not be able to obtain the proper angle of asynclitism, which sonographically appears as an inability to display the falx and thalami as midline structures. Instead, they appear too posterior or anterior in relation to the lateral skull walls. The use of the Trendelenberg position, in which the patient's head and torso are lowered and the lower body and legs raised, can allow the fetal head to move more superiorly in the maternal pelvis and thus allow an adequate measurement. Head shape variants can produce inaccurate BPD measurements. In **dolichocephaly** the lateral dimension of the skull is more narrow than normal and the posteroanterior dimension is wider than normal. This variation is rather common and often results from skull molding in relation to the breech presentation. In **brachycephaly** the posteroanterior dimension of the skull is smaller than normal, whereas the lateral dimension is larger than normal, resulting in a "round head" appearance. Brachycephaly does not occur as often as dolichocephaly nor does it effect the measurements as much as dolichocephaly. Based on the BPD measurement alone, dolichocephaly classically produces an erroneously younger gestational age estimate, whereas brachycephaly produces an erroneously older gestational age estimate.[11] In addition to the BPD, the use of the head circumference helps prevent inaccurate dating in the presence of these head-shape anomalies.

Head Circumference

As previously mentioned, the use of the head circumference for gestational dating helps prevent inaccurate estimates caused by head-shape anomalies. The same landmarks used for the BPD are used for this measurement—the cavum septum pellucidum and the thalamus. The actual measurement can be obtained by using one of two basic measurement techniques. For ultrasound units that have automatic obstetric calculation packages, the sonographer traces the head circumference along the outer border of the skull echo complex, and the computer program calculates the circumference and provides the corresponding gestational age. If this type of computer program is not available, the sonographer first obtains the BPD plane and places the calipers on the outer border of the near-field skull and the outer border of the far-field skull. The occipitofrontal diameter (OFD) is then measured by placing the calipers at the midline from the outer border of the anterior portion of the skull to the outer border of the posterior skull. These measurements are then used in the following formula to obtain the head circumference:

$$\text{Head circumference} = \frac{(\text{BPD}+\text{OFD})}{2} \times 3.14$$

To increase the accuracy of all these measurements, the sonographer must use the standard anatomic planes and landmarks, the standard caliper placement, and the same gestational calculation charts.[7] Even when these standard practices are followed, there is observer error whenever these measurements are obtained; that is, two different sonographers performing these calculations on the same patient will obtain slightly different measurements. Although this problem should not cause significant error in the gestational calculations, the use of the same sonographer to perform serial examinations on a patient will help ensure that observer error is statistically insignificant.[22]

Cephalic Index

The cephalic index provides another method to screen for head-shape anomalies and other abnormal conditions, such as intrauterine growth retardation. The sonographer obtains the BPD and OFD measurements and uses the following formula:

$$\text{Cephalic index} = \frac{\text{BPD}}{\text{OFD}} \times 100$$

The cephalic index has a normal range of 75 to 86; that is, if the cephalic index is greater than 86 or less than 75, the cephalic index is abnormally high or low, requiring further correlation and investigation. Many departments rely primarily on the head circumference and use the cephalic index as an adjunct or as a method of correlation with the head circumference.

Femur Length

The femur length achieves its highest accuracy for gestational dating when the gestational period is between 14 and 20 weeks. During this period this accuracy is as good as the BPD. To obtain the femur length the sonographer should initially perform a transverse scan through the fetal pelvis at the level of the urinary bladder to localize the head of the femur. The sonographer then rotates the transducer 90 degrees to display the length of the femur. For an alternate method, the sonographer should initially perform a longitudinal scan through the fetal pelvis and oblique the angle until the femoral shaft comes into view. However, the inexperienced sonographer may mistake the lower leg or even the humerus for the femur when using the latter technique, particularly in the third trimester when the fetal extremities are in close proximity to one another. For measurement purposes the optimum image should display the shaft of the femur as a homogeneous hyperechoic pattern that exhibits an even distal acoustic shadow (Fig. 18-25). The ends of the shaft should appear blunted or slightly thicker than the middle portion of the shaft. The measurement does not include the distal femoral cartilage or the femoral neck.[9] The near-field femur usually provides a more accurate estimate, since it is less affected by artifactual bowing. Recent studies have shown that there is no statistically significant rate of error between linear arrays and sector scanners when obtaining obstetric measurements.[21] However, a linear array can improve the image when the femur is in the extreme near field and when the use of a sector scanner will place the ends of the femur at the edge of the image frame. Underestimating the femoral length is more common than overestimating it. Causes for underestimating include an oblique or tangential scanning plane in relation to the true length of the femoral shaft, artifactual bowing (which is more evident in the far field), and a femur located in the extreme near field. Overestimating results when the femoral head or distal femoral cartilage is included. After 33 weeks LNMP the distal epiphysis ossifies, but there is a hypoechoic "break" between it and the femoral shaft, which allows correct identification and ensures that the sonographer does not include the cartilage in the femur measurement.

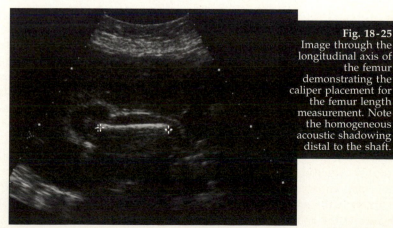

Fig. 18-25 Image through the longitudinal axis of the femur demonstrating the caliper placement for the femur length measurement. Note the homogeneous acoustic shadowing distal to the shaft.

SONOGRAPHIC MEASUREMENTS FOR EVALUATING FETAL GROWTH

Abdominal Circumference

Although the abdominal circumference is used to estimate gestational age, it is primarily used in conjunction with the head circumference for monitoring fetal growth and to estimate fetal weight. The standard plane for obtaining the abdominal circumference measurement is a transverse scan of the fetal abdomen at the level of the portal sinus in the liver (Fig. 18-26). Usually the fetal stomach lies in this plane and serves as an additional landmark, and usually this plane is slightly superior to the kidneys. Calipers are positioned on the outer border of the skin line, and the optimum image displays the entire skin line around the circumference of a true transverse, round abdomen. For consistency in measurement techniques, the calipers for the posteroanterior measurement are positioned first, coursing from the midline of the spine echo complex to the anterior abdominal wall, which bi-

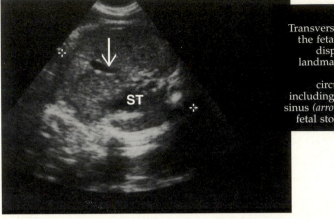

Fig. 18-26 Transverse image of the fetal abdomen displaying the landmarks for the abdominal circumference, including the portal sinus *(arrow)* and the fetal stomach *(ST)*.

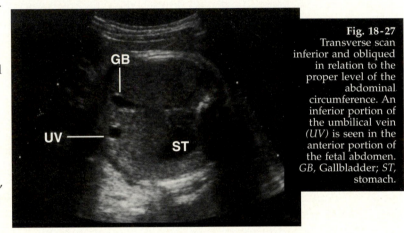

Fig. 18-27 Transverse scan inferior and obliqued in relation to the proper level of the abdominal circumference. An inferior portion of the umbilical vein *(UV)* is seen in the anterior portion of the fetal abdomen. *GB,* Gallbladder; *ST,* stomach.

sects the abdomen into equal halves. The calipers for the transverse diameter measurement are positioned in the midportion of the abdomen and form a 90-degree angle to the posteroanterior diameter. This technique ensures that the sonographer will obtain true posteroanterior and transverse measurements. The most common technical error is to obtain an oblique section through the abdomen, which displays the anterior portion of the umbilical vein and an elongated abdominal shape (Fig. 18-27). If the fetus is in the prone position, the acoustic shadowing from the spine may not allow confident identification of the portal sinus, and it may obscure the anterior skin line. The interpretation of an abdominal circumference obtained under these conditions should be done with caution, since the standard of error may be significant.[7] The use of a sector scanner and a more lateral scanning window may allow the sonographer to alleviate the spine shadowing and to identify the landmarks. A sector scanner usually provides a more accurate measurement during the third trimester, since the entire abdomen often fits in the image frame, decreasing the amount of estimation the sonographer must make when placing the calipers. The formula for obtaining the abdominal circumference using this method is:

$$\text{Abdominal circumference} = \frac{\text{(transverse diameter + posteroanterior diameter)}}{2} \times 3.14$$

If the ultrasound unit contains an obstetrical calculation program, the sonographer usually traces the abdominal circumference along the outer border of the skin. Of all the obstetric measurements, the abdominal circumference is the most difficult to reproduce and should never be used as the sole method for evaluating fetal growth.

Head Circumference/Abdominal Circumference Ratio

The head circumference/abdominal circumference (HC/AC) ratio provides one method for evaluating abnormal growth patterns. Asymmetric intrauterine growth retardation and fetal anomalies that include microcephaly, hydrocephalus, gastroschisis, and other abnormalities can cause the head circumference or abdominal circumference to be abnormally large or small. During the second trimester and the early part of the third trimester, the head circumference is slightly larger than the abdominal circumference, producing an HC/AC ratio between approximately 1.0 and 1.2. During the latter half of the third trimester, the deposition of adipose tissue in the abdomen starts to change the normal relationship between the head and abdomen, producing a ratio in the 1.0 range at approximately 32 weeks. By 38 weeks the ratio has decreased to a range of .97 to .99. These are approximate guidelines, and the sonographer should refer to the specific table currently used, which provides more precise ranges correlated with gestational age. Many computerized obstetric calculation programs will automatically indicate an abnormal ratio on the generated report. The effect of fetal anomalies and intrauterine growth retardation on the HC/AC ratio are discussed in later chapters.

Fetal Weight Estimation

The estimation of fetal weight is important information for the referring physician, but often the accuracy of this estimate is lower than other routine obstetric measurements. As mentioned previously, obtaining an optimum abdominal circumference can be technically difficult, which may lead to a greater margin of error in the calculation of gestational age and other parameters that use the abdominal circumference in the formula. Technical difficulties may also degrade the accuracy of the BPD, the head circumference measurement, and the femur length. Therefore the sonographer must carefully evaluate the quality and accuracy of the measurements and note when a measurement may not be valid as a result of technical difficulties, such as a prone measurement of the BPD or abdominal circumference. Another pitfall in estimating fetal weight, as well as other measurements, is the level of confidence in the patient's menstrual history and in the gestational age estimated during the first ultrasound examination. To improve the confidence in the age and growth estimates, the best conditions are a patient with a history of regular menstrual periods, knowledge of the exact date for the first day of the last menstrual period, and an initial ultrasound examination performed between 18 and 24 weeks. The sonographer should remember that this period provides the most accurate measurements, largely because of the fact that technical difficulties are not as common during this portion of the gestation. Another guideline in statistics is—the more variables used, the greater the potential to increase accuracy. However, the accuracy of the individual variables in the formula will also effect the accuracy of the estimate. A number of sonographers have undergone the experience of the referring physician coming to the department after the delivery of an infant and reporting that the fetal weight was underestimated or overestimated by as much as 1 pound. Depending on the formula used, the percentage of error in the estimate can range as high as plus or minus 20%.[19] To alleviate this problem, the sonographer should ensure that all fetal weight estimates include the percentage of error. In addition, the interpreting physician should caution the obstetrician when sources of error exist, such as technically suboptimal measurements, a patient with a poor menstrual history, or a patient who receives her first ultrasound examination during the third trimester of pregnancy. The fetal weight estimating formula, developed by R. E. Sabbagha and Associates,[17] factors in three variables: the gestational age in weeks, the AC/HC ratio, and the femur length. Also, there are three different formulas, one each for small-, normal-, and large-for-gestational age fetuses. The percentile ranking of the abdominal circumference determines the formula used. Again, these formulas can be no more accurate than the data used for the calculations. However, the proper use of these formulas can decrease the percentage of error to approximately 12%. Formulas derived by other researchers can also provide clinically useful information, as long as the sonographer remains aware of these limitations and always reports the weight estimate with the standard deviation or percentage of error.

ADDITIONAL MEASUREMENT TECHNIQUES

Intraorbital Distance

The intraorbital distance provides an alternative method for gestational-age estimates in cases where the BPD measurement is technically suboptimal, or when either the BPD or head circumference measurement causes an erroneous estimate of gestational age in the fetus with head anomalies, such as microcephaly or hydrocephalus. An additional use for this measurement occurs when the sonographer discovers fetal anomalies, such as skeletal dysplasia or trisomic syndromes associated with hypotelorism or hypertelorism. With these anomalies the long bone measurements will produce an inaccurate estimate of gestational age. For this measurement the sonographer should localize the BPD plane and move inferiorly to image the orbits. The face-up fetal position allows the easiest visualization. The calipers are placed at the lateral walls of the orbits through the widest dimension. Many of the computerized obstetric calculation programs do not calculate this measurement; hence the sonographer will have to refer to charts published in articles or textbooks.

Cerebellar Measurement

The cerebellum lies in the posterior and inferior portion of the skull. It is made up of butterfly-shaped hyperechoic halves connected by the hyperechoic vermis. The cisterna magna is located posterior to the cerebellum with the midbrain located anteriorly. To image the cerebellum the sonographer first localizes the BPD plane and then obliques the scanning plane, moving inferiorly (Fig. 18-28). Cerebellar width has been used to estimate gestational age, but its accuracy declines after 26 weeks.[20] Imaging the cerebellum also allows screening for congenital anomalies such as Dandy-Walker cysts, arachnoid cysts, and other anomalies that affect the posterior fossa. Also, the cisterna magna can be measured and evaluated for pathologic processes.

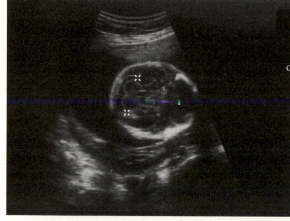

Fig. 18-28 Transverse scan of the cerebellum demonstrating the caliper placement for the cerebellar measurement (*X*).

Amniotic Fluid Index

For most routine examinations the sonographer makes a subjective determination regarding the amount of amniotic fluid. Excessive amniotic fluid, termed **polyhydramnios,** is classically defined as the presence of 2000 cc or more of fluid. The sonographer should suspect polyhydramnios if the amniotic fluid totally surrounds the fetus in the late second or third trimesters. A lack of amniotic fluid, termed **oligohydramnios,** is suspected when very little fluid is seen around the fetal body or extremities. To more accurately quantify and document these abnormalities, the sonographer should obtain an amniotic fluid index (AFI). The maternal abdomen is divided into four quadrants: right upper quadrant, right lower quadrant, left upper quadrant, and left lower quadrant. The sonographer should examine each quadrant and obtain an image of the largest pocket of amniotic fluid. Before measuring, the sonographer should use color-flow Doppler to ascertain if portions of the cord fill the pocket, since most departments will not include this area in the amniotic fluid calculations. The calipers are positioned vertically through the maximum depth of the amniotic fluid, and the four measurements added together form the index. Usually oligohydramnios is defined as the largest pocket measuring less than 2 to 3 cm, or an AFI of less than 8 cm.[16] The amount of fluid normally decreases during the late third trimester. However, the presence of oligohydramnios earlier in the pregnancy requires further clinical investigation and correlation.

TECHNICAL PITFALLS

Many student sonographers initially find the sonographic examination of the second- and third-trimester fetus frustrating. To identify all the anatomy and to achieve the correct scanning planes for the measurements, the sonographer must conceptualize the fetal lie and modify the scanning plane to achieve true transverse and longitudinal images of the organs and landmarks. Scanning experience will usually overcome this initial obstacle. Another common problem relates to the organization of the examination itself. The sonographer must remember the protocol and the routine images that are always obtained. Initially, a small index card summarizing the protocol can serve as a prompt while performing the examination. Another procedure many sonographers use is a quick survey scan through the transverse plane of the fetus, which allows identification of the fetal lie and a check for gross abnormalities, such as fetal nonviability, severe hydrocephalus, or multiple gestation. The sonographer can then perform a methodical study of the fetus organized by anatomic area, such as the head, or organized by organ system, such as the urinary tract. If the fetal position is not

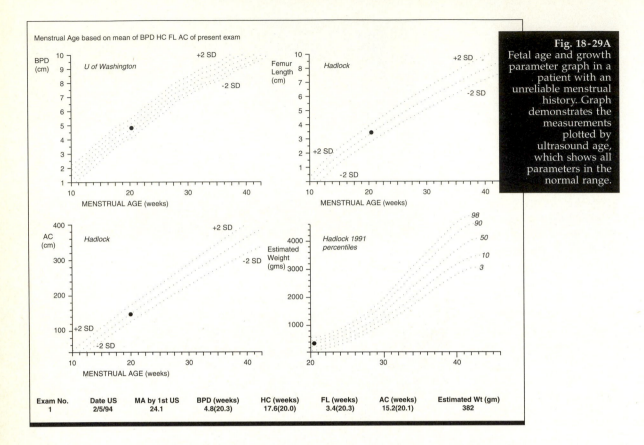

Menstrual Age based on mean of BPD HC FL AC of present exam

Fig. 18-29A
Fetal age and growth parameter graph in a patient with an unreliable menstrual history. Graph demonstrates the measurements plotted by ultrasound age, which shows all parameters in the normal range.

Exam No.	Date US	MA by 1st US	BPD (weeks)	HC (weeks)	FL (weeks)	AC (weeks)	Estimated Wt (gm)
1	2/5/94	24.1	4.8(20.3)	17.6(20.0)	3.4(20.3)	15.2(20.1)	382

optimal for certain views or measurements, the sonographer should proceed to another area for documentation and periodically recheck the suboptimal area. During the second trimester, simply asking the patient to lie on her side will often cause the fetus to change position. During the third trimester this is less likely to occur. However, during the third trimester the fetus may exert enough pressure on the maternal inferior vena cava when the mother is supine to cause symptoms such as shortness of breath and flushing. The sonographer should have the mother lie on her side for a few minutes; this will usually alleviate the symptoms. Allowing the mother to lie in a posterior oblique position will usually prevent the recurrence of symptoms.

Several of the technical pitfalls associated with measurement techniques are mentioned in previous sections of this chapter. An additional pitfall common to the inexperienced sonographer is obtaining a coronal view of the fetal skull and using it for the BPD and OFD measurements. To avoid this, the sonographer should move inferiorly to the fetus and examine the spine. If the cervical spine appears in its longitudinal plane, rotate 90 degrees to image the skull in the transverse plane.

With the advent of obstetric calculation packages, which automatically calculate the gestational age during the examination, many sonographers "fudge" the position of the calipers to obtain the same gestational age for all measurement parameters. This practice can mask abnormal growth patterns if the repositioning alters the gestational

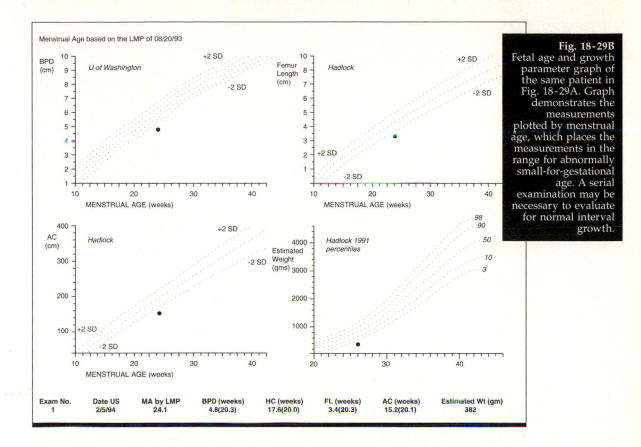

Menstrual Age based on the LMP of 08/20/93

Fig. 18-29B Fetal age and growth parameter graph of the same patient in Fig. 18-29A. Graph demonstrates the measurements plotted by menstrual age, which places the measurements in the range for abnormally small-for-gestational age. A serial examination may be necessary to evaluate for normal interval growth.

Exam No.	Date US	MA by LMP	BPD (weeks)	HC (weeks)	FL (weeks)	AC (weeks)	Estimated Wt (gm)
1	2/5/94	24.1	4.8(20.3)	17.6(20.0)	3.4(20.3)	15.2(20.1)	382

age by several weeks. The sonographer must evaluate the image and judge whether it is optimal and whether it demonstrates all landmarks. If the image is optimal, but there remains a 2-week gestational age discrepancy compared with other parameters, this discrepancy is suggestive of abnormal growth and requires serial sonographic examinations and clinical correlation. The patient with an unreliable menstrual history complicates the interpretation of gestational age and growth parameters. If the gestational age, as calculated by the ultrasound parameters, correlates to the gestational age by LNMP, graphing by either the LNMP or by the sonographic age will produce nearly identical graphs. However, if the sonographic age does not correlate with the menstrual age, the two graphs will be different (Fig. 18-29). The question now centers around the patient's clinical history. If the discrepancy is the result of an unreliable menstrual history or is caused by an abnormal growth pattern related to fetal or maternal factors, often the interpreting physician will request a serial examination to check for normal or abnormal interval growth. When performing serial examinations, the sonographer must always calculate the elapsed number of weeks between the examinations and use that date for graphing. For example, if the patient was graphed at 20 weeks at the time of the initial examination and she returns a month later, her gestational age for the second examination is 24 weeks. Serial examinations should be graphed simultaneously to enable the clinician to immediately perceive the growth patterns (Fig. 18-30).

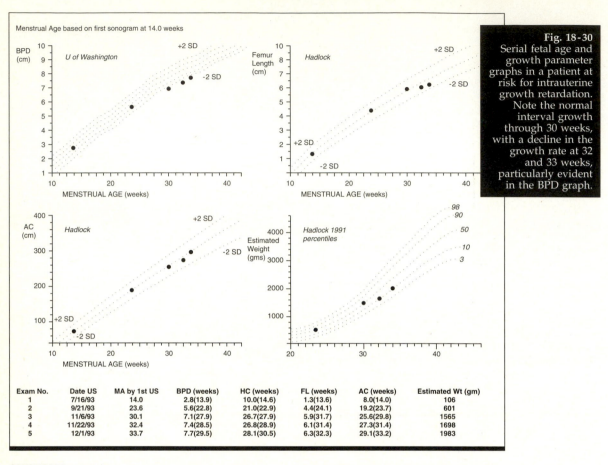

Menstrual Age based on first sonogram at 14.0 weeks

Fig. 18-30 Serial fetal age and growth parameter graphs in a patient at risk for intrauterine growth retardation. Note the normal interval growth through 30 weeks, with a decline in the growth rate at 32 and 33 weeks, particularly evident in the BPD graph.

Exam No.	Date US	MA by 1st US	BPD (weeks)	HC (weeks)	FL (weeks)	AC (weeks)	Estimated Wt (gm)
1	7/16/93	14.0	2.8(13.9)	10.0(14.6)	1.3(13.6)	8.0(14.0)	106
2	9/21/93	23.6	5.6(22.8)	21.0(22.9)	4.4(24.1)	19.2(23.7)	601
3	11/6/93	30.1	7.1(27.9)	26.7(27.9)	5.9(31.7)	25.6(29.8)	1565
4	11/22/93	32.4	7.4(28.5)	26.8(28.9)	6.1(31.4)	27.3(31.4)	1698
5	12/1/93	33.7	7.7(29.5)	28.1(30.5)	6.3(32.3)	29.1(33.2)	1983

SUMMARY

The sonographic examination of the second- and third-trimester pregnancy requires detailed knowledge of fetal anatomy and abnormal sonographic patterns. The sonographer must conduct a thorough evaluation of the technical quality of all fetal measurements. If all parameters display the proper landmarks and are technically optimal, any age or growth discrepancies should be brought to the attention of the interpreting physician. If the suspected or documented abnormality exceeds the skill level of the ultrasound department, the patient should be referred to a high-risk perinatal center that has the resources and experience to provide the patient with high-level care.

REFERENCES

1. American Institute of Ultrasound in Medicine: antepartum obstetrical examination guidelines, *AIUM*, Laurel, Md, 1988.
2. Barone CM, van Natra FC, et al: Sonographic diagnosis of fetal goiter, an unusual case of hydramnios, *J Ultrasound Med* 4:625, 1985.
3. Bowie J, Rosenberg E, et al: The changing sonographic appearance of fetal kidneys during pregnancy, *J Ultrasound Med* 2:505-507, 1988.
4. Chervenak FA, Berkowitz RL, et al: The diagnosis of fetal hydrocephalus, *Am J Obstet Gynecol* 147:703, 1983.

5. Copel JA, Pilu G, et al: Fetal echocardiographic screening for congenital heart disease: the importance of the four-chamber view, *Am J Obstet Gynecol* 157:648-655, 1987.

6. Cyr DR, Guntheroth WG, et al: A systematic approach to fetal echocardiography using real time/two-dimensional sonography, *J Ultrasound Med* 5:343-350, 1986.

7. Deter R, Harrist R, et al: Fetal head and abdominal circumferences: evaluation of measurement errors, *J Clin Ultrasound* 10:357-363, 1982.

8. Elejalde B, de Elejalde M, Heitman T: Visualization of fetal genitalia by ultrasonography: a review of the literature and analysis of its accuracy and ethical implications, *J Ultrasound Med* 4:630-639, 1985.

9. Goldstein RB, Filly RA, Simpson G: Pitfalls in femur length measurements, *J Ultrasound Med* 6:203-207, 1987.

10. Gray DL, Crane JP, Rudloff MA: Prenatal diagnosis of neural tube defects: origin of midtrimester vertebral ossification centers as determined by sonographic water-bath studies, *J Ultrasound Med* 7:421-427, 1988.

11. Hadlock FP, Deter RL, et al: Estimating fetal age: effect of head shape on BPD, *AJR* 137:83-85, 1981.

12. Hadlock FP, Deter RL, et al: Fetal biparietal diameter: rational choice of plane of section for sonographic measurement, *AJR* 138:871, 1982.

13. Hoddick W, Filly R, et al: Minimal renal pyelectasis, *J Ultrasound Med* 4:85-89, 1985.

14. McLeary RD, Kuhns LR, Barr M: Ultrasonography of the fetal cerebellum, *Radiology* 15:439-442, 1984.

15. Nyberg D, Mack L, et al: Fetal bowel: normal sonographic findings, *J Ultrasound Med* 6:3-6, 1987.

16. Phelan JP, Ahn MO, et al: Amniotic fluid index measurements during pregnancy, *J Reprod Med* 32:601-604, 1987.

17. Sabbagha RE, Minogue J, et al: Estimation of birth weight by the use of ultrasound formulas targeted to large-, appropriate-, and small-for-gestational age fetuses, *Am J Obstet Gynecol* 160:854, 1989.

18. Samuel N, Dicker D, Feldberg D: Ultrasound diagnosis and management of fetal intestinal obstruction and volvulus in utero, *J Perinat Med* 12:333-337, 1984.

19. Shepard MJ, Richards VA, et al: An evaluation of two equations of predicting fetal weight by ultrasound, *Am J Obstet Gynecol* 142:47, 1982.

20. Smith PA, Johannsson D, et al: Prenatal measurement of the fetal cerebellum and cisterna cerebellomedullaris by ultrasound, *Prenat Diagn* 6:133, 1986.

21. Winter J, Kimme-Smith C, King W III: Measurement accuracy of sonographic sector scanners, *AJR* 144:645-648, 1985.

22. Zador IE, Sokol RJ, Chik L: Interobserver variability: a source of error in obstetric ultrasound, *J Ultrasound Med* 7:245-249, 1988.

19

small-for-gestational age pregnancy

INSTRUCTIONAL OBJECTIVES

At the completion of this chapter, the reader will be able to:

1. Describe the clinical problems that are associated with the small-for-gestational age pregnancy.
2. Describe the clinical symptoms and pathologic basis for the various causes of intrauterine growth retardation, including maternal diabetes mellitus, hypertension, smoking, renal disease, poor nutrition, and cytotoxic agents, as well as causes of placental insufficiency and fetal conditions that may produce intrauterine growth retardation.
3. Define symmetric and asymmetric intrauterine growth retardation, and describe the sonographic criteria for diagnosing these conditions.
4. Describe the criteria used for the biophysical profile, including the scoring system and the differentiation of fetal distress from the normal fetus.
5. Discuss the use of pulsed and color-flow Doppler in the evaluation of intrauterine growth retardation.
6. Describe the sonographic features of fetal demise in the second and third trimesters.
7. Describe several technical pitfalls associated with the evaluation of the small-for-gestational age pregnancy.

THE CLINICAL PROBLEM

The small-for-gestational age (SGA) category covers a diverse group, including normally small fetuses, as well as those abnormally small. An SGA infant is defined as a baby at or below the 10th percentile of weight for gestational age. An average-for-gestational age (AGA) baby falls between the 10th and 90th percentiles.[4] The clinician should evaluate the patient's fundal height and correlate it with the gestational age according to the last normal menstrual period (LNMP), as well as evaluate the patient's current weight gain during the pregnancy. This information is further correlated with the patient's clinical history. If the patient has a poor menstrual history, the obstetrician will have difficulty in evaluating normal or abnormal fetal growth. This type of patient also poses a problem when obtaining an accurate sonographic determination of the gestational age. The patient often requires serial sonographic examinations to evaluate normal or abnormal interval growth. In addition, serial examinations assists the clinician in determining if the date used for the LNMP is inaccurate, or if the fetus is a normal SGA baby or is at risk for intrauterine growth retardation (IUGR). Since the diagnosis of IUGR is based primarily on the interpretation of the gestational age and fetal growth measurements, the sonographer must ensure that the measurements are as accurate as possible. Once diagnosed, the clinician can alter the clinical management of the patient, based on the underlying cause of the aberrant growth. However, the cause remains unknown or idiopathic in approximately 50% of cases.

Another cause for the clinical category of SGA is oligohydramnios. Congential anomalies (such as renal agenesis) and genetic conditions (such as trisomy 13) can be related to oligohydramnios. This condition is also associated with fetal demise, although other clinical symptoms may raise the suggestion of this diagnosis.

CAUSES OF INTRAUTERINE GROWTH RETARDATION

IUGR causes the largest percentage of fetal morbidity; only premature births have a higher rate of fetal mortality. IUGR is clinically diagnosed when the neonatal birth weight is at or below the 5th percentile or when the baby is born after 36 weeks and weighs less than 2.5 kg (approximately 5.5 lbs.).[4] One of the most common fetal effects of IUGR is a decrease in mental alertness and function. Three main categories cause IUGR: maternal disease states, primary placental pathology, and fetal congenital anomalies and infections.

Maternal Factors

Maternal disease states include severe diabetes mellitus, chronic renal disease, chronic hypertension, smoking, poor nutrition, ingestion of cytotoxic agents, and uteroplacental insufficiency secondary to maternal vascular disease. **Diabetes mellitus,** a metabolic disorder related to decreased insulin levels, is one of the most significant medical complications of pregnancy. The American College of Obstetricians and Gynecologists categorize diabetes mellitus according to the severity of the symptoms. The disease occurs in two forms: type I, which is insulin-dependent, and type II, which is non–insulin-dependent.[5] If the onset occurs before pregnancy, the disease is further categorized according to the length and severity of the metabolic disorder (Table 19-1). Gestational diabetes, more correctly known as glucose intolerance of pregnancy, can cause symptoms ranging from mild, which may be controlled by diet, to severe, which

TABLE 19-1   CLASSIFICATION OF DIABETES MELLITIS

CLASS	AGE AT ONSET	DURATION	MANAGEMENT	OTHER
A	Any age	Varies	Diet restrictions	
B	Over 20 years old	Less than 10 years	Insulin	
C	10 to 19 years old	10 to 19 years	Insulin	
D	Less than 10 years old	20 years plus	Insulin	Chronic hypertension, retinopathy

requires insulin supplementation. However, the glucose levels return to within the normal range after delivery. Juvenile-onset diabetes or the presence of severe symptoms, such as renal or heart disease, are contraindications for pregnancy, since the maternal and fetal morbidity and mortality are higher. If the diabetes affects the patient's vascular system, this condition can lead to uteroplacental insufficiency and the consequent development of IUGR. Diabetes can affect the fetus in other ways, including the development of macrosomia, which is discussed in Chapter 20, and congenital anomalies, which are discussed in Chapter 21.

Preeclampsia-eclampsia, also known as toxemia of pregnancy, is characterized by the development of hypertension during pregnancy. A patient with preeclampsia, the less severe form, presents with hypertension, edema, proteinuria, sudden and excessive weight gain, and headaches. The criteria for diagnosing hypertension usually includes a systolic increase over 30 mm Hg, although a diastolic increase is a more reliable sign. In eclampsia the preeclamptic patient experiences one or more convulsions and may slip into a coma. The clinician should initiate treatment with the first symptoms of preeclampsia to decrease the patient's risk of developing eclampsia. These symptoms usually affect primigravid patients and develop during the latter half of the third trimester. The effects of this disease on the pregnancy include IUGR (when the onset of hypertension occurs in the second trimester or in the early part of the third trimester), prematurity, an increased incidence of abruptio placenta and placental infarcts, and an abnormally thin placenta. Patients with preexisting, moderate-to-severe hypertension are often advised against pregnancy, since the risk of maternal and fetal morbidity and mortality are high. This type of patient has a higher risk of developing IUGR, as well as developing the other complications associated with preeclampsia.[6]

If the patient smokes or suffers from poor nutrition during pregnancy, these factors can cause placental insufficiency and the development of IUGR. However, if the patient quits smoking or if the maternal nutrition is improved, the detrimental effects on the fetus may be lessened. Many **cytotoxic agents** may cause IUGR, including alcohol, narcotics (such as heroin and cocaine), steroids, and many other drugs.[4]

Placental Causes

Primary placental pathology, which may lead to IUGR, includes infarctions and neoplasms. Since these occurrences are not related to underlying maternal disease, the incidence of primary placental pathology is uncommon.[4] Examples of neoplasms include chorioangioma. Placental pathology is discussed in Chapter 23.

Fetal Causes

Fetal congenital anomalies and infections may also lead to the development of IUGR. These abnormalities include congenital heart disease, anomalies of the central nervous system and genitourinary tract, and chromosomal anomalies such as trisomy 13, 18, and 21. These conditions are discussed in Chapter 21.

SCANNING PROTOCOLS AND TECHNIQUES

Standard Sonographic Examination

When screening for IUGR, the scanning protocol for the sonographic examination during the second and third trimesters follows the guidelines outlined in Chapter 18. The following section summarizes the standard protocol:

Fetal Age and Growth Parameters
1. BPD
2. Head circumference or cephalic index
3. Abdominal circumference
4. Femur length
5. Estimation of fetal weight

Fetal Anatomy
1. Cerebral ventricles to rule out hydrocephaly
2. Four-chamber heart and heart position within the thoracic cavity
3. Spine to rule out spina bifida
4. Stomach to assess function and rule out anomalies
5. Kidneys to rule out anomalies and obstruction
6. Urinary bladder to assess renal function and rule out obstruction
7. Umbilical cord insertion to rule out abnormalities of the anterior abdominal wall
8. Three-vessel cord
9. Fetal lie in relation to maternal longitudinal axis

Placenta and Maternal Anatomy
1. Anatomic location and grade
2. Position of placenta in relation to internal cervical os
3. Amount of amniotic fluid
4. Uterus for fibroids and other abnormalities
5. Adnexal areas to rule out masses

Sonography plays a crucial role in the detection of IUGR, and the sonographer must document the gestational age as accurately as possible. The fetal weight estimate must allow the clinician to distinguish normal SGA and AGA babies from those fetuses experiencing aberrant growth. The normal range for most sonographic growth estimates is two standard deviations around the average, which corresponds to a range between the 10th and 90th percentiles. Thus aberrant growth may be indicated when the fetus falls at or below the 10th percentile or above the 90th percentile for large-for-gestational age (LGA) fetuses.[4] Since the head and abdominal circumferences are used for the fetal weight estimate and since this estimate can have a rather large percentage of error, the sonographer must pay particular attention to obtaining optimal images for these parameters. The sonographer should obtain a good clinical history, including the LNMP, ascertain maternal weight gain, and ask screening questions for maternal disorders. The primary growth parameters used for IUGR screening include the head circumference, abdominal circumference, and femur length. The biparietal diameter (BPD) should not be included. Because of head-shape anomalies (see Chapter 18), the BPD is not as accurate as the head circumference, and the fetal weight estimating formulas should not use it.[8] Sonographic signs most suggestive of IUGR include:

1. Lack of normal interval growth on serial examinations
2. Asymmetry between head and abdomen sizes
3. Small-or advanced-grade placenta
4. Decrease in amniotic fluid (oligohydramnios); pocket less than 1 to 2 cm; amniotic fluid index equal to or less than 5 cm
5. Depressed fetal activity on evaluation of biophysical profile and non-stress test
6. Identification of fetal anomaly

Chapter 18 contains additional information on computing the amniotic fluid index (AFI). Although severe oligohydramnios with IUGR has a reported incidence of approximately 25%, (Fig. 19-1) this sign has serious consequences for the fetus, particularly since the interaction of the amniotic fluid with the fetal lungs assists lung development.[9] A discussion of the non-stress test and stress test is included in Chapter 15, and placental grading and pathology is discussed in Chapter 23.

Biophysical Profile

The most widely used tests for evaluating fetal condition are the non-stress test and the stress test. A reactive finding is usually an indication of fetal well being, whereas a nonreactive finding indicates possible fetal distress. The biophysical profile consists of the sonographic evaluation of typically five criteria: the results of the non-stress test, fetal breathing, gross body movements, tone, and the amount of amniotic fluid. The sonographer also evaluates the fetal heart rate in comparison with the normal range of 120 to 140 beats per minute in the second and third trimesters. Fetal heart rate variation often occurs and can be a normal finding if the incident is short in duration or if the heart rate variation is only slightly beyond the normal range. Pronounced and prolonged **bradycardia,** a slow heart rate, is a poor prognostic sign and should always require further clinical investigation. Moderate to severe **tachycardia,** an excessively rapid action of the

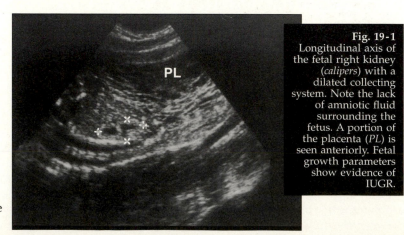

Fig. 19-1
Longitudinal axis of the fetal right kidney (*calipers*) with a dilated collecting system. Note the lack of amniotic fluid surrounding the fetus. A portion of the placenta (*PL*) is seen anteriorly. Fetal growth parameters show evidence of IUGR.

heart, and cardiac arrhythmias are not as common, but both also require further clinical workup at a center specializing in high-risk obstetrics.[1]

The current method and scoring system for the biophysicial profile is based on the initial work of Manning and Associates.[2] The scoring system ranges from 2 to 0 for each parameter; 2 is assigned when the fetus displays all aspects in relation to the parameter, and 0 is assigned when the fetus does not exhibit all of the related criteria for the category. Generally a score of 8 is an indication of fetal well being. Since it is equivocal, a score of 6 requires a repeat profile 12 to 24 hours later. A score below 6 usually indicates fetal distress. Generally a biophysical profile is performed on high-risk patients from 24 to 40 weeks LNMP. However, the reliability of the profile criteria can vary with gestational age. For example, fetal breathing becomes less consistent between approximately 21 to 26 weeks, but it becomes progressively stronger and of longer duration as the gestation progresses through the third trimester. Fetal breathing, as well as body movements and tone, are also affected by the fetal sleep-wake cycle. The sonographer can perform the **motor provocation test** by applying slight pressure on the maternal abdomen to awaken the sleeping fetus, particularly if the mother notes that the fetus is most active at night. The current standard observation time for the biophysical profile is 30 minutes. The sonographic criteria for each category include:[2]

- **Non-stress test**—Reactive is assigned a score of 2; nonreactive is assigned a score of 0.
- **Fetal respirations**—the sonographer evaluates diaphragmatic and intercostal muscular movement on a longitudinal or transverse view of the right hemidiaphragm and chest area. A score of 2 is assigned if a minimum of one 30-second period of sustained fetal breathing is observed during the 30-minute observation period; a score of 0 is assigned if less than 30 seconds of breathing is observed or if no breathing is noted.
- **Gross fetal movements**—the observation of at least three separate fetal movements of the extremities or trunk, with the simultaneous movement of the trunk and extremities, is recorded as one episode. A score of 2 is assigned if three episodes are observed during the 30-minute observation period; a score of 0 is assigned if two or less episodes are observed.
- **Fetal tone**—to assign a score of 2, the fetal extremities are fully flexed and the head is flexed. The sonographer should observe a minimum of one episode of extremity extension with a full return of flexion or an extension of the spine with a return to flexion. A score of 0 is assigned if the extremities remain in extension or in partial flexion or if fetal extension is not followed by complete flexion.
- **Amniotic fluid**—a pocket that measures greater than 2 cm or an AFI greater than 5 cm should receive a score of 2. A score of 0 is assigned if a pocket measures 2 cm or less or if the AFI is 5 cm or less (the AFI is the preferred method).

The absence of fetal breathing usually indicates a chronic hypoxic state. If repeat biophysical profiles demonstrate a decreased frequency in body movements, or if the body movements are slow but persist on serial biophysical profile examinations, both are indications of less severe distress. However, if a lack of fetal movement persists over serial profiles, a more severe compromise is indicated, particularly if the fetus does not react to stimuli, such as the motor provocation test.

Umbilical Vessel Doppler Evaluation

The umbilical cord is made up of three vessels: the umbilical vein, which transports oxygen and nutrients to the fetus, and the two umbilical arteries, which return blood to the placenta. Under normal circumstances the fetus receives an overabundance of oxygen from the placenta, since the oxygen saturation level of the blood in the umbilical arteries is usually above 50%. As a result, initial oxygen deprivation will decrease this oxygen saturation level. A pulsed Doppler evaluation of the amount of blood flow and its resistance can indirectly assess the physiologic status of the fetal system. Current clinical indications for umbilical Doppler studies include the presence of maternal diseases, such as hypertension and diabetes, clinically suggestive cases of IUGR, umbilical cord anomalies or pathology, fetal anomalies, or a history of previous fetal demise.

Many departments use duplex sonography with pulsed Doppler to perform this evaluation. Most protocols require the computation of the systolic/diastolic (S/D) ratio, the pulsatility index, or the resistive index to interpret normal and abnormal fetal states (Fig. 19-2). Since most ultrasound units automatically calculate these values, the sonographer needs only to ensure that the sample used for these formulas is optimum. However, the calculation of flow is angle dependent, and it is technically difficult to obtain a good Doppler angle.[10] Since the indices are independent of the Doppler angle, the sonographer needs to place the sample volume in the middle of the umbilical artery on a transverse or longitudinal plane of section. The optimum spectral analysis should demonstrate a strong signal with discrete systolic- and diastolic-flow components. Blood flow in the umbilical vein normally courses in the opposite direction. Placing the patient in a posterior oblique position will minify the effects of maternal hypotension. The sonographer should not obtain a sample during fetal breathing or during periods of fetal bradycardia or tachycardia, since these factors will change the spectral analysis. The sample should be obtained as close to the placental insertion site as possible, since flow resistance is greater near the fetal cord insertion.

TYPES OF INTRAUTERINE GROWTH RETARDATION

Symmetric

Symmetric IUGR, also called the low-profile group, usually occurs before the twenty-eighth week of gestation and includes both head and body growth lag. Causes of symmetric IUGR include genetic anomalies, maternal or fetal infections, and maternal malnutrition or ingestion of cytotoxic agents. Oxygen deprivation occurs before the end of organogenesis, resulting in a decrease in

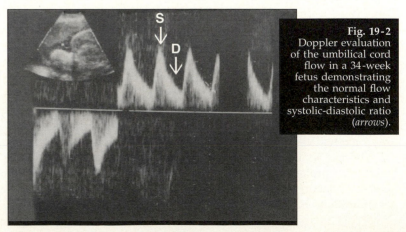

Fig. 19-2
Doppler evaluation of the umbilical cord flow in a 34-week fetus demonstrating the normal flow characteristics and systolic-diastolic ratio (*arrows*).

cell count in many organs, including the brain. This type of aberrant growth accounts for approximately 25% of all IUGR cases. The detection of symmetric IUGR can pose problems to the clinician and the sonography team. As mentioned in a previous chapter, the head circumference/abdominal circumference (HC/AC) ratio allows a comparison of the growth rates. The sonographer should look for an abnormal ratio. However, in the symmetric type the head and body often decrease at approximately the same rate; consequently, the ratio appears within the normal range. If the patient has a good menstrual history, the interpreting physician may determine that the fetal head and body correspond to a younger gestational age than the LNMP, which is suggestive of IUGR. In these cases, serial examinations are usually necessary.[9] If the patient has a poor menstrual history, several examinations are usually required to provide a baseline, but interpretation will remain difficult. Accurate measurements may demonstrate poor interval growth, which narrows the clinical diagnosis. Fig. 19-3 illustrates the sonographic findings for symmetric IUGR.

Asymmetric

Asymmetric IUGR has a later onset than the symmetric type, usually occurring in the latter portion of the second trimester and in the third trimester. Maternal diseases, such as hypertension or placental insufficiency, are among the causes for this type of IUGR.

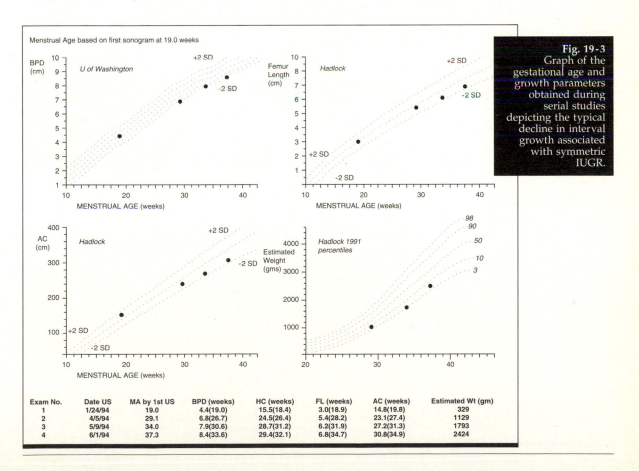

Fig. 19-3 Graph of the gestational age and growth parameters obtained during serial studies depicting the typical decline in interval growth associated with symmetric IUGR.

Exam No.	Date US	MA by 1st US	BPD (weeks)	HC (weeks)	FL (weeks)	AC (weeks)	Estimated Wt (gm)
1	1/24/94	19.0	4.4(19.0)	15.5(18.4)	3.0(18.9)	14.8(19.8)	329
2	4/5/94	29.1	6.8(26.7)	24.5(26.4)	5.4(28.2)	23.1(27.4)	1129
3	5/9/94	34.0	7.9(30.6)	28.7(31.2)	6.2(31.9)	27.2(31.3)	1793
4	6/1/94	37.3	8.4(33.6)	29.4(32.1)	6.8(34.7)	30.8(34.9)	2424

Because of the unique properties of fetal circulation, the oxygen supply to the brain remains strong while the oxygen to other fetal structures declines. This mechanism is referred to as "brain-sparing." It causes a characteristic loss of normal growth in the body and extremities, but the head retains a relatively normal growth pattern. Because this type occurs after the end of major organogenesis, the oxygen deprivation initially results in a reduction of cell size, but severe compromise can still cause cell loss.[4] The classic growth pattern in asymmetric IUGR reveals an abnormal HC/AC ratio. Since the head circumference usually stays in the normal range and the abdominal circumference decreases, the HC/AC ratio becomes larger than the normal ratio for the specific gestational age. Again, more severe cases of asymmetric IUGR may exhibit oligohydramnios and placental changes, such as advanced grading and a smaller than normal size. Fig. 19-4 illustrates a typical case of asymmetric IUGR.

Some researchers feel that Doppler evaluation of the umbilical artery may provide additional information that may lead to an earlier diagnosis of this condition than is allowed by the estimation of the fetal weight.[7] The normal S/D ratio should be close to 3.0. In asymmetric IUGR the brain receives more blood supply as a result of a decrease in the resistance in the carotid and cerebral arteries and because of an increase in resistance in the fetal aorta and the umbilical arteries. This increase in vascular resistance in the umbilical arteries decreases the amount of diastolic flow; consequently, the S/D ratio becomes higher than the normal value. Occasionally the

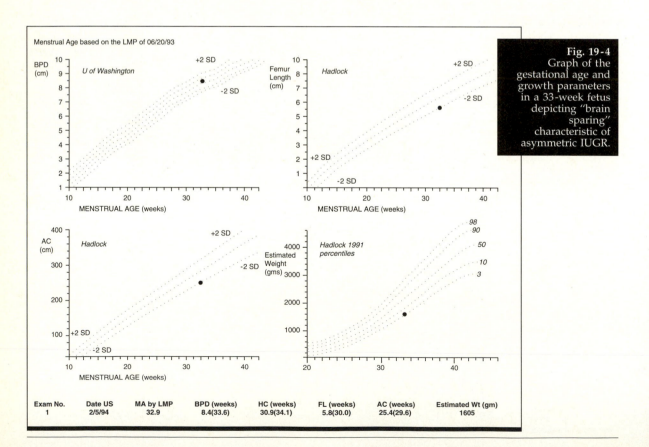

Fig. 19-4 Graph of the gestational age and growth parameters in a 33-week fetus depicting "brain sparing" characteristic of asymmetric IUGR.

Exam No.	Date US	MA by LMP	BPD (weeks)	HC (weeks)	FL (weeks)	AC (weeks)	Estimated Wt (gm)
1	2/5/94	32.9	8.4(33.6)	30.9(34.1)	5.8(30.0)	25.4(29.6)	1605

resistance becomes so high that no diastolic flow is present, or there may be a flow reversal. These findings have been associated with increased risk of fetal morbidity and mortality.[7] The more advanced Doppler examination of the fetal cerebral circulation includes a sampling of the internal cerebral artery that is located anterior to the thalamus. The resistance in the cerebral circulation decreases, resulting in an abnormally low S/D ratio.[11] Color flow allows easy identification of these small intracerebral vessels.

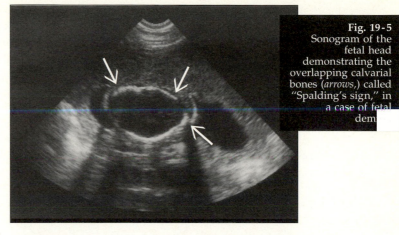

Fig. 19-5 Sonogram of the fetal head demonstrating the overlapping calvarial bones (*arrows,*) called "Spalding's sign," in a case of fetal demise.

FETAL DEMISE IN THE SECOND AND THIRD TRIMESTERS

There are many causes for fetal demise in the second and third trimesters. These include severe congenital anomalies, severe IUGR, and a disruption of the fetal oxygen supply from a nuchal cord. The typical clinical symptoms of fetal demise are failure of interval growth and a lack of fetal movement felt by the mother.[3]

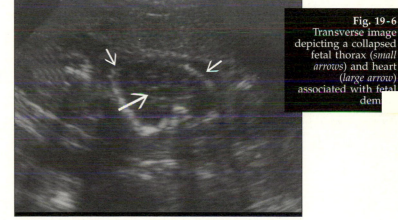

Fig. 19-6 Transverse image depicting a collapsed fetal thorax (*small arrows*) and heart (*large arrow*) associated with fetal demise.

The primary sonographic sign of fetal demise is a lack of heart motion. Depending on the time interval from fetal death to the sonographic examination, the sonographer may note several additional patterns. Because the fetus is the primary regulator of amniotic fluid volume in the second and third trimesters, oligohydramnios usually develops several days after death. This leads to a compression and an overlapping of the calvarial bones, producing the "Spalding sign" (Fig. 19-5). The fetal chest and abdomen may also appear collapsed and distorted (Fig. 19-6). The sonographer should have the findings verified by the interpreting physician before the patient leaves the department.

TECHNICAL PITFALLS

As mentioned previously, the accuracy of all fetal measurements is crucial to the diagnosis of IUGR. The sonographer must inform the interpreting physician when any measurement is technically suboptimal. Also, discrepancies in the 2-week range require careful evaluation of the measurements, using the standard criteria discussed in Chapter 18 to determine if this discrepancy could indicate fetal pathology.

Several pitfalls relate to the biophysical profile. Inexperienced sonographers may misidentify the fetal movement in response to maternal respirations as fetal respirations. This is particularly common in thin patients. The sonographer should scan other portions of the fetus to determine if they are also moving, as well as observe the maternal respiration rate and confirm when all these movements coincide. The sonographer should ask the mother to hold her breath. Evidence of fetal respirations near the fetal heart can also cause the misidentification of transmitted heart motion to the left hemidiaphragm. To allow a confident identification, the sonographer should observe the fetal chest wall for what appears to be "panting movements." Experience will usually eliminate this pitfall.

SUMMARY

Sonography plays an important role in the evaluation of the SGA pregnancy. The sonographer must obtain technically optimal measurements to increase the specificity and sensitivity for detecting IUGR. The use of the biophysical profile and Doppler evaluation of the umbilical cord can also enhance the diagnosis of fetal distress. All the examinations discussed in this chapter can allow the referring physician to implement clinical strategies to improve the prognosis of the SGA fetus.

REFERENCES

1. Freeman RE, Anderson G, Dorcester W: A prospective multi-institutional study of ante-partum fetal heart-rate monitoring: I. Risk of perinatal mortality and morbidity according to ante-partum fetal heart-rate test results, *Am J Obstet Gynecol* 143:771, 1982.
2. Manning FA, Morrison I, et al: Fetal assessment based on fetal biophysical profile screening: experience in 12,620 referred high-risk pregnancies: perinatal mortality by frequency and etiology, *Am J Obstet Gynecol* 151:343-350, 1985.
3. Pernoll ML, Benson RC, editors: *Current obstetric and gynecologic diagnosis and treatment,* Norwalk, Conn, 1987, Appleton and Lange, p 168.
4. Pernoll ML, Benson RC, editors: *Current obstetric and gynecologic diagnosis and treatment,* Norwalk, Conn, 1987, Appleton and Lange, pp 311-317.
5. Pernoll ML, Benson RC, editors: *Current obstetric and gynecologic diagnosis and treatment,* Norwalk, Conn, 1987, Appleton and Lange, pp 332-339.
6. Pernoll ML, Benson RC, editors: *Current obstetric and gynecologic diagnosis and treatment,* Norwalk, Conn, 1987, Appleton and Lange, pp 340-351.
7. Rochelson BL, Schulman H, et al: The significance of absent end-diastolic velocity in umbilical artery velocity waveform, *Am J Obstet Gynecol* 156:1213-1218, 1987.
8. Sabbagha RE, Minogue J, et al: Estimation of birth weight by the use of ultrasound formulas targeted to large-, appropriate-, and small-for-gestational age fetuses, *Am J Obstet Gynecol* 160:854, 1989.
9. Tejani N, Mann LI, Weiss RR: Antenatal diagnosis and management of the small-for-gestational age fetus, *Obstet Gynecol* 47:31, 1976.
10. Trudinger BJ, Giles WB, Cook CM: Flow velocity waveforms in the maternal uteroplacental and fetal umbilical placental circulation, *Am J Obstet Gynecol* 152:163, 1985.
11. Wladimiroff JW, Tonge HM, Stewart PA: Doppler ultrasound assessment of cerebral blood flow in the human fetus, *Br J Obstet Gynaecol* 93:471-475, 1986.

20

large-for-gestational age pregnancy

INSTRUCTIONAL OBJECTIVES

At the completion of this chapter, the reader will be able to:

1. Describe the clinical problems that are typical reasons for the sonographic evaluation of the large-for-gestational age pregnancy.
2. Describe the clinical symptoms and pathologic basis for the various causes of a large-for-gestational age pregnancy, including maternal diabetes, Rh isoimmunization, nonimmune hydrops, polyhydramnios, and the major fetal anomalies associated with a large-for-gestational age pregnancy.
3. Identify on sectional sonograms the above-mentioned pathologic processes in relation to the large-for-gestational age pregnancy, based on the sonographic appearance, the clinical history, and the results of other diagnostic procedures.
4. Describe several technical pitfalls associated with the sonographic examination of the large-for-gestational age pregnancy.

THE CLINICAL PROBLEM

The large-for-gestational age (LGA) pregnancy is defined as a fetus whose growth parameters are above the 90th percentile. An accurate clinical evaluation of the patient with a LGA pregnancy includes the menstrual history, pertinent clinical history, a review of maternal weight gain, and the estimation of the fundal height. A patient with a history of irregular periods or without a precise date for the last normal menstrual period (LNMP) broadens the clinical differential diagnosis. Initially the sonographer should consider that the patient may be simply further along in her pregnancy. Even with a reliable menstrual history, the differential diagnosis for an LGA pregnancy includes multiple gestation, fetal macrosomia, polyhydramnios caused by the development of fetal hydrops or other fetal congenital anomalies, or a large maternal pelvic mass. A sonographic examination can usually narrow the differential diagnosis and often accurately identify the abnormality. This chapter discusses a number of the causes that produce an LGA pregnancy, including maternal diabetes, immune and nonimmune hydrops, and the development of polyhydramnios associated with fetal congenital anomalies. Chapter 21 includes a more complete discussion of the fetal anomalies.

SCANNING PROTOCOLS AND TECHNIQUES

When screening for an LGA pregnancy, the scanning protocol for the sonographic examination during the second and third trimesters follows the guidelines outlined in Chapter 18. The following section summarizes the standard protocol:

Fetal Age and Growth Parameters
1. BPD
2. Head circumference or cephalic index
3. Abdominal circumference
4. Femur length
5. Estimation of fetal weight

Fetal Anatomy
1. Cerebral ventricles to rule out hydrocephaly
2. Four-chamber heart and heart position within the thoracic cavity
3. Spine to rule out spina bifida
4. Stomach to assess function and rule out anomalies
5. Kidneys to rule out anomalies and obstruction
6. Urinary bladder to assess renal function and to rule out obstruction
7. Umbilical cord insertion to rule out abnormalities of the anterior abdominal wall
8. Three-vessel cord
9. Fetal lie in relation to maternal longitudinal axis

Placenta and Maternal Anatomy
1. Anatomic location and grade
2. Position of placenta in relation to internal cervical os
3. Amount of amniotic fluid

4. Uterus for fibroids and other abnormalities
5. Adnexal areas to rule out masses

The following sections discuss the clinical signs and symptoms and sonographic patterns of the major abnormalities that cause an LGA pregnancy.

FETAL MACROSOMIA

Fetal macrosomia is defined as a birth weight over 4000 g, or approximately 9 lbs, which exceeds the 90th percentile. The macrosomic infant is at high risk for complications, such as stillbirth and intrapartum trauma. The incidence of macrosomia in obese patients is greater than it is in patients of average weight. As mentioned in Chapter 19, maternal diabetes mellitus is one of the most significant medical complications of pregnancy, since it can cause intrauterine growth retardation, the development of macrosomia, or congenital anomalies. Although the incidence of diabetes is greater in obese patients, most cases of macrosomia do not involve diabetes. Postmature infants can receive good nourishment and present as LGA babies at their delayed birth. Other causes of macrosomia include multiparity, maternal height, and the sex of the fetus. Through the fifth pregnancy, fetal weight increases an average of 80 to 120 g for each successive pregnancy. Birth weight also correlates with maternal height. Taller women give birth to larger babies. Typically, male fetuses gain more weight during the third trimester than female fetuses and are approximately 150 g heavier at birth. In fact, approximately 65% of macrosomic babies are boys. Several congenital syndromes may produce macrosomia, such as Beckwith-Wiedemann syndrome, which is usually the result of hyperplasia of the islet cells in the pancreas. Insulin can act as a growth hormone in the fetus.[6]

The primary sonographic diagnosis of fetal macrosomia relies on the interpretation of the growth parameters—the head circumference, abdominal circumference, femur length, and estimated fetal weight. With macrosomia these parameters are above the 90th percentile. Additional sonographic features depend on the underlying cause. In maternal diabetes the sonographer may also demonstrate polyhydramnios, typically developing in the third trimester (Fig. 20-1). Studies indicate that approximately 80% of all cases of polyhydramnios are associated with maternal diabetes.[6] Patients with mild to moderate diabetes may present with a grade 0 or 1 placenta in the third trimester. In the nonvascular categories of the disease the placental thickness may increase, measuring greater than 4 cm. In maternal diabetes the fetus should also receive a thorough examination for anomalies, particularly the heart, the central nervous system, and the genitourinary and

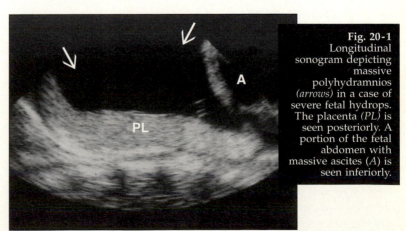

Fig. 20-1 Longitudinal sonogram depicting massive polyhydramnios (arrows) in a case of severe fetal hydrops. The placenta (PL) is seen posteriorly. A portion of the fetal abdomen with massive ascites (A) is seen inferiorly.

gastrointestinal tracts. The sonographer should note the amount of amniotic fluid to exclude polyhydramnios from the diagnosis and perform an anomaly screen to eliminate diabetes as a possible cause of the macrosomia.

FETAL HYDROPS

Fetal hydrops can occur from a variety of causes and are divided into two major categories—immune and nonimmune. In immune hydrops an antigen incompatibility between the mother and fetus typically leads to the development of complications that include hydrops. The fetal signs of this disease differ according to the severity of the case. The fetal physiologic changes cause fetal-fluid overload. The classic sonographic signs of hydrops include ascites, pleural effusions, and skin edema. Normal fetal skin thickness should not exceed 3 mm. Hydrops is the most common cause of fetal ascites, followed by ascites as a result of urinary tract leakage or rupture.[3] The following subsections discuss each of these categories in detail.

Immune Hydrops

Because a fetus receives half of its genetic material from each parent, the fetal blood type can differ from the maternal blood type. Various types of antigens travel in the red blood cells. If the blood antigens are different and the fetal blood mixes with the maternal circulatory system, the mother may produce antibodies in response to the fetal antigen. Some of these antibodies can pass through the placental barrier and interact with the fetal red blood cells, causing hemolytic anemia, which leads to the development of **erythroblastosis fetalis. Rh-factor incompatibility** is the cause for a majority of the cases of immune hydrops, although other factors include Kell, Duffy, and Kidd.[5]

In Rh isoimmunization the Rh-negative mother develops antibodies if her blood mixes with Rh-positive red blood cells. This development can occur from an incompatible blood transfusion or from fetomaternal hemorrhage, either during pregnancy or at the time of delivery. Causes of fetomaternal hemorrhage range from a prior induced or spontaneous abortion to placenta previa or abruptio placenta to amniocentesis and maternal abdominal trauma. Other causes include a cesarean section and the manual removal of the placenta. However, approximately 30% of Rh-negative mothers never become sensitive after exposure to the opposite antigen. Currently all obstetric patients are typed for the Rh factor. If they are Rh negative, the clinician will perform antibody screening periodically during the pregnancy and give the patient Rh-immune globulin (RhIgG). If the result is positive, the clinician manages the patient as if she were Rh sensitized and monitors the fetus for evidence of adverse reactions.[5]

Mild fetal effects from Rh incompatibility include anemia and the resulting hyperbilirubinemia at birth. More serious signs include the development of hepatosplenomegaly. In severe cases the fetus develops congestive heart failure, which can cause the formation of pleural effusions, ascites, and skin edema (Fig. 20-2). Other signs of more severe effects include the development of an enlarged placenta (Fig. 20-3), polyhydramnios, and umbilical vein dilatation. The clinician can monitor the severity of the disease by performing serial amniocentesis procedures. The clinical laboratory can assay the fetal bilirubin levels, which abnormally increase proportionately to the severity of the liver failure. If the case is severe, the obstetrician may perform an intrauterine transfusion to save the fetus.[7]

Nonimmune Hydrops

The causes of nonimmune hydrops are many and linked together by the production of increased fetal venous pressure. Many of the conditions that cause hydrops present no discrete sonographic patterns to enable their identification. Examples of fetal abnormalities detectable by sonography include cardiovascular anomalies, cystic adenomatoid (CAM) formation, pulmonary hyperplasia, diaphragmatic hernia, trisomy 18 or 21, cystic hygroma, maternal diabetes mellitus, and preeclampsia-eclampsia. Of these conditions, cardiovascular anomalies are the most common cause of nonimmune hydrops in the United States. Although a few of these underlying abnormalities can be treated at birth, many cases of nonimmune hydrops are fatal.[2]

The sonographic signs for nonimmune hydrops initially include those listed for immune hydrops—fetal pleural effusions, ascites, and skin edema. If the clinical history does not support a preliminary diagnosis of immune hydrops, the sonographer should perform an extensive anomaly screen to determine the cause of the hydrops, beginning with a thorough examination of the heart. Some of the cardiac anomalies associated with hydrops are hypoplastic left-heart syndrome and dysrhythmias. Fig. 20-4 illustrates a case of fetal hydrops caused by a cystic hygroma.

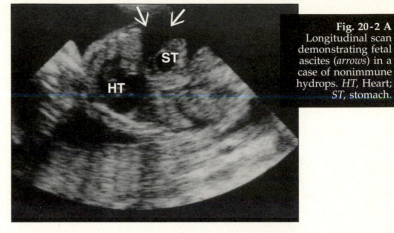

Fig. 20-2 A Longitudinal scan demonstrating fetal ascites (*arrows*) in a case of nonimmune hydrops. *HT,* Heart; *ST,* stomach.

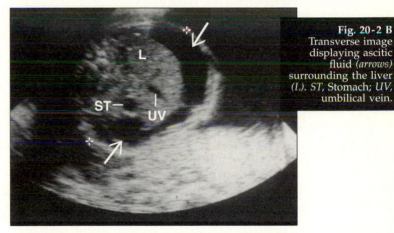

Fig. 20-2 B Transverse image displaying ascitic fluid (*arrows*) surrounding the liver (*L*). *ST,* Stomach; *UV,* umbilical vein.

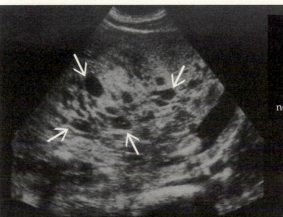

Fig. 20-3 Transverse image depicting a placenta that is enlarged and contains numerous anechoic areas (*arrows*), in a case of nonimmune hydrops.

POLYHYDRAMNIOS

Polyhydramnios, an excess of amniotic fluid, exists when the amniotic fluid volume exceeds 2000 cc. This limit correlates with an amniotic fluid index (AFI) of greater than 20 to 24 cm.[1] In the latter half of the second trimester and during the third trimester, the sonographer should suspect polyhydramnios if the amniotic fluid totally surrounds the fetus. As mentioned in a previous section, the most common cause of polyhydramnios is a diabetic pregnancy. Approximately 20% of cases have fetal congenital anomalies, with central nervous system anomalies having the highest frequency of polyhydramnios.[4] Other anomalies associated with polyhydramnios include abnormalities of the gastrointestinal tract involving the esophagus, stomach, and/or small bowel, as well as a number of skeletal anomalies, such as dwarfism. Multiple gestations frequently develop polyhydramnios, and often the cause remains unknown or idiopathic. The sonographer should remember that polyhydramnios is also associated with fetal hydrops. When polyhydramnios is discovered, the sonographer must perform a complete anomaly screen to narrow the clinical differential diagnosis by eliminating a number of the major anomalies detectable by sonography.

OTHER CAUSES OF A LARGE-FOR-GESTATIONAL PREGNANCY

The pathologic processes mentioned in the previous sections

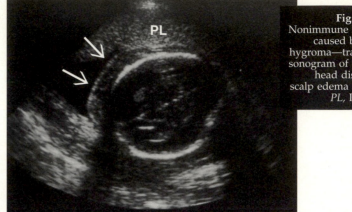

Fig. 20-4 A Nonimmune hydrops caused by cystic hygroma—transverse sonogram of the fetal head displaying scalp edema *(arrows)*. *PL*, Placenta.

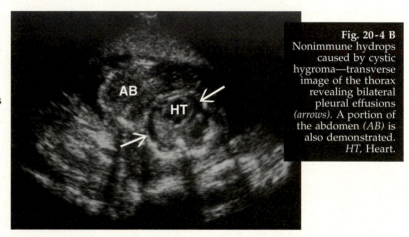

Fig. 20-4 B Nonimmune hydrops caused by cystic hygroma—transverse image of the thorax revealing bilateral pleural effusions *(arrows)*. A portion of the abdomen *(AB)* is also demonstrated. *HT*, Heart.

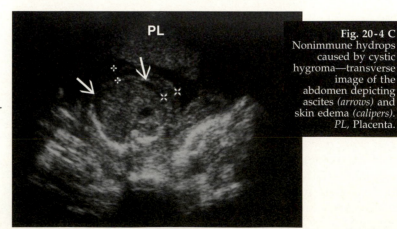

Fig. 20-4 C Nonimmune hydrops caused by cystic hygroma—transverse image of the abdomen depicting ascites *(arrows)* and skin edema *(calipers)*. *PL*, Placenta.

represent the most common causes of an LGA pregnancy during the second and third trimesters. Other types of pathology that may result in an LGA pregnancy are the hydatidiform mole and maternal pelvic masses. However, the hydatidiform mole has additional clinical symptoms, such as vaginal bleeding and an elevated β-hCG, which allows the clinician to reorder the differential diagnosis. Pelvic masses during pregnancy (discussed in Chapter 17) can

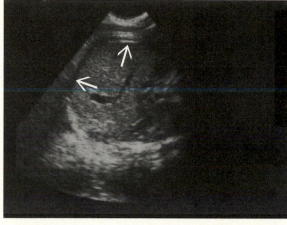

Fig. 20-5 Transverse image of a normal fetal abdomen demonstrating the hypoechoic ring *(arrows)*, which may be mistaken for fetal ascites.

remain asymptomatic and undetectable on an early pelvic examination and can become symptomatic during the second trimester. The serous cystadenoma and large uterine fibroids provide examples of maternal pathology that could result in an LGA pregnancy.

TECHNICAL PITFALLS

As mentioned in previous chapters, the sonographer must ensure that all gestational measurements are as accurate as possible and inform the interpreting physician of any suboptimal measurements. Examining the fetus, the amniotic fluid volume, and the placenta provides additional clues to narrow the differential diagnosis.

An additional pitfall relates to the determination of fetal ascites. At the level of the liver, the abdominal wall musculature can appear hypoechoic, producing a pattern similar to minimal ascites. This "pseudoascites" differs from pathologic ascites wherein fluid is seen in other peritoneal recesses, such as between bowel loops (Fig. 20-5). Another pitfall can occur as the sonographer inspects the shape of the abdomen. Particularly in the third trimester and with the LGA fetus, the fetal abdomen may appear distorted as a result of normal compression by the uterine walls. This condition may mimic pathology such as an omphalocele. The sonographer must remember that an omphalocele often occurs with other anomalies and that this technical artifact should be included in the differential diagnosis if no other abnormal patterns are demonstrated.

SUMMARY

The sonographer must consider a number of conditions when a patient for sonographic examination is LGA. The list ranges from a normal multiple gestation to serious conditions, such as fetal hydrops and other congenital anomalies. If multiple abnormalities are detected or if the differential diagnosis is unclear, the patient should be referred to a high-risk perinatal lab for further evaluation and treatment.

REFERENCES

1. Dunnihoo DR: *Fundamentals of gynecology and obstetrics,* ed 2, Philadelphia, 1992, JB Lippincott, p 303.
2. Dunnihoo DR: *Fundamentals of gynecology and obstetrics,* ed 2, Philadelphia, 1992, JB Lippincott, pp 259-260.

3. Fleischer AC, Killam AP, et al: Hydrops fetalis: sonographic evaluation and clinical implications, *Radiology* 141:163-168, 1981.
4. Pernoll ML, Benson RC, editors: *Current obstetric and gynecologic diagnosis and treatment,* Norwalk, Conn, 1987, Appleton and Lange, p 247.
5. Pernoll ML, Benson RC, editors: *Current obstetric and gynecologic diagnosis and treatment,* Norwalk, Conn, 1987, Appleton and Lange, pp 273-278.
6. Pernoll ML, Benson RC, editors: *Current obstetric and gynecologic diagnosis and treatment,* Norwalk, Conn, 1987, Appleton and Lange, pp 318-320.
7. Seeds JW, Watson AB: Ultrasound-guided fetal intravascular transfusion in severe rhesus immunization, *Am J Obstet Gynecol* 154:1105-1107, 1986.

congenital anomalies

INSTRUCTIONAL OBJECTIVES

At the completion of this chapter, the reader will be able to:

1. Describe the clinical problems that are typical reasons for a sonographic evaluation of fetal congenital anomalies.
2. Describe the clinical laboratory tests used for anomaly screening, including testing for abnormal alpha-fetoprotein levels.
3. Describe the clinical symptoms and pathologic basis for anomalies of the central nervous system, including ventriculomegaly and hydrocephalus; anencephaly, microcephaly, holoprosencephaly, hydranencephaly, and iniencephaly; agenesis of the corpus callosum; Dandy-Walker syndrome and other congenital neoplasms and cysts; and spina bifida and meningocele.
4. Describe the clinical symptoms and pathologic basis for the anomalies of the gastrointestinal tract, including esophageal, duodenal, and small bowel atresias, a tracheal-esophageal fistula, colon malformations, omphalocele, umbilical hernias, gastroschisis, and meconium peritonitis.
5. Describe the clinical symptoms and pathologic basis for the anomalies of the genitourinary system, including renal agenesis, infantile polycystic disease, multicystic kidney disease, hydronephrosis, posterior urethral valve syndrome, and neoplasms.
6. Describe the clinical symptoms and pathologic basis for the anomalies of the skeletal system, including thanatophoric and camptomelic dysplasias, osteogenesis imperfecta, achondroplasia and achondrogenesis, and amniotic band syndrome.
7. Describe the clinical symptoms and pathologic basis for the anomalies of the thoracic cavity, including cystic adenomatoid malformation, diaphragmatic hernia, pleural effusion, other cystic and solid neoplasms, and contour or proportion abnormalities.
8. Describe the clinical symptoms and pathologic basis for the major anomalies of the heart, including atrial and ventricular septal defects, hypoplastic left-heart syndrome, and transposition of the great vessels.

9. Describe the clinical symptoms and pathologic basis for the major anomalies of the face and neck, including hypertelorism and hypotelorism, cleft lip and palate, and cystic hygroma, teratoma, and other neoplasms.
10. Describe the clinical symptoms and pathologic basis for umbilical cord anomalies, including single umbilical artery, cysts, thrombosis, hemangioma and hematoma, cord prolapse, and velamentous insertion.
11. Describe the clinical symptoms and pathologic basis of the major trisomic conditions, including trisomy 13, 18, and 21.
12. Identify on sectional sonograms the above-mentioned fetal congenital anomalies, based on the sonographic appearance, the clinical history, and the results of other diagnostic procedures.
13. Describe several technical pitfalls associated with the sonographic evaluation for fetal anomalies.

THE CLINICAL PROBLEM

The obstetrician evaluates a number of factors to determine if a patient is at risk for fetal malformations. These factors include a family history of genetic anomalies, maternal age, which may increase the risk for trisomic conditions like Down's syndrome, or a previous infant born with congenital anomalies. Other maternal factors that increase the risk of birth defects include a number of viral infections, drug administration during the first trimester (which is considered teratogenic), and alcohol or drug abuse. Maternal diseases, such as diabetes, increase the risk of anomalies. Multiple gestations are also at higher risk for malformations. The clinician must also include congenital anomalies in the differential diagnosis when a patient presents either as a small-for-gestational age (SGA) or large-for-gestational age (LGA) pregnancy. Polyhydramnios may develop with anomalies of the central nervous system, the gastrointestinal tract, and the skeletal system. Severe bilateral renal dysfunction can cause oligohydramnios. Some major anomalies cause no suspicious clinical symptoms and are diagnosed as incidental findings during a routine sonographic examination performed for gestational dating. The sonographer must possess an extensive knowledge of the anomalies detectable by sonography. The discovery of one malformation requires a thorough examination of all other fetal structures, since a single major anomaly is rare. In addition, a more extensive and advanced evaluation is necessary to determine the presence of various syndromes and trisomic conditions.

CLINICAL LABORATORY TESTS

The fetal liver produces alpha-fetoprotein (AFP), which constitutes the major protein in the fetal serum. After birth, the presence of AFP is always an abnormal finding. Normal AFP levels are higher in the fetal serum, but lower levels are found in the amniotic fluid and the maternal serum. A number of fetal conditions will cause an abnormal elevation of AFP in both the maternal serum and the amniotic fluid. With an open neural tube defect, AFP leaks into the amniotic fluid, producing an elevated AFP value, as well as an elevated maternal AFP. This elevation is usually present by the eighteenth gestational week.[2] Although a multiple pregnancy can cause a false-positive elevation, sonography can readily document a normal multiple gestation as the cause of the elevation. Another factor that can produce a false-positive elevation is an incorrect gestational age, since normal AFP levels are correlated with gestational age. Besides open neural tube defects, other causes for AFP elevation include gastrointestinal obstructions, omphalocele, cystic hygroma, missed abortion, fetal distress, fetal death, and severe immune hydrops. Low AFP levels have been associated with Down's syndrome and other trisomic conditions.[18] In all cases of abnormal AFP values, the fetus should receive a full anomaly screen to refine the differential diagnosis.

RELATED IMAGING PROCEDURES

Plain-film radiography can play a role in the differential diagnosis of fetal skeletal abnormalities. This examination can identify short extremities, poor ossification, and the narrow chest associated with a number of the major skeletal dysplasias. Radiography can also verify anencephaly, fetal acrania, and other types of pathologic abnormalities that affect the size and shape of the calvaria. However, this technique will not allow the diagnosis of most major abnormalities involving the soft-tissue organs of the fetus. In some instances, magnetic resonance imaging (MRI) is used to provide greater detail of soft-tissue structures, particularly when the sonographic examination does not provide the information needed for an accurate diagnosis.

SCANNING PROTOCOLS AND TECHNIQUES

Chapter 18 discusses the examination protocol for second- and third-trimester pregnancies. This protocol includes routine imaging of major fetal anatomy, which should provide a screening for the most common fetal abnormalities. The following section summarizes the routine examination:

Fetal Age and Growth
1. BPD
2. Head circumference or cephalic index
3. Abdominal circumference
4. Femur length
5. Estimation of fetal weight

Fetal Anatomy
1. Cerebral ventricles to rule out hydrocephaly
2. Four-chamber heart and heart position within the thoracic cavity
3. Spine to rule out spina bifida
4. Stomach to assess function and rule out anomalies
5. Kidneys to rule out anomalies and obstruction
6. Urinary bladder to assess renal function and rule out obstruction
7. Umbilical cord insertion to rule out abnormalities of the anterior abdominal wall
8. Three-vessel cord
9. Fetal lie in relation to maternal longitudinal axis

Placenta and Maternal Anatomy
1. Anatomic location and grade
2. Position of placenta in relation to internal cervical os
3. Amount of amniotic fluid
4. Uterus for fibroids and other abnormalities
5. Adnexal areas to rule out masses

An ultrasound department can expand the basic protocol, based on the risk factors of its patient population and on the level of expertise of the interpreting physicians and sonographers. The sonographer must also expand the examination when an abnormality is evident during a routine examination. Examples include measuring the nuchal fold, evaluating the fetal extremities, examining for a cleft lip and palate, measuring the orbits for the presence of hypotelorism or hypertelorism, and performing a full fetal cardiac evaluation.

The sonographer must continually monitor changes in fetal position to obtain the proper plane necessary to depict the anatomy. In the third trimester, acoustic shadowing from the ribs can interfere with the proper visualization of the heart and abdominal organs. As in abdominal sonography in the infant or adult, the sonographer must find an acoustic window that avoids the fetal spine and ribs. In some cases, placing the mother in an oblique position will allow a more detailed examination of fetal anatomy.

ABNORMAL SONOGRAPHIC PATTERNS

Anomalies of the Central Nervous System

Ventricles of the brain. The cerebrospinal fluid is produced by the choriod plexus in the **lateral ventricles.** The ventricles are numbered, starting superiorly. The lateral ventricles, also known as the first and second ventricles, are positioned within the cerebral hemispheres. Each lateral ventricle is made up of the frontal (or temporal) horn, the body (or atria), and the occipital horn. The region where the body and occipital horns meet is called the **trigone.** The slitlike **third ventricle** lies between the right and left thalami. The cerebrospinal fluid normally courses from the lateral ventricle through the third ventricle via the **foramen of Monro.** The **cerebral aqueduct,** or the aqueduct of Sylvius, connects the third and fourth ventricle. The fluid then courses from the **fourth ventricle** into the **subarachnoid space** via the **foramen of Luschka** and the **foramen of Magendie.**

Hydrocephaly. An enlargement of the ventricles is called **ventriculomegaly.** Severe ventriculomegaly can cause an enlargement of the entire head, termed **hydrocephalus.** Causes vary from infections, stenosis, metabolic disorders, and neoplasms to chromosomal abnormalities. The ratio of the lateral ventricle/cerebral hemisphere width changes during the normal course of pregnancy. At 15 weeks gestation, the lateral ventricles are prominent, as well as the choriod plexus, and the ratio may reach 80%. It decreases rather quickly until 25 weeks gestation, attaining a 30% ratio, which remains fairly constant until term.[16]

Classifications. There are two types of hydrocephalus, based on the location of the obstruction. **Noncommunicating hydrocephalus,** the more common type, occurs when the obstruction causes dilatation of the ventricular system. Since the cerebrospinal fluid is produced in the lateral ventricles and courses inferiorly, the ventricular system will dilate superior to the level of obstruction. The occipital horns usually enlarge before the other portions of the lateral ventricles. Displacement of the medial wall of the lateral ventricle usually occurs before lateral displacement.[22] The most frequent cause is **aqueductal stenosis,** which is a narrowing of the aqueduct of Sylvius. In approximately 50% of cases, the stenosis is caused by an infection, such as mumps or toxoplasmosis. Other causes include embryonic malformation or an X-linked recessive trait, with a 25% incidence of recurrence.[44]

The other type, **communicating hydrocephalus,** accounts for approximately 38% of cases of congenital hydrocephalus. The obstruction occurs external to the ventricular system, which causes ventricular dilatation and an enlargement of the subarachnoid space. Typically, all four ventricles appear enlarged, although the fourth ventricle is usually the least affected. The subarachnoid space between the calvaria and the brain fills with fluid, although this may become less prominent as the gestation progresses.[37]

Clinical signs and sonographic patterns. The patient may present clinically as a LGA pregnancy or have an elevated AFP value. However, polyhydramnios does not usually develop until the latter part of the second trimester or during the third trimester. In aqueductal stenosis the sonographic examination typically reveals dilatation of the lateral and third ventricles, but the fourth ventricle is normal (Fig. 21-1). In communicating hydrocephalus the sonographic examination may demonstrate both ventriculomegaly and a dilated subarachnoid space. However, documentation of this space is technically difficult as a result of reverberation artifacts from the calvaria. Severe enlargement of the ventricles may also mask the dilatation of the subarachnoid space.

The sonographer should always document the level of obstruction, as well as conduct a careful evaluation for other related abnormalities, including spina bifida, meningocele, and encephalocele. Asymmetric hydrocephalus can be caused by cerebral neoplasms, such as teratoma or tumors of the face and neck. In addition, the amount of amniotic fluid should be carefully evaluated for evidence of polyhydramnios.

Anencephaly. Normally the neural tube closes by the twenty-eighth day after conception. Anencephaly develops when the superior portion of the neural groove fails to close. This failure causes either a large symmetric calvarial defect or a complete absence of the calvarium. The base of the skull and the facial features are not affected. In an anencephalic fetus the cerebral hemispheres are absent, and the remainder of the brain is typically malformed. However, there is always functional neural tissue, which may allow the fetus to have intact autonomic nervous function, display a heart beat, and even some muscular motion. This condition is uniformly fatal, with death occurring perinatally or several days after birth.[44]

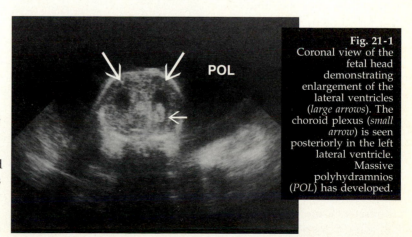

Fig. 21-1 Coronal view of the fetal head demonstrating enlargement of the lateral ventricles (*large arrows*). The choroid plexus (*small arrow*) is seen posteriorly in the left lateral ventricle. Massive polyhydramnios (*POL*) has developed.

Clinical history. The patient may present an elevated AFP value, since this is an open neural tube defect. The clinician may note that the fetal head is not palpable on physical examination. The patient may appear LGA in the latter portion of the second trimester and during the third trimester, since polyhydramnios develops in approximately 50% of cases.

Sonographic patterns. The suggested view for documenting anencephaly is a longitudinal view of the spine that demonstrates only the base of the skull (Fig. 21-2). A coronal view of the face will demonstrate intact facial structures with no frontal bone superior to the orbits (Fig. 21-3). If the initial examination is performed in the third trimester, an endovaginal examination may be necessary to document anencephaly if the fetal head is located considerably inferior and posterior in the maternal pelvis. The Trendelenburg position may also reposition the fetal head and allow adequate visualization.[12] The sonographer should always evaluate the amniotic fluid volume for signs of polyhydramnios. Since spina bifida, meningocele, and myelomeningocele occur in approximately 50% of anencephalic patients, the sonographer should perform a careful examination of the spine.[15]

Microcephaly. Microcephaly develops with a variety of disorders and is suspected when the biparietal diameter (BPD), head cirumference, and cephalic index fall below three standard devia-

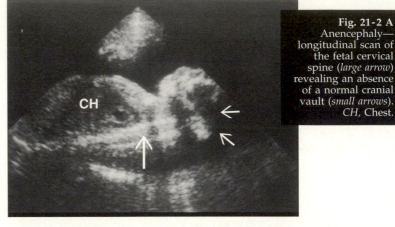

Fig. 21-2 A
Anencephaly—longitudinal scan of the fetal cervical spine (*large arrow*) revealing an absence of a normal cranial vault (*small arrows*). *CH*, Chest.

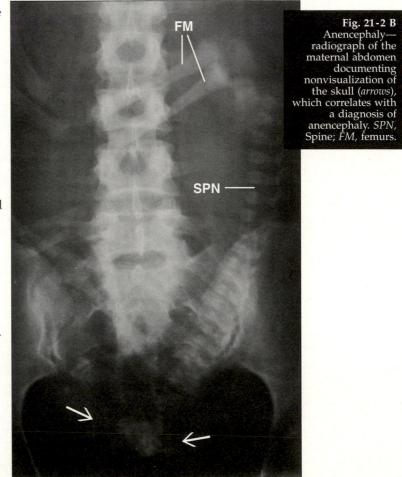

Fig. 21-2 B
Anencephaly—radiograph of the maternal abdomen documenting nonvisualization of the skull (*arrows*), which correlates with a diagnosis of anencephaly. *SPN*, Spine; *FM*, femurs.

tions, but other measurements, such as the abdominal circumference and femur length, fall within the normal range. Causes of microcephaly include infections, such as rubella and toxoplasmosis; teratogens, such as alcohol and heroin; metabolic disorders, including phenylketonuria (PKU); and genetic conditions, such as trisomy 13 and 18. A large cystic hygroma may also lead to microcephaly. **Craniosynostosis,** the premature closure of the cranial sutures, can develop with a variety of genetic syndromes. Asymmetric closure, or closure of only some of the paired sutures, will lead to abnormal head shapes, as well as microcephaly. Premature closure of all sutures may not produce a prominent head-shape deviation, but may only display microcephaly.[44]

Primarily the sonographer depends on the evaluation of the fetal head measurements to suspect microcephaly. The head circumference and cephalic index provide more accurate statistical measurements, since the BPD

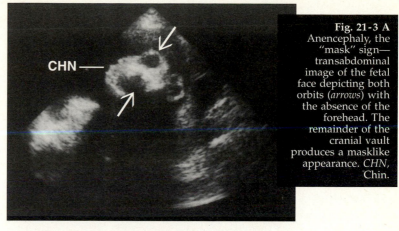

Fig. 21-3 A Anencephaly, the "mask" sign— transabdominal image of the fetal face depicting both orbits (*arrows*) with the absence of the forehead. The remainder of the cranial vault produces a masklike appearance. *CHN,* Chin.

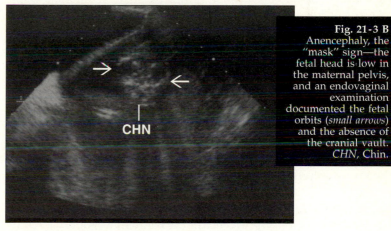

Fig. 21-3 B Anencephaly, the "mask" sign—the fetal head is low in the maternal pelvis, and an endovaginal examination documented the fetal orbits (*small arrows*) and the absence of the cranial vault. *CHN,* Chin.

does not differentiate normal head-shape anomalies from other pathologic conditions. Consequently, the sonographer should perform a careful examination for other anomalies.

Holoprosencephaly. Holoprosencephaly occurs with the failure of normal forebrain and/or facial development during the third week of embryologic development. This anomaly is frequently associated with trisomy 13, but the cause remains unknown in a number of patients. This condition has two classifications, lobar and alobar. The alobar is the more severe variety and often includes facial anomalies, such as cyclopia with a proboscis superior to the orbit, hypotelorism, and cleft lip and palate. As a result of the deficits produced by abnormal forebrain development, severe mental retardation often occurs.[44]

In alobar holoprosencephaly, abnormal development of the midline brain structures leads to the development of a large sickle-shaped monoventricle in the posterior portion of the lateral ventricles and a dorsal sac at the level of the posterior fossa.[38] In lobar holoprosencephaly the brain development is not as abnormal, typically producing ventriculomegaly with the presence of occipital and temporal horns. The sonographer should examine the fetal face for signs of cyclopia, hypotelorism, and cleft lip and palate, since the severity of the facial anomalies alters the clinical management and prognosis of the abnormality.

Hydranencephaly. Hydranencephaly is the complete or near-complete destruction of the cerebral cortex and basal ganglia, probably as a result of an infection or a vascular abnormality. The lower portions of the brain, such as the cerebellum, generally remain intact. Because of the absence of the cerebral hemispheres, the prognosis is uniformly fatal.[44]

Sonographically, the classic pattern is a cranial vault filled with cerebrospinal fluid and the depiction of some echogenic cerebellar tissue inferiorly.[28] The patient may develop polyhydramnios.

Iniencephaly. Similarly to anencephaly, iniencephaly is also related to an incomplete closure of the neural tube during the first month of gestation. Incomplete closure of the occipital, cervical, and thoracic portions of the neural tube produces gross hyperextension of the fetal head and fusion of the occiput to the cervical spine. In some cases the brain may prolapse into the spinal cavity. This condition is more rare than anencephaly and its cause often remains idiopathic. This condition is usually an open neural tube defect (no epithelial covering), which typically produces elevated AFP levels.[44]

The typical sonographic pattern for iniencephaly includes a hyperextension of the fetal neck and an abnormal cervical and thoracic vertebrae, which may appear as either hypoechoic and more widely spaced or totally absent. The sonographer should search for evidence of hydrocephalus and spina bifida or meningocele in the inferior portions of the spine.[15]

Agenesis of the corpus callosum. The corpus callosum is located superior to the atria of the lateral ventricles. The absence of the corpus callosum leads to the displacement of surrounding brain structures. The agenesis may be partial or total. Agenesis of the corpus callosum may be associated with other conditions, such as trisomy 8, 13, 15, and 18, as well as Dandy-Walker syndrome.[20,43,44]

The typical sonographic pattern for near-total agenesis of the corpus callosum is a superiorly deviated, enlarged third ventricle. The bodies of the lateral ventricles appear more laterally located than normal (Fig. 21-4). If total agenesis is present, the cavum septum pellucidi are also absent.[14] The sonographer

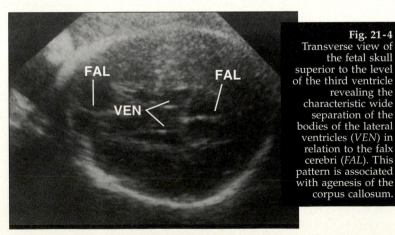

FAL   FAL

VEN

Fig. 21-4 Transverse view of the fetal skull superior to the level of the third ventricle revealing the characteristic wide separation of the bodies of the lateral ventricles (*VEN*) in relation to the falx cerebri (*FAL*). This pattern is associated with agenesis of the corpus callosum.

should perform a full anomaly screen, since this abnormality is associated with a number of trisomic conditions.

Dandy-Walker syndrome. Dandy-Walker syndrome is the abnormal development of the cerebellum and fourth ventricle. An **arachnoid cyst,** less common and not as serious as Dandy-Walker syndrome, displaces the cerebellum but does not separate it. The classic sonographic pattern is a dilated fourth ventricle that often enlarges to occupy the posterior fossa (called the "Dandy-Walker cyst"), separating the cerebellar hemispheres.[20] The superior portions of the ventricular system should be evaluated for ventriculomegaly, and the sonographer should look for signs of agenesis of the corpus callosum.

Encephalocele. The encephalocele, the least common open neural tube defect, occurs with the failure of the surface epithelium to separate from the neuroectoderm, resulting in a calvarial defect that allows the herniation of the meninges and/or neural tissue through the defect. A **meningocele** occurs with herniation of the meninges and contains cerebrospinal fluid. A **meningomyelocele** forms when both the meninges and the brain tissue protruded through the calvarial defect. For patients in the United States, the most common location for an encephalocele is the occipital region. However, people of Asian descent have a higher incidence of frontal encephaloceles. In these cases the defect is midline. If an asymmetric defect is seen, this may be associated with amniotic band syndrome. Encephalocele is associated with other anomalies, including hydrocephalus, Dandy-Walker syndrome, agenesis of the corpus callosum, and Meckel's syndrome. **Meckel's syndrome** consists of polycystic kidneys, polydactyly, microcephaly, and encephalocele. Since this is an open neural tube defect, the most common clinical symptom is elevated AFP levels.[44]

To confirm the presence of an encephalocele and eliminate other anomalies (such as cystic hygroma), the sonographer should demonstrate the calvarial defect. This primary sonographic sign can present a technical challenge, since it can be difficult to attain the proper scanning window and angle necessary to reduce artifact production and acoustic shadowing.[25] A meningocele typically appears as a cystic structure adjacent to the fetal skull. A meningomyelocele typically produces a complex pattern, with variable amounts of brain tissue herniated into the sac (Fig. 21-5). Moderate to severe brain herniation can lead to microcephaly. The sonographer should perform a full anomaly screen, particularly searching for evidence of hydrocephalus and Meckel's syndrome.

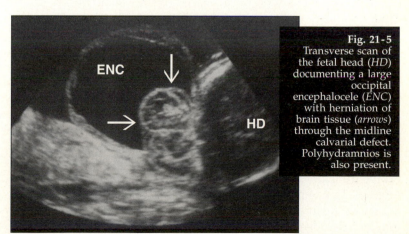

Fig. 21-5 Transverse scan of the fetal head (*HD*) documenting a large occipital encephalocele (*ENC*) with herniation of brain tissue (*arrows*) through the midline calvarial defect. Polyhydramnios is also present.

Choroid plexus cysts. Choroid plexus cysts, a rather common occurrence, are usually demonstrated sonographically between 16 and 21 weeks as cystic structures adjacent to the choroid plexus in the lateral ventricles (Fig. 21-6). They may develop singly or in multiples and may contain debris as they resolve. Typically they regress by 25 or 26 weeks. Several case reports have associated choroid plexus cysts with chromosomal abnormalities.[35] If regression and resolution is not apparent by 25 to 26 weeks, the patient may be referred for genetic screening.

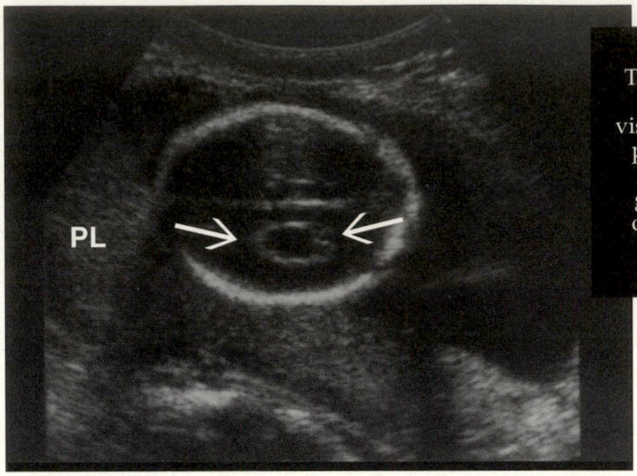

Fig. 21-6
Transverse image of the fetal skull visualizing a choroid plexus cyst (*arrows*) at 20 weeks gestational age. No other abnormalities were noted. *PL,* Placenta.

Brain neoplasms. Congenital neoplasms of the brain are rare. The teratoma is the most common and typically displays sonographically as a complex mass. It may produce asymmetric hydrocephalus.

Spina bifida. Spina bifida refers to an incomplete closure of the neural tube and is related to anencephaly and encephalocele. There are several classifications related to the severity of the defect.

Classifications. **Spina bifida occulta,** the most mild form, involves an incomplete closure of only one vertebral arch and causes no neurologic deficits. The only clinical indication of this condition may be a tuft of hair over a slight skin depression posterior to the abnormality. A more severe defect involves several vertebrae and causes the formation of a **meningocele,** which is a sac that usually protrudes posteriorly and contains the meninges and cerebrospinal fluid. This slightly more severe form may cause some neurologic problems. Since this is an open neural defect, it typically causes an elevation of the maternal serum AFP. With a **myelomeningocele,** the most severe form, the sac also contains a portion of the spinal cord and nerve roots. This herniation usually causes the medulla and part of the cerebellum to become displaced inferiorly into the superior portion of the spinal canal, which typically causes hydrocephalus. This condition is called the **Arnold-Chiari malformation.**[7] The most common location for spina bifida is the sacrolumbar region, although they may occur anywhere along the course of the spine. In rare cases most of the spine fails to fuse, and this condition is called **rachischisis.**

Sonographic patterns. The sonographer must evaluate the spine in all three body planes—coronal, transverse, and longitudinal—to rule out smaller meningoceles and a widening of ossification centers. In the transverse imaging plane the abnormal separation of the ossification centers creates a U-shaped configuration (Fig. 21-7) and may also reveal a meningocele or myelomeningocele. A meningocele tends to contain only fluid, whereas the myelomeningocele appears complex. However, this distinction can be difficult to demonstrate. Real-time examination of the fetal extremities, which reveals a lack of movement, an unusual position, or a prolapse of the foot, may allow a more confident diagnosis of a myelomeningocele. Longitudinal views reveal the skin line and the identification of the saclike defect (Fig. 21-8). The coronal view allows identification of a widening of the ossification centers and the diagnosis of small, more subtle defects.[26] The sonographer should always evaluate the fetal head for signs of Arnold-Chiari malformation. The displacement of the medulla and cerebellum leads to the "banana sign," which is a banana-shaped cerebellum.[33] (Fig. 21-9). This distortion also causes a unique calvarial molding called the "lemon sign," usually affecting the anterior portion of the skull (Fig. 21-10). The sonographer should carefully check for any signs of ventriculomegaly. In the case of small defects or a suboptimal fetal position for visualizing the spine, these sonographic signs in the fetal head can lead to the mention of a possible myelomeningocele in the interpreting physician's report.

Anomalies of the Gastrointestinal Tract

Esophageal atresia. Esophageal atresia develops during the early part of the first trimester when a portion of the esophagus fails to form. Because the esophagus and trachea evolve from the same precursor tissue, approximately 90% of cases of esophageal atresia also develop a fistulous tract between the esophagus and trachea, which is called a tracheoesophageal fistula. This condition appears to be an embryologic malformation, although it occasionally occurs with Down's syndrome. Other associated anomalies include genitourinary, other gastrointestinal, and cardiac anomalies. The AFP levels may

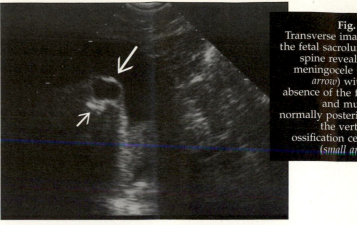

Fig. 21-7
Transverse image of the fetal sacrolumbar spine revealing a meningocele (*large arrow*) with an absence of the fascia and muscles normally posterior to the vertebral ossification centers (*small arrow*).

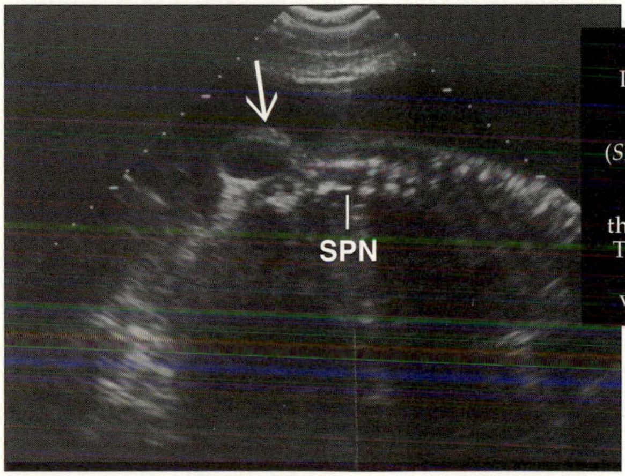

Fig. 21-8
Longitudinal image of the fetal sacrolumbar spine (*SPN*) demonstrating a meningocele (*arrow*) disrupting the normal skin line. The maternal serum alpha-fetoprotein value was elevated.

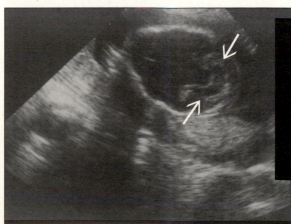

Fig. 21-9
Transverse scan of the fetal head demonstrating the elongated appearance of the cerebellum, the "banana" sign (*arrows*). The fetus has a myomeningocele in the sacrolumbar region.

be normal or increased. Because this malformation disrupts the normal fetal intake of amniotic fluid, many patients develop polyhydramnios.[11]

In the small number of cases of esophageal atresia, the sonographic criteria for diagnosis include nonvisualization of the fetal stomach and polyhydramnios. The sonographer should image the superior portion of the esophagus and document its course to the atretic portion. However, the vast majority of

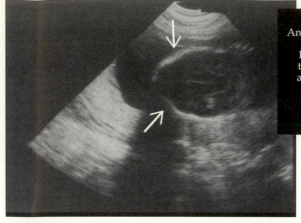

Fig. 21-10
An image of the fetal head illustrated in Fig. 21-9 depicting the skull moulding associated with the depression of the cerebellum, called the "lemon" sign (*arrows*).

cases have a fistulous tract, which makes the sonographic diagnosis very difficult, since some fluid is usually in the stomach. Serial examinations may document a consistently small stomach and the development or progression of polyhydramnios. The sonographer should perform a complete anomaly survey to exclude other anomalies, particularly those associated with polyhydramnios.

Duodenal atresia. Duodenal atresia, the most common small bowel atresia, results from a malformation of the duodenum during the first trimester. This malformation is associated with several genetic conditions, including Down's syndrome, which has a reported incidence of approximately 33%. Other associated abnormalities include additional bowel anomalies, skeletal anomalies, such as supernumerary ribs, sacral agenesis and hemivertebrae, and cardiac anomalies.[43] The AFP levels may be normal or increased. As a result of the disruption of normal amniotic fluid intake to the fetus, polyhydramnios typically develops.

The classic sonographic pattern for duodenal atresia is the visualization of the "double bubble" sign, which is made up of the fluid-filled stomach and the first portion of the duodenum[32] (Fig. 21-11). To accurately identify this condition, a transverse scan through the fetal abdomen will prevent mistaking a prominent fetal stomach and antrum for duodenal atresia. The typical presence of polyhydramnios also aids the differential diagnosis. The sonographer should perform a full anomaly screen, including measuring the nuchal fold in the second trimester for Down's syndrome and screening for skeletal, other gastrointestinal, and cardiac anomalies. If this type of detailed examination is beyond the capabilities of the initial ultrasound department, the patient should be referred to a high-risk perinatal center.

Bowel atresias. Atresias can occur in the inferior portions of the small bowel and are usually the result of a disruption of the vascular supply during the fetal period, or they may be associated with an inherited pattern of multiple bowel atresias. Atresias involving the duodenum and jejunum are usually associated with polyhydramnios. In the absence of a higher gastrointestinal obstruction, colon atresias are less common and are not typically associated with polyhydramnios, since one of the primary functions of the colon is water reabsorption.[11] Anal atresia is difficult to diagnose because it rarely produces distended bowel loops. Since the fetus does not normally excrete meconium until after birth, the presence of meconium in the rectum of a third-trimester fetus may be a normal finding. The presence of multiple, fluid-filled bowel loops in the third trimester may be entirely normal; consequently, the diagnosis of bowel obstruction during this period is difficult.

The typical sonographic pattern for a bowel obstruction is multiple fluid-filled loops of bowel that usually contain echogenic meconium (Fig. 21-12) and the evidence of polyhydramnios. The upper limits of normal for a transverse section of the small bowel diameter is 7 mm.[34] Typically, real time demonstrates active peristalsis. Anal atresia in the third trimester may present as distal, dilated bowel loops in the fetal pelvis, without polyhydramnios.

Meconium ileus. Meconium ileus is associated with cystic fibrosis, with an incidence of approximately 15%. In this bowel anomaly, abnormally thick meconium causes an obstruction at the level of the ileocecal valve, causing a dilatation of the ileum. The typical sonographic pattern consists of a dilated loop, which contains a rather homogeneous echogenic pattern of meconium.[11]

Meconium peritonitis. Meconium peritonitis develops when a small bowel atresia or, more rarely, a meconium ileus perforates or leaks, leading to peritonitis and the deposition of calcific deposits in the fetal

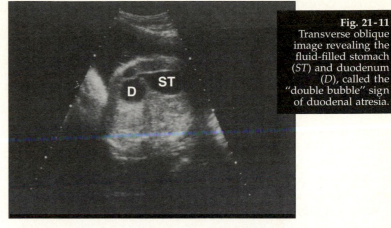

Fig. 21-11 Transverse oblique image revealing the fluid-filled stomach (*ST*) and duodenum (*D*), called the "double bubble" sign of duodenal atresia.

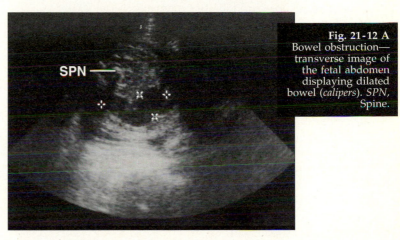

Fig. 21-12 A Bowel obstruction—transverse image of the fetal abdomen displaying dilated bowel (*calipers*). *SPN,* Spine.

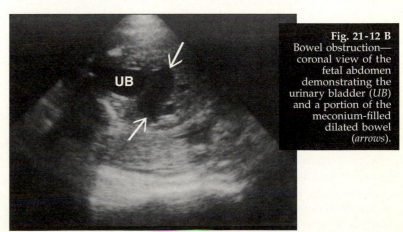

Fig. 21-12 B Bowel obstruction—coronal view of the fetal abdomen demonstrating the urinary bladder (*UB*) and a portion of the meconium-filled dilated bowel (*arrows*).

peritoneal cavity.[10] The perforation usually heals without treatment. On sonographic examination one or more hyperechoic calcifications in any of the potential peritoneal spaces suggest this pathologic process (Fig. 21-13). Additional sonographic signs include fetal ascites and polyhydramnios.

Anomalies of the Genitourinary Tract

Oligohydramnios. In many obstetric examinations the first abnormality that the sonographer notices is too much or too little amniotic fluid. In the case of oligohydramnios the sonographer should immediately consider severe renal dysfunction as the fetal cause for this condition.

The causes for oligohydramnios are more limited than those for polyhydramnios and include severe, bilateral fetal renal dysfunction, premature rupture of membranes, intrauterine growth retardation (IUGR), postmaturity, and fetal demise. The lack of amniotic fluid leads to fetal compression, which causes additional complications that include the development of Potter facies, positional defects of the limbs, IUGR, and pulmonary hypoplasia. To evaluate fetal urinary tract function, the sonographer primarily relies on imaging the fetal urinary bladder, since a lack of amniotic fluid compromises the ability to attain a good acoustic window to evaluate fetal soft-tissue organs for evidence of anomalies.[3] The normal fetal bladder fills and/or empties approximately every hour.

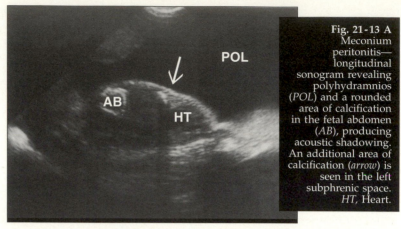

Fig. 21-13 A Meconium peritonitis—longitudinal sonogram revealing polyhydramnios (*POL*) and a rounded area of calcification in the fetal abdomen (*AB*), producing acoustic shadowing. An additional area of calcification (*arrow*) is seen in the left subphrenic space. *HT*, Heart.

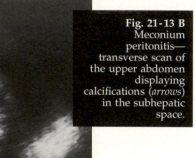

Fig. 21-13 B Meconium peritonitis—transverse scan of the upper abdomen displaying calcifications (*arrows*) in the subhepatic space.

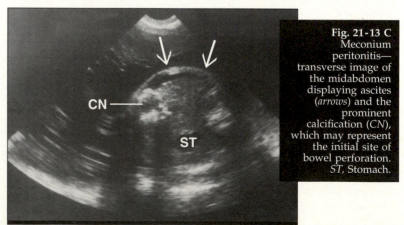

Fig. 21-13 C Meconium peritonitis—transverse image of the midabdomen displaying ascites (*arrows*) and the prominent calcification (*CN*), which may represent the initial site of bowel perforation. *ST*, Stomach.

Renal agenesis. Bilateral renal agenesis is the cessation of renal development in the early first trimester. This condition may present as an isolated anomaly or in association with chromosomal disorders such as Fraser syndrome, which consists of bilateral renal agenesis, anomalies of the external genitalia, and cleft palate. Other associated anomalies found with renal agenesis include cardiac, gastrointestinal, and central nervous system malformations. This condition is uniformly fatal, since functional renal tissue does not typically exist, and the oligohydramnios leads to severe pulmonary hypoplasia. The affected fetus develops **Potter facies,** which typically includes folds of dehydrated skin, hypertelorism, a flat nose, low-set ears, and a small chin.[19]

This condition usually produces pronounced oligohydramnios in the second trimester, which should immediately suggest renal agenesis. The most reliable sonographic sign is nonvisualization of the fetal bladder over the course of 60 to 90 minutes. The renal fossa may be difficult to visualize if severe oligohydramnios is present. If the renal fossa are demonstrated, the sonographer must not mistake the prominent fetal adrenal glands for renal tissue. If possible the sonographer should evaluate the heart, spine, and gastrointestinal system for signs of other abnormalities.

Infantile polycystic kidney disease. Infantile polycystic kidney disease is an inherited autosomal recessive condition, with a 25% chance of recurrence in successive offspring. On the basis of patient age at the time clinical symptoms develop, this condition has four classifications: perinatal, neonatal, infantile, and juvenile. In the perinatal classification, fetal renal failure typically develops during pregnancy or at birth, and death usually occurs shortly after birth. This condition develops in response to a defect in the formation of the collecting tubules with the resultant formation of small cysts in the low millimeter range. Both kidneys are always affected, but the distal urinary tract is usually normal. Depending on the severity of renal dysfunction, oligohydramnios develops, and fetal urinary output is absent.[40]

On sonographic examination the sonographer typically finds evidence of oligohydramnios, nonvisualization of the urinary bladder, and bilateral, hyperechoic fetal kidneys (Fig. 21-14). Because the multiple cysts are small, resolution limitations may not allow the demonstration of the anechoic cyst interior; only the hyperechoic walls may be seen. The sonographer should also examine the fetal liver, because this disease may also cause the development of cysts in this organ. Infantile polycystic kidney disease is also associated with **Meckel-Gruber syndrome,** a lethal condition. As a result, the sonographer should search for signs of an occipital encephalocele and polydactyly. Severe oligohydramnios, however, will make identification of these other anomalies difficult.

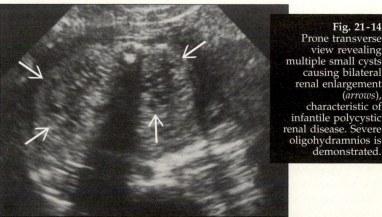

Fig. 21-14 Prone transverse view revealing multiple small cysts causing bilateral renal enlargement (*arrows*), characteristic of infantile polycystic renal disease. Severe oligohydramnios is demonstrated.

Multicystic dysplastic kidney disease. Multicystic dysplastic kidney (MCDK) can present as a unilateral or bilateral process or may affect only a portion of one kidney. This condition relates to the malformation of the collecting tubules, which dilate to form multiple cysts. Although MCDK is a developmental anomaly, it can occur with genetic conditions, such as Dandy-Walker syndrome. If the disease causes severe, bilateral renal dysfunction, oligohydramnios can occur with its associated fetal effects. Bilateral MCDK is typically fatal.[5]

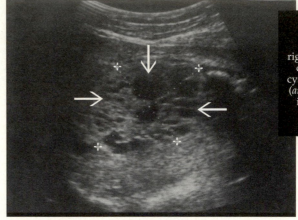

Fig. 21-15 Longitudinal sonogram of the right kidney (*calipers*) displaying multiple cysts of varying sizes (*arrows*). This pattern is consistent with a multicystic, dysplastic kidney.

Unlike infantile polycystic disease, MCDK usually presents sonographically as discrete cysts in one or both kidneys (Fig. 21-15). The sonographer should evaluate the effects on renal function by documenting the fetal urinary bladder. If the disease is unilateral, examine the opposite kidney for signs of hydronephrosis or other complications. If the disease is bilateral, the sonographer should perform an anomaly screen for other associated conditions, including the heart, the head for hydrocephalus and anencephaly, a diaphragmatic hernia, spina bifida, and cleft lip and palate.

Hydronephrosis. Obstruction of the fetal urinary tract can occur as either a unilateral or bilateral process. Although the site of obstruction can vary, the ureteropelvic junction (UPJ) is the most common site. Bilateral obstruction can result in renal dysfunction severe enough to cause oligohydramnios, but unilateral involvement is not typically associated with a decrease in the amniotic fluid.[47] Massive dilatation can cause a leak or rupture of the urinary tract, which produces **urinary ascites,** the second most common cause of fetal ascites, following hydrops.

The typical sonographic pattern for fetal hydronephrosis is a dilated renal pelvis and calyces (Fig. 21-16). If the posteroanterior measurement of the renal pelvis exceeds 10 mm, the possibility of hydronephrosis should be included in the differential diagnosis.[3] However, the third-trimester fetus may have physiologic hydronephrosis as a result of the normal intake of a bolus of amniotic fluid. Usually the renal calyces are dilated, as well as the renal pelvis, if the dilitation is caused by obstructive uropathy. The presence of renal cortical cysts suggests renal dysfunction. The sonographer should perform a full anomaly screen to rule out other anomalies, particularly those associated with the heart, the gastrointestinal tract, and neural tube defects.

Posterior urethral valve outlet obstruction. Posterior urethral valve outlet obstruction is typically a developmental anomaly related to the formation of the urethral valve, which leads to urinary tract obstruction. This condition affects male infants, and a severe obstruction can lead to progressive hydronephrosis, which may cause severe dysplasia and dysfunction. This condition can occur with trisomy 13 and 18 and other associated anomalies that affect the cardiac and skeletal systems and the urinary tract.[43]

The sonographic criteria for posterior urethral valve outlet obstruction are an enlarged urethra and urinary bladder, producing the "keyhole sign" on a longitudinal scan (Fig. 21-17). Other signs include dilated ureters, bilateral hydronephrosis, and cortical cysts in the case of severe renal dysfunction.[23] Determining that the fetus is a boy further refines the diagnosis. Oligohydramnios may occur with severe renal dysfunction. The sonographer should perform a full anomaly screen, particularly of the heart. However, the presence of oligohydramnios may interfere with a complete anomaly evaluation.

Renal neoplasms. Congenital renal neoplasms are rare and include the mesoblastic nephroma and Wilms' tumor. The **mesoblastic nephroma** is usually a benign, unilateral neoplasm that generally has no other associated anomalies. Occasionally this condition may occur in association with other genitourinary tract anomalies. The sonographer should also search for evidence of gastrointestinal abnormalities and hydrocephalus. This tumor is typically associated with polyhydramnios. **Wilms' tumor** is a malignant neoplasm that usually affects only one kidney and is capable of both local and distant metastasis. On sonography both neoplasms present as an echogenic renal mass, which makes a specific diagnosis difficult.

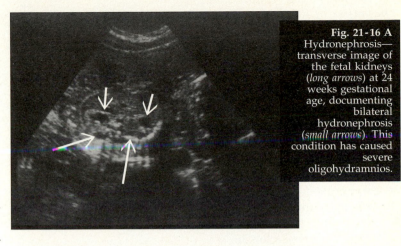

Fig. 21-16 A Hydronephrosis—transverse image of the fetal kidneys (*long arrows*) at 24 weeks gestational age, documenting bilateral hydronephrosis (*small arrows*). This condition has caused severe oligohydramnios.

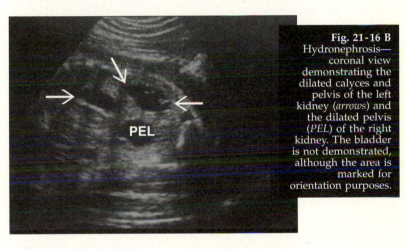

Fig. 21-16 B Hydronephrosis—coronal view demonstrating the dilated calyces and pelvis of the left kidney (*arrows*) and the dilated pelvis (*PEL*) of the right kidney. The bladder is not demonstrated, although the area is marked for orientation purposes.

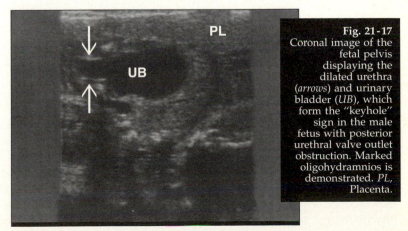

Fig. 21-17 Coronal image of the fetal pelvis displaying the dilated urethra (*arrows*) and urinary bladder (*UB*), which form the "keyhole" sign in the male fetus with posterior urethral valve outlet obstruction. Marked oligohydramnios is demonstrated. *PL*, Placenta.

Anomalies of the Skeletal System

Thanatophoric dysplasia. Thanatophoric dysplasia, or dwarfism, is a fatal condition that affects boys more often than girls. Most cases do not demonstrate a genetic link, although some are associated with autosomal recessive conditions. Distinguishing features include a narrow chest, protuberant abdomen, marked symmetric shortening of the limbs, large head with a cloverleaf skull, and hypertelorism. The small chest leads to the development of pulmonary hypoplasia, which is usually the cause of death.[6,44]

Sonographic examination usually reveals polyhydramnios, and a longitudinal scan through the fetus will display the small chest and protuberant abdomen (Fig. 21-18). Thoracic and abdominal circumferences will provide further documentation. All long-bone measurements are small for the gestational age (Fig. 21-19), and an examination of the skull may reveal a cloverleaf shape. The sonographer should also check for the presence of hydrocephalus.

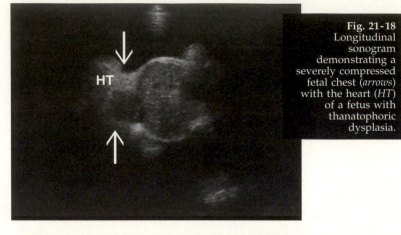

Fig. 21-18 Longitudinal sonogram demonstrating a severely compressed fetal chest (*arrows*) with the heart (*HT*) of a fetus with thanatophoric dysplasia.

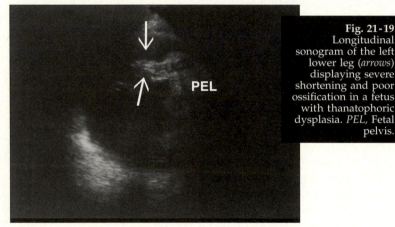

Fig. 21-19 Longitudinal sonogram of the left lower leg (*arrows*) displaying severe shortening and poor ossification in a fetus with thanatophoric dysplasia. *PEL,* Fetal pelvis.

Camptomelic dysplasia. Camptomelic dysplasia is a rare autosomal recessive condition characterized by a large dolichocephalic head, shortened and bowed extremities (especially the lower extremities), hypoplastic scapulae, cleft palate, hypertelorism, and a short chest and protuberant abdomen. The prognosis is usually poor.[44]

The primary sonographic feature, which increases the suggestion of this condition, is moderate to severe bowing of the bones of the lower extremities.[4,21] However, bowing can occur with other types of skeletal abnormalities. The discovery of associated anomalies, including cardiac defects, hydronephrosis, and hypoplastic scapulae, can narrow the differential diagnosis.

Achondrogenesis. Achondrogenesis is a lethal autosomal recessive condition that consists of two types. In Type I the vertebral column does not ossify, the pelvic bones are poorly ossified, and the skull may show signs of irregular ossification. The long bones are symmetrically short, and the thoracic cavity is short with poor rib ossification. In Type II the skull exhibits more normal ossification and displays smoother borders, the ribs are slightly more ossified, the limbs are symmetrically short, and the vertebral column is not ossified. Radiographic evaluation can usually distinguish between these two types.[24]

In a general ultrasound department, distinguishing the types may be difficult. The sonographic features suggesting achondrogenesis include an absence of the hyperechoic ossification centers of the vertebral column, a less hyperechoic skull pattern, and symmetric long-bone shortening (Fig. 21-20). The sonographer may find polyhydramnios.

Achondroplasia. Achondroplasia is the most common type of short-limbed dwarfism. The most common predisposing factor is maternal age, although some cases have an autosomal dominant link. Typically all limbs appear foreshortened, although the upper extremities are usually more seriously effected. The head is large with a brachycephalic shape and a bulging forehead.

On sonographic examination, long-bone growth typically appears normal until the third trimester, before measurements reveal aberrant growth and a bowed shape.[21] Longitudinal scans of the abdomen and thorax may display a disproportionate small thorax compared with the

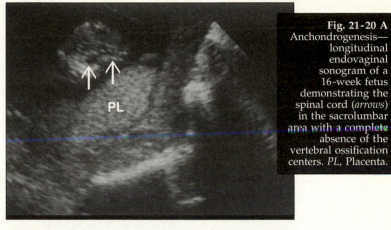

Fig. 21-20 A Anchondrogenesis— longitudinal endovaginal sonogram of a 16-week fetus demonstrating the spinal cord (*arrows*) in the sacrolumbar area with a complete absence of the vertebral ossification centers. *PL,* Placenta.

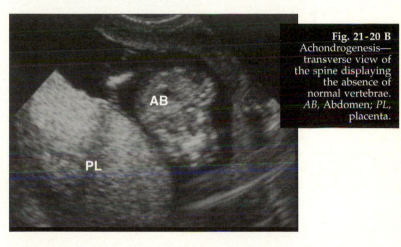

Fig. 21-20 B Achondrogenesis— transverse view of the spine displaying the absence of normal vertebrae. *AB,* Abdomen; *PL,* placenta.

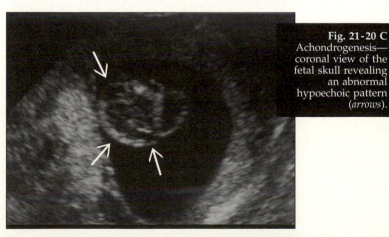

Fig. 21-20 C Achondrogenesis— coronal view of the fetal skull revealing an abnormal hypoechoic pattern (*arrows*).

abdomen. Since several cases of hydrocephalus have been associated with this condition, the sonographer should evaluate the ventricular system.

Osteogenesis imperfecta. Osteogenesis imperfecta is a genetic collagen disease that consists of four major types. Type II, the most common, presents poorly mineralized bones that are susceptible to numerous intrauterine fractures, particularly of the long bones and ribs. Radiography reveals the presence of wormian bones with poor ossification in the skull. The other types do not experience intrauterine fractures as frequently and, as a result, are not diagnosed as often with sonography. Type II is uniformly lethal.[46]

The classic sonographic pattern in Type II osteogenesis imperfecta is multiple fractures in the long bones, which appear less hypoechoic than normal, with unusual angles at the site of the fractures. If healing has started the sonographer may see localized hyperechoic areas at the fracture sites. Examination of the skull may reveal an irregular hypoechoic/hyperechoic pattern.

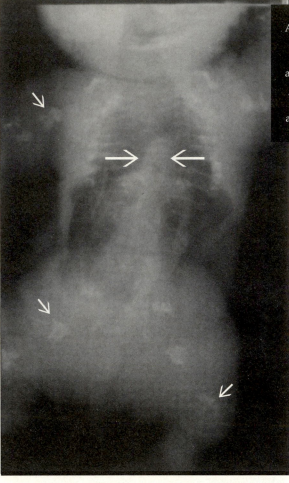

Fig. 21-20 D Achondrogenesis—a postmortem radiograph documenting the absence of vertebrae (*large arrows*) and visualizing severely abnormal bones in all extremities (*small arrows*).

Amniotic band syndrome. Amniotic band syndrome is probably the result of a rupture of the amnion, which can occur during any stage of pregnancy. This disruption can lead to a separation of the amnion from the chorion, producing bands that may attach to the embryo or fetus. Generally, earlier disruptions more severely affect the embryo. These bands can cause visceral defects, such as gastrochisis or omphalocele, asymmetric encephaloceles, and unusual cleft palates. Bands attaching to the extremities may only cause a ringlike depression in the soft tissues of the extremity. More serious consequences include disrupted bone growth, necrosis, and amputations. The prognosis depends on the severity and number of anomalies.[29]

Sonographic clues for this condition include asymmetric foreshortening of the extremities, limb amputations, asymmetric and often multiple encephaloceles, and other unusual deformities that do not fit a pattern for known genetic syndromes. The demonstration of the hyperechoic band attached to the effected body part provides a more definitive sonographic sign (Fig. 21-21). However, this may be technically difficult to visualize, particularly if amniotic fluid levels are decreased or if the sonographer cannot achieve the proper scanning angle to visualize the thin band.

Anomalies Related to the Abdominal Wall

Omphalocele. The omphalocele is the result of a malformation of the anterior abdominal wall caused by the failure of the lateral folds to close. These folds normally close to form the umbilicus. This failure causes a midline defect in the abdominal wall, which allows the abdominal contents to herniate into the base of the umbilical cord; the herniated contents then become enclosed in a peritoneal membrane. This anomaly can occur as a developmental malformation, but numerous genetic conditions are associated with omphalocele development, including trisomies 13 and 18, Beckwith-Wiedemann syndrome, and Pentrology of Cantrell. Omphalocele is associated with elevated AFP levels. The prognosis for an omphalocele directly correlates with the presence of these syndromes and their related, overall prognosis.[43]

The classic sonographic appearance of an omphalocele is a midline mass, which may contain liver and bowel, covered by a hyperechoic membrane.[30] (Fig. 21-22). The sonographer should demonstrate the umbilical cord

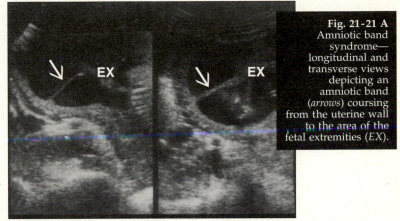

Fig. 21-21 A Amniotic band syndrome—longitudinal and transverse views depicting an amniotic band (*arrows*) coursing from the uterine wall to the area of the fetal extremities (*EX*).

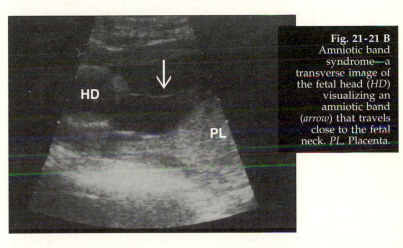

Fig. 21-21 B Amniotic band syndrome—a transverse image of the fetal head (*HD*) visualizing an amniotic band (*arrow*) that travels close to the fetal neck. *PL*, Placenta.

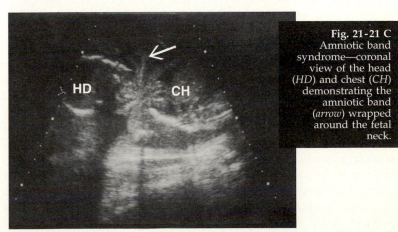

Fig. 21-21 C Amniotic band syndrome—coronal view of the head (*HD*) and chest (*CH*) demonstrating the amniotic band (*arrow*) wrapped around the fetal neck.

inserting into the mass, which is a very definitive diagnostic sign. With a large omphalocele, the abdominal circumference will measure small for the gestational age. The sonographer should always perform a full anomaly screen, since this condition is related to other genetic syndromes. The primary sonographic abnormalities include cardiac anomalies, renal malformations, and related intestinal atresias.

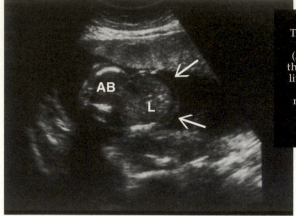

Fig. 21-22 Transverse image of the fetal abdomen (*AB*) demonstrating the herniation of the liver (*L*) surrounded by a hyperechoic membrane (*arrows*). This pattern is characteristic of an omphalocele.

Umbilical Hernia. Umbilical hernias are less serious than omphalocele, because the defect in the abdominal wall closure at the level of the umbilicus is typically smaller. Because of the smaller size of the defect, the hernia usually contains peritoneum, and rarely does the omentum or bowel enter the hernia.

Gastroschisis. Gastroschisis is a developmental anomaly where typically a 2- to 4-cm portion of the anterior abdominal wall is absent. This defect most often occurs on the right, producing bowel herniation, which is not encapsulated by a peritoneal layer. The liver does not usually experience herniation. The umbilical cord insertion is normal. Because this defect is not related to genetically linked conditions, other associated bowel anomalies include only atresias and malrotations. Gastroschisis usually produces elevated AFP levels. The prognosis varies depending on the extent of the herniation and the effects of the amniotic fluid on the bowel, which can lead to permanent damage that impedes function after birth.[30]

Sonography typically reveals loops of bowel floating in the amniotic fluid with no covering membrane. Additional differentiation from the omphalocele is the demonstration of a normal cord insertion[39] (Fig. 21-23). The sonographer should look for evidence of bowel obstruction and other types of bowel anomalies. As bowel function decreases, the sonographer often finds evidence of polyhydramnios.

Anomalies of the Thoracic Cavity

Cystic adenomatoid malformation. Cystic adenomatoid malformation (CAM) is the replacement of normal pulmonary tissue with cysts of various sizes. This disease typically affects only one lung field, although extensive cyst formation may compress the opposite lung field and initially appear as a bilateral process. CAM may cause the development of nonimmune hydrops and associated polyhydramnios. This relatively uncommon condition consists of three major types. Type I presents single or multiple cysts measuring greater than 2 cm. In type II the cysts measure less than 1 cm, and there is a high incidence of associated renal and gastrointestinal anomalies. A large, solid mass that often causes a mediastinal shift characterizes the type III category.[36]

The sonographic pattern usually includes multiple cysts involving the right or left thoracic cavity (Fig. 21-24). The solid type of mass is more rare. The sonographer should search for signs of hydrops, because this development affects the postnatal complication rate and the overall prognosis. The sonographer should also look for signs of renal and gastrointestinal anomalies.

Diaphragmatic hernia. Diaphragmatic hernia occurs when the diaphragm fails to close, allowing the herniation of abdominal contents into the thoracic cavity. The most common location for this defect is the left side, although it may develop on the right. This condition may occur as a developmental anomaly related to maternal ingestion of teratogenic agents, or it may develop in relation to genetically linked conditions, such as Beckwith-Wiedemann syndrome. The prognosis depends on the size of the herniation and the extent of pulmonary hypoplasia that is the result of the compression of lung tissue by the displaced abdominal contents.[1]

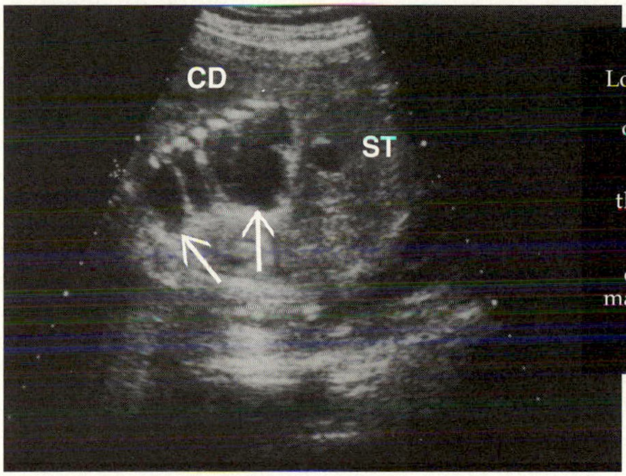

Because this defect usually occurs on the left side, the typical sonographic pattern is the

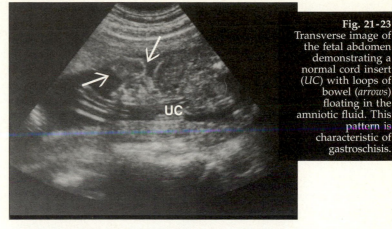

Fig. 21-23 Transverse image of the fetal abdomen demonstrating a normal cord insert (*UC*) with loops of bowel (*arrows*) floating in the amniotic fluid. This pattern is characteristic of gastroschisis.

Fig. 21-24 Longitudinal view of the fetal chest displaying multiple large cystic masses (*arrows*) in the left thoracic cavity. This pattern is characteristic of cystic adenomatoid malformation, type I. *ST*, Stomach; *CD*, chest.

nonvisualization of the stomach in its normal position and a cystic mass adjacent to a deviated heart. Herniated bowel loops may appear as cystic, complex, or solid masses in the chest. The abdominal circumference will usually measure small for the gestational age and will correspond to the extent of the herniation. The sonographer should also search for signs of polyhydramnios, which often develop in the latter half of the second trimester and into the third trimester.

Major Anomalies of the Heart

The detection and differentiation of cardiac malformations are the subspecialty of fetal cardiac sonography in obstetric sonography. These skills require advanced study and experience, which typically are found in a high-risk obstetrics department. As mentioned previously, the use of a four-chamber heart view serves as the initial screening for cardiac abnormalities in a routine sonographic protocol. In the case of high-risk patients for cardiac anomalies or when a cardiac defect is suspected after a routine examination, the patient should be referred to a high-risk center for further evaluation, unless the sonographer performing the initial examination possesses the required skill and experience to proceed with a comprehensive study.

Scanning protocol for cardiac anomalies. The prime time for the evaluation of the fetal heart ranges between 18 and 28 weeks. Six basic images will allow the identification of most major cardiac defects. These views are the standard four-chamber view, a longitudinal scan of the left ventricular outflow tract (LVOT), the short axis or transverse view of the right ventricular outflow tract (RVOT), a longitudinal scan of the RVOT, and the short and long axis views of the aortic arch. The anatomy and types of anomalies visualized are summarized below:

- *Four-chamber view* is obtained by scanning perpendicular to the intraventricular and atrial septum to rule out septal defects. This view also allows a comparison of chamber size and the position of the heart with surrounding structures.
- *Long axis of LVOT* will demonstrate the left ventricle, aortic root, aortic valve, and ascending aorta. This view will demonstrate transposition of the great vessels and stenosis of the ascending aorta.
- *Short and long axis of RVOT* will demonstrate the main pulmonary artery, pulmonary valve, and ductus arteriosus. This view will often visualize transposition of the great vessels and pulmonic stenosis.
- *Short and long axis of aortic arch* will demonstrate the aortic arch superior to the aortic valve and will demonstrate truncus arteriosis, coarctation of the aorta, and transposition of the great vessels.

Factors that place the pregnancy at high risk for cardiac anomalies include maternal diabetes, a history of congenital heart disease, fetal arrythmias, the development of nonimmune hydrops, and the discovery of a fetal anomaly. The following sections discuss several major cardiac anomalies.

Cardiac septal defects. Because of the unique anatomy and physiology in the fetal circulatory system, cardiac septal defects do not usually cause a change in the normal hemodynamics but generally become symptomatic in the neonatal period. The **ventricular septal defect (VSD)** is the most common cardiac anomaly. The discovery of a VSD requires a full cardiac evaluation, since a VSD can occur with other associated anomalies, such as transposition of the great vessels and Fallot's tetrology. **Atrial septal defects (ASD)** range from small defects adjacent to the foramen ovale to an almost complete absence of the septum. An **atrioventricular septal defect (AVSD)** involves both the atrial and ventricular septa. If this defect involves both atrioventricular orifices, it will cause the formation of one common orifice containing a five-leaflet valve, referred to as a complete AVSD. If two atrioventricular orifices are present, the condition is termed an incomplete AVSD. These abnormalities are associated with other cardiac anomalies, such as pulmonary stenosis and transposition of the great vessels.[44]

Sonographically these defects demonstrate as a disruption in the normal echogenic pattern of the atrial and ventricular septa. The sonographer must attain a 90-degree angle to the septa to accurately assess its continuity. A subcostal view of the atrial septum may be necessary to achieve this angulation. The sonographer must not misidentify the normal foramen ovale for an atrial defect. The movement of the valve into the left atrium allows its proper identification.

Hypoplastic left-heart syndrome.
Hypoplastic left-heart syndrome is made up of a small left ventricle and aorta with an underdeveloped mitral valve. This condition has a high mortality rate if not treated early in the neonatal period. Sonographic examination reveals a small left ventricle and LVOT (Fig. 21-25). This abnormality can cause congestive heart failure and the development of nonimmune hydrops.

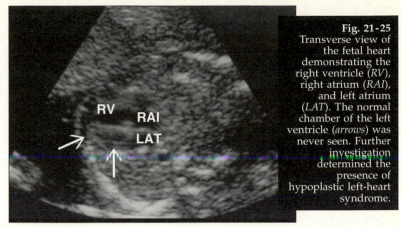

RV RAI
LAT

Fig. 21-25
Transverse view of the fetal heart demonstrating the right ventricle (*RV*), right atrium (*RAI*), and left atrium (*LAT*). The normal chamber of the left ventricle (*arrows*) was never seen. Further investigation determined the presence of hypoplastic left-heart syndrome.

Transposition of the great vessels. Complete transposition of the great vessels is an anomaly in which the aorta originates from the right ventricle and the pulmonary artery originates from the left ventricle. This condition is associated with a number of other cardiac anomalies, including atrial and ventricular septal defects and pulmonic stenosis. The sonographic diagnosis relies on the demonstration of the abnormal originations of the aorta and pulmonary arteries, which requires a high level of technical skill and a fetus in a position that allows a technically satisfactory examination.

Major Anomalies of the Face and Neck

Cleft lip and palate. Cleft lip occurs when the primary palate fails to close, and cleft palate occurs when the secondary palate does not fuse at the midline. Either condition can develop alone or together. Cleft lip and palate may occur as an isolated developmental anomaly or in conjunction with a number of genetic abnormalities that include, most frequently, trisomy 18 and Robert's syndrome and, less frequently, Meckel-Gruber syndrome and triploidy. Usually these basic deformities can be surgically corrected, but the long-term prognosis depends on the presence of other congenital anomalies.[43]

The best sonographic view for cleft lip and palate is a coronal plane section through the face. The best method for localizing this plane is to initially determine the plane of section for the BPD, move the transducer inferiorly until the orbits come into view, and then rotate 90 degrees. A more anterior plane will demonstrate the fetal lips and nares, which normally appear as homogeneously hyperechoic structures displaying bilateral symmetry. Cleft lip will appear as a hypoechoic to anechoic area disrupting the normal surrounding tissue (Fig. 21-26). A more posterior scanning plane will allow the examination of the palate, which normally appears as a homogeneously hyperechoic area. Cleft palate will also appear as a hypoechoic to anechoic area (Fig. 21-27). Further documentation of cleft palate may be observed on a longitudinal section, which demonstrates the fetal tongue traveling superiorly into the nasal passages during swallowing.[38] These abnormalities may be unilateral or bilateral and range from a small to a very large defect. The sonographer should perform a full anomaly screen to rule out genetic conditions and other abnormalities, including cardiac malformations, renal anomalies, and omphalocele.

Hypotelorism and hypertelorism. Hypotelorism, abnormally close-set eyes, and hypertelorism, abnormally wide-set eyes, develop with numerous genetic abnormalities. These conditions are determined by performing intraorbital distance measurements, but severe cases are apparent during a routine sonographic evaluation of the face. Hypertelorism develops frequently with craniosynostosis, triploidy, and Robert's syndrome. Hypotelorism occurs frequently with holoprosencephaly, trisomy 13 and 20, and some types of dwarfism.[43] The diagnosis of these conditions usually occurs in a high-risk obstetrics department in conjunction with a more accurate determination of multiple congenital anomalies.

Cystic hygroma. The cystic hygroma, or lymphangioma, normally results from a failure of the lymphatic system to form the normal primitive lymph sacs, which obstruct and expand with lymphatic fluid. These predominantly benign neoplasms typi-

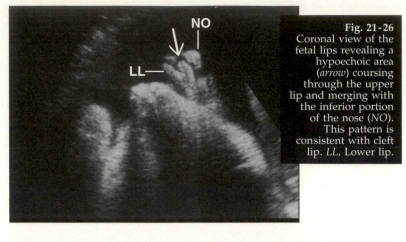

Fig. 21-26 Coronal view of the fetal lips revealing a hypoechoic area (*arrow*) coursing through the upper lip and merging with the inferior portion of the nose (*NO*). This pattern is consistent with cleft lip. *LL,* Lower lip.

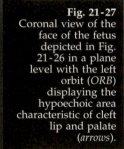

Fig. 21-27 Coronal view of the face of the fetus depicted in Fig. 21-26 in a plane level with the left orbit (*ORB*) displaying the hypoechoic area characteristic of cleft lip and palate (*arrows*).

cally develop in the posterior cervical region, although they may occur anteriorly or laterally in the neck or in other anatomic regions. This condition is associated with elevated AFP levels. Although they may develop as an isolated anomaly, the cystic hygroma has a high rate of incidence with a number of genetic syndromes, including Turner's syndrome (the most common) and trisomies 13, 18, and 21. The sizes range from small to quite large, and may totally envelope the fetal head. Large hygromas may cause the development of nonimmune hydrops, which is an extremely poor prognostic sign. Small, isolated cystic hygromas may regress spontaneously.[13,43]

On sonographic examination the typical cystic hygroma appears as a septated cystic mass adjacent to the posterior aspect of the head (Fig. 21-28). The sonographer should evaluate the fetal thorax, upper extremities, and neck for signs of skin edema, as well as search for evidence of fetal hydrops. Because of the high incidence of other abnormalities, a full anomaly screen should be obtained to rule out cardiac anomalies, omphalocele, and other major malformations.

Other Fetal Neoplasms and Anomalies

Teratoma. A teratoma is made up of elements from all three primary germ layers. The most common location is in the sacro-coccygeal region, although they may develop along the spine and in the brain and other organs. Most of these neoplasms are benign, but malignancy normally correlates with the stage of development. The risk of malignancy increases if the neoplasms begin to develop after the sixth month of gestation. An elevated AFP is suggestive of malignancy.[42]

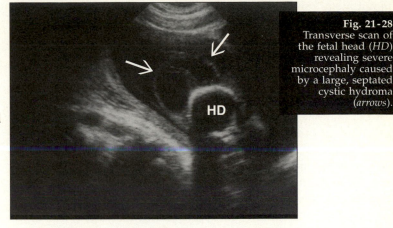

Fig. 21-28 Transverse scan of the fetal head (*HD*) revealing severe microcephaly caused by a large, septated cystic hydroma (*arrows*).

The sonographic pattern of the teratoma ranges from complex to solid, and the sonographer will often note the presence of polyhydramnios. Rarely, hydrops will develop. Depending on the size of the mass, other abnormalities in adjacent structures may be visualized. There are no other true associated anomalies.

Choledochal cyst. The choledochal cyst is an abnormal congenital dilatation of the extrahepatic biliary system, usually the common bile duct, which results in the formation of a cystic mass. This is a rare developmental anomaly with no known genetic link. The cyst is often located medial to the gallbladder and adjacent to the pancreas, and may be mistaken for duodenal atresia. The sonographer must demonstrate that the mass is not continuous with the gallbladder, bowel, or stomach.[17]

Cholelithiasis. Fetal cholelithiasis, although uncommon, can be an incidental finding on sonography. The sonographic criterion is the same as in an adult—hyperechoic, intraluminal mass(es) exhibiting acoustic shadowing.[8] (Fig. 21-29).

Cystic abdominal masses. Cystic abdominal masses can pose a challenge for the accurate identification of the organ of origin. Renal cysts are generally located posterior to and in close proximity of the fetal spine[3] (Fig. 21-30). The sonographer must evaluate the renal sinus to rule out hydronephrosis with a distended renal pelvis. Rarely, the sonographer may visualize an adrenal mass or hemorrhage (Fig. 21-31). Mesentric cysts tend to originate more anteriorly. In female fetuses an ovarian cyst can develop in response to maternal hormonal stimulation. Because of the small size of the fetal pelvis, an ovarian cyst may be located in the upper abdomen (Fig. 21-32). Determining the fetal sex can narrow the differential diagnosis of the cystic abdominal mass.

Trisomic and Triploidic Conditions

Triploidy. Genetic syndromes and conditions are classified by evaluating the fetal karyotype and visually inspecting for chromosomal abnormalities. This evaluation will not identify all genetic conditions, because some involve an abnormal deoxyribonucleic acid (DNA) sequence imbedded in a chromosome, which requires more advanced testing, or because current research levels have not identified the exact nature of the abnormality. However, the two common genetic aberrations that are often confused by the sonographer are trisomy and triploidy. In the normal condition each human cell contains 22 pairs of chromosomes (called autosomes) plus one set of sex chromosomes (XX in the female fetus and XY in the male). When complete **trisomy** occurs, there are three chromosomes instead of two. For example, in trisomy 21 the twenty-first autosome contains three chromosomes. Triploidy is the most common form of polyploidy. **Polyploidy** occurs when the embryologic cells contain multiples of the normal haploid complement of chromosomes, which each parent contributes at conception, instead of the normal complete set of 23 chromosomes. In **triploidy** the embryo has 69 chromosomes. This condition is not as common as the various trisomic conditions, and most triploidic embryos abort early in the pregnancy. The sonographer may observe this condition in the rare instance of hydatidiform mole with a coexistent fetus, since the fetus is often triploidic. The most typical abnormalities that may be demonstrated sonographically include a large, hydropic placenta,

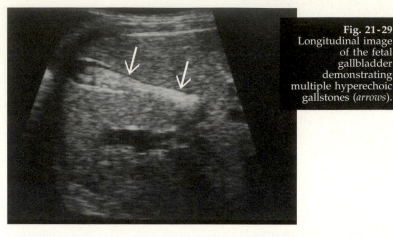

Fig. 21-29
Longitudinal image of the fetal gallbladder demonstrating multiple hyperechoic gallstones (*arrows*).

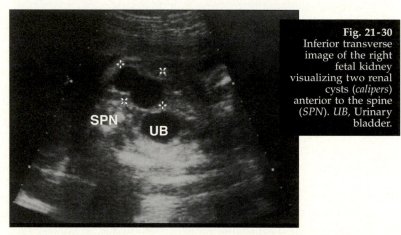

Fig. 21-30
Inferior transverse image of the right fetal kidney visualizing two renal cysts (*calipers*) anterior to the spine (*SPN*). *UB*, Urinary bladder.

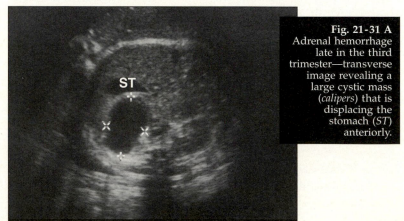

Fig. 21-31 A
Adrenal hemorrhage late in the third trimester—transverse image revealing a large cystic mass (*calipers*) that is displacing the stomach (*ST*) anteriorly.

disproportionate growth with skeletal and body growth lag, cardiac septal defects, hydro-cephalus, and holoprosenceph-aly.[43]

There are a number of tri-somic conditions that are either rare or do not demonstrate readily identifiable sonographic patterns. Other conditions re-quire examination by experi-enced physicians, typically work-ing in high-risk perinatal departments. The following sec-tions discuss the three most common trisomies and their re-lated sonographic patterns. The sonographer must remember that none of the current sonographic patterns for these conditions are present in all effected fetuses. Some of the patterns are quite subtle and require a higher level of experience and skill. Most pa-tients require a genetic amnio-centesis to obtain a definitive diagnosis.

Trisomy 21—Down's syndrome. Down's syndrome, the most common pattern of malformation in humans, increases in fre-quency with advancing maternal age. A mother over the age of 45 faces a risk factor of 1 in 25 of conceiving an infant with Down's syndrome.[43] This in-creased risk is associated with all autosomal trisomies and is the major factor for the widespread practice of performing a genetic amniocentesis on patients over the age of 40. Down's syndrome has also been associated with an abnormally low maternal serum alpha-fetoprotein (AFP).[18]

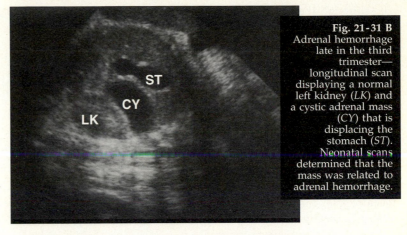

Fig. 21-31 B Adrenal hemorrhage late in the third trimester—longitudinal scan displaying a normal left kidney (*LK*) and a cystic adrenal mass (*CY*) that is displacing the stomach (*ST*). Neonatal scans determined that the mass was related to adrenal hemorrhage.

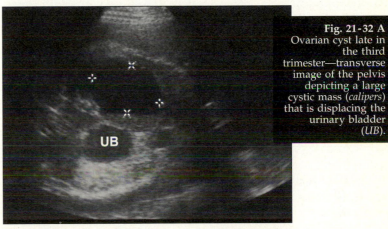

Fig. 21-32 A Ovarian cyst late in the third trimester—transverse image of the pelvis depicting a large cystic mass (*calipers*) that is displacing the urinary bladder (*UB*).

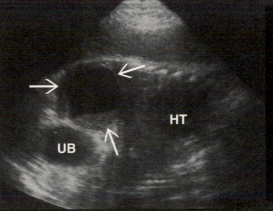

Fig. 21-32 B Ovarian cyst late in the third trimester—longitudinal view demonstrating debris in the cyst (*arrows*). *UB*, Urinary bladder; *HT*, heart. An examination several weeks after birth showed a reduction in the size of the cyst, suggestive of a physiologic origin in response to maternal hormonal stimulation.

Although the physical characteristics are quite obvious in infants and children, research continues to determine specific sonographic characteristics that can identify the effected fetus in a majority of cases. To date, the most consistent sonographic feature of trisomy 21 is abnormal nuchal skin thickening at the base of the skull (Fig. 21-33). In a normal infant this fold should measure less than 5 mm between 15 and 20 weeks. This measurement begins to lose specificity

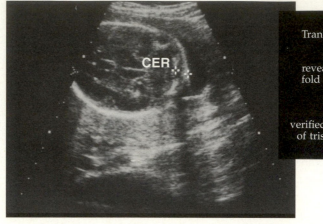

Fig. 21-33 Transverse scan of the head of a 23-week fetus revealing a nuchal fold thickness of 8 mm (*calipers*). Genetic amniocentesis verified the presence of trisomy 21. *CER,* Cerebellum.

after 20 weeks, and the accuracy progressively decreases as the pregnancy advances into the third trimester. Approximately 80% of newborns with Down's syndrome have a thickened nuchal fold. However, a normal infant, particularly in the third trimester, can deposit additional adipose tissue in this same area. Cardiac anomalies, such as septal defects, occur in approximately 40% of cases. Duodenal atresia occurs in approximately 33% of infants with Down's syndrome. More rare defects detectable by sonography include hydrocephalus, nonimmune hydrops, diaphragmatic hernia, and posterior urethral valves.[43]

Trisomy 18—Edwards' syndrome. Trisomy 18, the second most common pattern of malformation, develops three chromosomes on the eighteenth autosome. Again the risk increases with advancing maternal age. This condition is more common in female fetuses than male. This syndrome may also cause a decreased maternal serum AFP level.[31] Recent research has reported that the best indication of this condition is clenched fetal hands with the index finger over the third and fourth fingers, which are not extended during the examination. However, other initial abnormal sonographic patterns have already increased the suggestion of this chromosomal abnormality. The presenting sonographic patterns frequently include polyhydramnios, a single umbilical artery, and an abnormally small placenta. The fetus is often small for the gestational age. Cardiac anomalies occur in over 50% of cases, as well as cryptorchidism and inguinal or umbilical hernia. Less frequently seen anomalies include cleft lip and/or palate, microcephaly, omphalocele, Meckel's diverticulum, and horseshoe kidney.[43]

Trisomy 13—Patau's syndrome. Trisomy 13 affects the thirteenth pair of autosomes and has an occurrence of approximately 1 in 5000 births. The prognosis is poor, with approximately 70% dying in the first 6 months of life. Common abnormalities include holoprosencephaly, microcephaly, cleft lip and/or palate, polydactyly of the hands, cardiac anomalies, single umbilical artery, cryptorchidism in boys, and bicornuate uterus in girls. Less common anomalies include hypotelorism, agenesis of the corpus callosum, cyclopia, omphalocele, and polycystic kidney.[43]

Anomalies of the Umbilical Cord

Single umbilical artery. The detection of a single umbilical artery (SUA) causes clinical concern as a result of its high association with congenital anomalies, a greater risk of perinatal mortality, and an increased risk of IUGR. Multiple gestations have a significantly higher risk for SUA than singleton pregnancies, and this condition affects more male fetuses than female (Fig. 21-34). The list of associ-

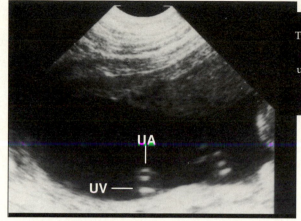

Fig. 21-34 Transverse image of the umbilical cord demonstrating the umbilical vein (*UV*) and a single umbilical artery (*UA*).

ated anomalies is long, but many of these defects are not currently detectable with sonography.[45] The most common anomalies detected by sonography include cardiac malformations, velamentous cord insertion, spina bifida, hydrocephalus and other brain anomalies, cystic hygroma, esophageal atresia, diaphragmatic hernia, cleft lip and/or palate, and renal anomalies.[44] The routine scanning protocol for fetal anatomy should enable the identification of most of these anomalies. Because of the high rate of cardiac anomalies, the patient often receives a detailed cardiac examination.

Umbilical cord masses. Although rare, umbilical cord masses always require Doppler evaluation and serial examinations to ascertain any increase in mass size or a decrease in umbilical venous flow, which could produce fetal hypoxia, IUGR, or fetal demise.[9] Several cystic masses can develop, including the omphalomesenteric cyst and the allantoid cyst. Usually both masses lie near the fetus. Sonographic differentiation is difficult.[41] Cord hematomas present as either solid or complex masses located in Wharton's jelly. Hemangioma classically appears as a hyperechoic, discrete mass, which may produce surrounding edema. The sonographer should check for fetal hydrops, if this type of mass is demonstrated. Teratomas rarely develop in the umbilical cord and display the typical complex sonographic pattern.

Cord prolapse. The presentation of the umbilical cord as the presenting part is always a concern to the obstetrician, because the risk of serious maternal bleeding and fetal hypoxia increase. The typical sonographic pattern is loops of umbilical cord between the internal cervical os and the presenting fetal part (Fig. 21-35). When this condition is seen in the late third trimester, the patient may require a cesarean section.[27]

Velamentous cord insertion. In velamentous cord insertion the umbilical cord attaches to the amniotic membrane instead of inserting into the placental substance. The sonographer should demonstrate the cord terminating at the amnion. Color Doppler can evaluate the cord flow, since this condition can disrupt the normal vascular supply, resulting in the development of IUGR. The sonographer should perform a full anomaly screen, since this abnormality can develop with other anomalies, such as trisomies.[43] Serial examinations are usually required to monitor fetal effects.

TECHNICAL PITFALLS

One of the most common technical pitfalls relates to the fetal position during the anomaly screen. The sonographer and interpreting physician should never report that an organ or area is normal if the fetal position is suboptimal for proper visualization. For example, the spine cannot be completely examined if the fetus is supine, since the weight of the fetus can compress a meningocele. Resolution always suffers degradation in the far field, so evaluating the ossification centers is usually suboptimal. A prone fetus prevents the proper examination of the anterior abdominal wall; consequently, gastroschisis or omphalocele cannot be excluded. In one instance a fetus was prone during the entire examination, and no abnormality was demon-

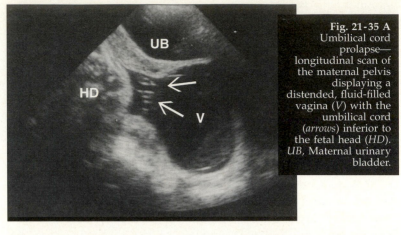

Fig. 21-35 A Umbilical cord prolapse—longitudinal scan of the maternal pelvis displaying a distended, fluid-filled vagina (*V*) with the umbilical cord (*arrows*) inferior to the fetal head (*HD*). *UB*, Maternal urinary bladder.

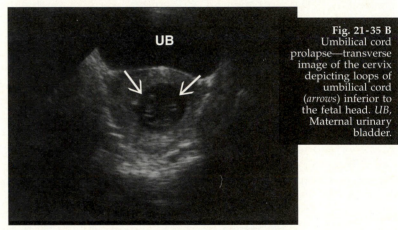

Fig. 21-35 B Umbilical cord prolapse—transverse image of the cervix depicting loops of umbilical cord (*arrows*) inferior to the fetal head. *UB*, Maternal urinary bladder.

strated. At delivery, the baby had gastroschisis with moderate bowel herniation. After viewing the sonograms retrospectively, the fetal body had compressed the bowel and the abnormality remained undetected. The sonographer can change the fetal position by applying some pressure to the fetus with the transducer, placing the mother in a decubitus position, or allowing the patient to walk for several minutes. If these techniques fail, a repeat examination is necessary to improve the confidence in the diagnosis.

SUMMARY

As mentioned previously, a general sonography department may not have the expertise to accurately diagnose all of these anomalies. It is important to recognize these limitations and refer the patient to a high-risk perinatal center when evidence of abnormalities is visualized. The sonographer must remember that normal fetal physiologic processes can mimic abnormalities, such as hydronephrosis and bowel obstruction, particularly in the third trimester. The sonographer must remember to

TABLE 21-1 FETAL ANOMALIES – Maternal Serum Alpha Fet-Protein Correlation	
CONDITION	*MATERNAL SERUM ALPHA FETO-PROTEIN*
ARNOLD-CHIARI MALFORMATION	Increased
ANENCEPHALY	Increased
INIENCEPHALY	Increased
ENCEPHALOCOELE	Increased
SPINA BIFIDA	Increased when open defect
ESOPHAGEAL ATRESIA	Normal to increased
DUODENAL ATRESIA	Normal to increased
OMPHALOCELE	Increased
GASTROSCHISIS	Increased
CYSTIC HYGROMA	Increased
TRISOMY 21	Normal to decreased
TRISOMY 18	Normal to decreased

always evaluate the amount of amniotic fluid; if the finding is abnormal, this increases the possibility of a true pathologic state rather than normal physiologic processes. Table 21-1 contains a summary of fetal conditions associated with abnormal AFP values.

REFERENCES

1. Adzick N, Harrison M, et al: Diaphragmatic hernia in the fetus: prenatal diagnosis and outcome in 94 cases, *J Pediatr Surg* 20:357, 1985.
2. Allen LC, Doran TA, et al: Ultrasound and amniotic fluid alpha-fetoprotein in the prenatal diagnosis of spina bifida, *Obstet Gynecol* 60:169, 1982.
3. Arger PH, Coleman BG, et al: Routine fetal genitourinary tract screening, *Radiology* 156:485, 1985.
4. Balcar I, Bieber FR: Sonographic and radiographic findings in camptomelic dysplasia, *AJR* 141:481, 1985.
5. Bateman BG, Brenbridge ANAG, Buschi AJ: In utero diagnosis of multicystic kidney disease by sonography, *J Reprod Med* 25:256, 1980.
6. Beetham FGT, Reeves JS: Early ultrasound diagnosis of thanatophoric dwarfism, *J Clin Ultrasound* 12:43, 1984.
7. Bell JE, Gordon A, Maloney AFJ: The association of hydrocephalus and Arnold-Chiari malformation with spina bifida in the fetus, *Neuropathol Appl Neurobiol* 6:29, 1980.
8. Beretsky I, Lankin D: Diagnosis of fetal cholelithiasis using real-time high-resolution imaging employing digital detection, *J Ultrasound Med* 2:381, 1983.
9. Bjoro K Jr: Vascular anomalies of the umbilical cord: I. obstetric implications, *Early Hum Dev* 8:119, 1983.
10. Blumenthal DH, Rushovich AM, et al: Prenatal sonographic findings of meconium peritonitis with pathologic correlation, *J Clin Ultrasound* 10:350, 1982.

11. Bovicelli L, Rizzo N, et al: Prenatal diagnosis and management of fetal gastrointestinal abnormalities, *Semin Perinatol* 7:109, 1983.
12. Campbell S, Johnstone FD, et al: Anencephaly: early ultrasonic diagnosis and active management, *Lancet* 2:1226, 1972.
13. Chervenak FA, Isaacson G, Torrora M: A sonographic study of fetal cystic hygroma, *J Clin Ultrasound* 5:311, 1985.
14. Comstock CH, Culp D, et al: Agenesis of the corpus callosum in the fetus: its evolution and significance, *J Ultrasound Med* 4:613, 1985.
15. David TJ, Nixon A: Congenital malformations associated with anencephaly and iniencephaly, *J Med Genet* 13:263, 1976.
16. Denkhaus H, Winsberg P: Ultrasonic measurement of the fetal ventricular system, *Radiology* 131:781, 1979.
17. Dewbury K, Aluwihare M, at al: Prenatal ultrasound demonstration of a choledochal cyst, *Br J Radiol* 53:906, 1980.
18. Dimaio MS, Baumgarten A, et al: Screening for fetal Down's syndrome in pregnancy by measuring maternal serum alpha-fetoprotein levels, *N Engl J Med* 317:342, 1987.
19. Dubrins PA, Kurtz AB, et al: Renal agenesis: spectrum of in utero findings, *J Clin Ultrasound* 9:189, 1981.
20. Fileni A, Colosimo C, et al: Dandy-Walker syndrome: diagnosis in utero by means of ultrasound and CT correlations, *Neuroradiology* 24:233, 1983.
21. Filly RA, Golbus MS, et al: Short-limbed dwarfism: ultrasonographic diagnosis by mensuration of fetal femoral length, *Radiology* 130:653, 1981.
22. Fiske CE, Fily RA, Callen PW: Sonographic measurement of lateral ventricular width in early ventricular dilation, *J Clin Ultrasound* 9:303, 1981.
23. Glaser GM, Filly RA, Callen PW: The varied sonographic appearance of the urinary tract in the fetus and newborn with urethral obstruction, *Radiology* 144:563, 1982.
24. Glenn LW, Teng SSK: In utero sonographic diagnosis of achondrogenesis, *J Clin Ultrasound* 13:195, 1985.
25. Graham D, Johnson TR, et al: The role of sonography in the prenatal diagnosis and management of encephalocele, *J Ultrasound Med* 1:111, 1982.
26. Gray DL, Crane JP, Rudloff MA: Prenatal diagnosis of neural tube defects: origin of midtrimester vertebral ossification centers as determined by sonographic water path studies, *J Ultrasound Med* 7:421, 1988.
27. Lange IR, Manning FA, et al: Cord prolapse: is antenatal detection possible? *Am J Obstet Gynecol* 151:1083, 1985.
28. Lee TG, Warren BH: Antenatal diagnosis of hydranencephaly by ultrasound: correlation with ventriculography and computed tomography, *J Clin Ultrasound* 5:271, 1977.
29. Mahoney BS, Filly RA, et al: The amniotic band syndrome: antenatal sonographic diagnosis and potential pitfalls, *Am J Obstet Gynecol* 152:63, 1985.
30. Mann L, Ferguson-Smith MA, et al: Prenatal assessment of anterior abdominal wall defects and their prognosis, *Prenat Diagn* 4:427, 1984.
31. Milunsky A, Wands J, et al: First trimester maternal serum alpha-fetoprotein screening for chromosome defects, *Am J Obstet Gynecol* 159:1209, 1988.
32. Nelson LH, Clark LE, et al: Value of serial sonography in the in utero detection of duodenal atresia, *Obstet Gynecol* 59:657, 1982.
33. Nicolaides KM, Campbell S, et al: Ultrasound screening for spina bifida: cranial and cerebellar signs, *Lancet* 2:72, 1986.
34. Nyberg DA, Mack LA, et al: Fetal bowel: normal sonographic findings, *J Ultrasound Med* 6:3, 1987.
35. Ostlere SJ, Irving HC, Lilford RJ: Choriod plexus cysts in the fetus, *Lancet* 1:1491, 1987.
36. Pezzuti RT, Isler RJ: Antenatal ultrasound detection of cystic adenomatoid malformation of the lung: report of a case and review of the recent literature, *J Clin Ultrasound* 11:342, 1983.
37. Pilu G, DePalma L, et al: The fetal subarachnoid cisterns: an ultrasound study: with report of a case of communicating hydrocephalus, *J Ultrasound Med* 5:365, 1986.
38. Pilu G, Romero R, et al: Criteria for the antenatal diagnosis of holoprosencephaly, *Am J Perinatol* 4:41, 1987.
39. Redford DHA, McNay MB, Whittle MJ: Gastroschisis and exomphalos: precise diagnosis by mid-pregnancy ultrasound, *Br J Obstet Gynaecol* 92:54, 1985.
40. Romero R, Cullen M, et al: The diagnosis of congenital renal anomalies with ultrasound. II. infantile polycystic kidney disease, *Am J Obstet Gynecol* 150:259, 1984.

41. Sachs L, Fourcroy JL, et al: Prenatal detection of umbilical cord allantoic cyst, *Radiology* 145:445, 1982.

42. Sheth S, Nussbaum A, et al: Prenatal diagnosis of sacrococcygeal teratoma: sonographic-pathologic correlation, *Radiology* 169:131, 1988.

43. Smith DW, editor: *Recognizable patterns of human malformation: genetic, embryonic, and clinical aspects,* ed 3 Philadelphia, 1982, WB Saunders, pp 10-33.

44. Smith DW, editor: *Recognizable patterns of human malformation: genetic, embryonic, and clinical aspects,* ed 3 Philadelphia, 1982, WB Saunders, pp 460-463.

45. Tortora M, Chervenak FA, et al: Antenatal sonographic diagnosis of single umbilical artery, *Obstet Gynecol* 63:693, 1984.

46. White RD, Lewis PE, Sanders, RC: Prenatal sonographic diagnosis of osteogenesis imperfecta: case reports, *Va Med* 3:218, 1984.

47. Wladimiroff JW, Campbell S: Fetal urine-production rates in normal and complicated pregnancy, *Lancet* 1:151, 1974.

22

multiple gestation

INSTRUCTIONAL OBJECTIVES

At the completion of this chapter, the reader will be able to:

1. Describe the clinical symptoms and complications that are typical reasons for a sonographic evaluation of a multiple gestation.
2. Define dizygotic and monozygotic twinning and describe the embryologic development of each, including the classification of monozygotic twinning on the basis of the division of the amnion and chorion.
3. Describe the use of maternal serum alpha-fetoprotein and human placental lactogen in the diagnosis of multiple gestation and related complications.
4. Describe the scanning protocols and techniques for the examination of the multiple gestation.
5. Describe the clinical symptoms and pathologic basis for the major complications of the multiple gestation, including intrauterine growth retardation, twin-to-twin transfusion syndrome, conjoined twins, intrauterine demise, and other associated congenital anomalies.
6. Identify on sectional sonograms the above-mentioned pathologic or anomalous conditions of a multiple gestation, based on the sonographic appearance, the clinical history, and the results of other diagnostic procedures.
7. Describe several technical pitfalls associated with the sonographic evaluation of a multiple gestation.

THE CLINICAL PROBLEM

With the widespread use of fertility drugs, the number of multiple gestation pregnancies have increased. Besides the use of fertility drugs, other clinical findings will cause the clinician to consider the possibility of a multiple gestation, including a history of dizygotic twins in the family and a patient who is clinically large-for-gestational age (LGA). During the second and third trimesters, the obstetrician can palpate two fetal heads or hear two fetal heart beats. However, these signs are more difficult to diagnose if the patient is obese, if the placenta is located anteriorly in the uterus, or if polyhydramnios is present. During the first trimester the physician may order a sonographic examination because of an elevated alpha-fetoprotein (AFP). A multiple gestation produces a false-positive AFP elevation, when compared with the levels normally found in the standard singleton pregnancy. A true elevation of AFP may indicate that the pregnancy is at higher risk to terminate in abortion or stillbirth, that one twin has died, or that one or both twins have a neural tube defect.

A multiple gestation is categorized as a high-risk pregnancy, since the obstetrician must monitor the patient for a number of potential complications that can occur during the pregnancy. These complications include[3]:

1. Premature delivery with low birth weight
2. Intrauterine growth retardation, particularly in monozygotic twinning
3. Twin-to-twin transfusion syndrome in monozygotic twins
4. Placental infarcts
5. Congenital anomalies, which occur twice as frequently when compared with a singleton pregnancy
6. Maternal hypertension
7. Abruptio placentae
8. Placenta previa
9. Polyhydramnios

A sonographic evaluation can screen for the development of most of these complications. Many patients receive serial examinations if abnormalities are detected. Because of these risk factors, the sonographer must perform a detailed, high-quality examination. One of the most important diagnostic criterion is the determination of monozygotic twins, since they are at a higher risk for many of these complications.

EMBRYOLOGIC DEVELOPMENT

Dizygotic Twins

Dizygotic twins develop when more than one ovum is fertilized. This type of twinning is called fraternal twins, because the fetuses are not identical and may be the same or opposite sex. Each fetus has separate amniotic and chorionic cavities and, therefore, separate placentae (Fig. 22-1). How-

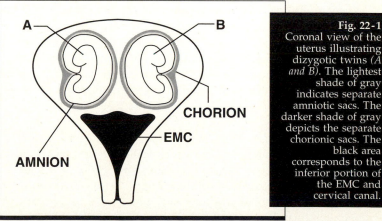

Fig. 22-1 Coronal view of the uterus illustrating dizygotic twins (*A and B*). The lightest shade of gray indicates separate amniotic sacs. The darker shade of gray depicts the separate chorionic sacs. The black area corresponds to the inferior portion of the EMC and cervical canal.

ever, the placentae may course adjacent to each other and appear to be fused. Sonography can distinguish a multiple gestation as early as 5 weeks, using the endovaginal technique. However, a definite diagnosis must include documentation of two embryos with cardiac activity, which more typically corresponds to 6 to 6½ gestational weeks. At this early stage the separate chorionic and amniotic cavities produce a thick interface between the two gestational sacs (Fig. 22-2). By the second trimester the membranes fuse, producing the appearance of one membrane. If the determination of the number of layers in the membrane is crucial to the differential diagnosis, the sonographer can use a 5.0 MHz transducer. The sonographer should use a 90-degree scanning angle in relation to the membrane in order to use axial resolution. The depiction of four layers narrows the differential diagnosis to dizygotic twins or monozygotic, dichorionic, diamniotic twins.[9] Imaging the membrane adjacent to the cord insert allows easier identification of the layers, because they are slightly wider apart in this region.

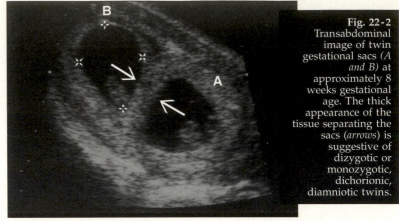

Fig. 22-2 Transabdominal image of twin gestational sacs *(A and B)* at approximately 8 weeks gestational age. The thick appearance of the tissue separating the sacs *(arrows)* is suggestive of dizygotic or monozygotic, dichorionic, diamniotic twins.

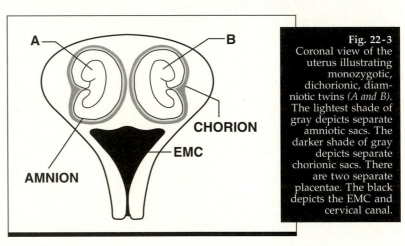

Fig. 22-3 Coronal view of the uterus illustrating monozygotic, dichorionic, diamniotic twins *(A and B)*. The lightest shade of gray depicts separate amniotic sacs. The darker shade of gray depicts separate chorionic sacs. There are two separate placentae. The black depicts the EMC and cervical canal.

Other multiple-gestation categories, such as **triplets** or **quadruplets,** always involve multiple zygotes, particularly with artificial hormonal stimulation. However, monozygotic twinning can also occur, which may result in triplets that develop from one set of monozygotic twins with one additional zygote. The sonographer must demonstrate the membranes and the number of layers to determine the number of initial zygotes, which helps to establish the risk factors for the pregnancy.

Monozygotic Twins

Monozygotic twins develop when one fertilized zygote divides into two embryos during early development. These are identical twins and therefore are always the same sex. The classification system for monozygotic twins is based on the number of membranes and placentae. If splitting occurs between the second and fifth day of embryologic development, the embryos will reside in two separate chorionic and amniotic cavities and are called **dichorionic, diamniotic, monozygotic twins** (Fig. 22-3).

This type of twinning is sono-graphically indistinguishable from dizygotic twins, because both have separate sacs and pla-centae.

If the division occurs be-tween the fifth and tenth days of development, the chorion has already formed. The result is two embryos in separate amni-otic cavities but with the same chorionic cavity, called **mono-chorionic, diamniotic, monozy-gotic twins** (Fig. 22-4). This is the most common type of monozygotic twinning. Examina-tion of the early gestation will typically reveal a thinner mem-brane, since it has only two lay-ers (Fig. 22-5). Because they share the chorionic sac, the fe-tuses will share a common pla-centa and are at risk for the de-velopment of twin-to-twin transfusion syndrome (see p. 383).

Division of one fertilized zygote between the tenth and fourteenth days will produce two embryos in a common chorionic and amniotic sac. This condition is called **monochori-onic, monoamniotic, monozy-gotic twins** (Fig. 22-6), the rarest form of monozygotic twin-ning. A sonographic examination will reveal the lack of a mem-brane separating the fetuses (Fig. 22-7). This type of twinning has a high mortality rate, usually caused by a tangling of the um-bilical cords, which may result in vascular compromise to one or both twins. Incomplete separa-tion of the embryonic disk re-sults in conjoined twins[3] (see p. 384).

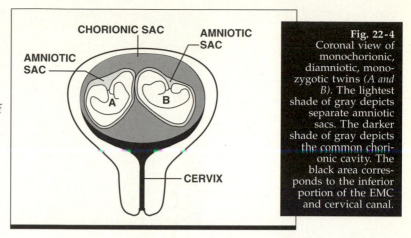

Fig. 22-4 Coronal view of monochorionic, diamniotic, mono-zygotic twins (A and B). The lightest shade of gray depicts separate amniotic sacs. The darker shade of gray depicts the common chori-onic cavity. The black area corres-ponds to the inferior portion of the EMC and cervical canal.

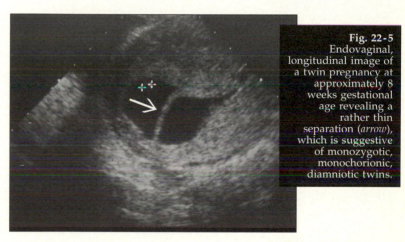

Fig. 22-5 Endovaginal, longitudinal image of a twin pregnancy at approximately 8 weeks gestational age revealing a rather thin separation (*arrow*), which is suggestive of monozygotic, monochorionic, diamniotic twins.

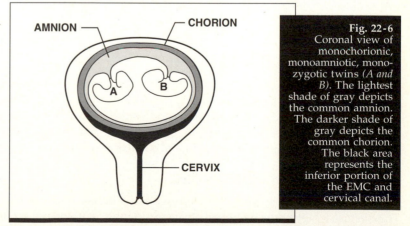

Fig. 22-6 Coronal view of monochorionic, monoamniotic, mono-zygotic twins (A and B). The lightest shade of gray depicts the common amnion. The darker shade of gray depicts the common chorion. The black area represents the inferior portion of the EMC and cervical canal.

CLINICAL LABORATORY TESTS

As mentioned in previous chapters, maternal serum AFP is used as a screening method for congenital anomalies and trisomic conditions. In the unsuspected multiple gestation, initial serum levels generally appear elevated when compared with the ranges found in the normal singleton pregnancy. If the AFP values are elevated beyond the normal multiple range, the pregnancy is at higher risk to terminate in abortion or stillbirth. Other causes of an elevated AFP include the intrauterine death of one twin, one or both twins with an open neural tube defect, or other congenital anomalies.[4] An abnormally low AFP level may indicate a trisomic condition or inaccurate pregnancy dating.

Evaluating the levels of **human placental lactogen (HPL)**, a protein hormone produced by the placenta, provides a method to monitor placental function. HPL values can also appear abnormally high in a multiple gestation. After the thirtieth week of gestation, serial HPL values can be used to monitor for signs of fetal distress. Normal values slowly build throughout the pregnancy, reaching 7 μg/ml by term. If the value is only 4 μg/ml after the thirtieth week, the clinician should suspect fetal distress.[5] Correlation with non-stress tests and the biophysical profile provides additional documentation.

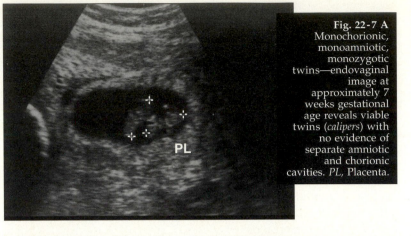

Fig. 22-7 A Monochorionic, monoamniotic, monozygotic twins—endovaginal image at approximately 7 weeks gestational age reveals viable twins (*calipers*) with no evidence of separate amniotic and chorionic cavities. *PL*, Placenta.

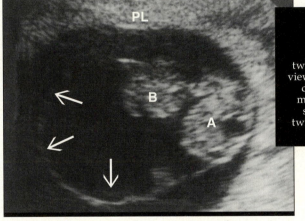

Fig. 22-7 B Monochorionic, monoamniotic, monozygotic twins—a magnified view demonstrates a common amniotic membrane (*arrows*) surrounding both twins (*A and B*). *PL*, Placenta.

RELATED IMAGING PROCEDURES

Although seldom used today, a radiographic examination of the maternal abdomen can verify the number of fetuses and their position. Likewise, magnetic resonance imaging can provide greater detail of anatomy and may be indicated in cases of suspected conjoined twins. However, sonography remains the primary imaging method of choice for the diagnosis of multiple gestation and related abnormal conditions.

SCANNING PROTOCOLS AND TECHNIQUES

The sonographer must initially determine the number and position of the fetuses. Transverse survey scans will prevent the misidentification of one active fetus as twins.

Scans demonstrating both fetal heads or trunks on the same image serve as definitive documentation. The sonographer must classify the presentation for each fetus (breech, vertex, transverse) and the location of each fetus in relation to maternal anatomy (maternal left or right). The sonographer should label each fetus with a number or letter. For example, for a particular set of twins, baby A is in the vertex position located on the maternal left, and baby B is in the breech position located on the maternal right (Fig. 22-8). This labeling is used when obtaining all the measurements and anatomic images for each fetus. The sonographer must periodically recheck the fetal positions to ensure that movement has not resulted in erroneously labeling measurements and images as belonging to baby A when, in fact, they correspond to baby B. The position of the fetus in relation to the membrane, if present, serves as an additional landmark. Labeling poses a greater problem in cases involving triplets, quadruplets,

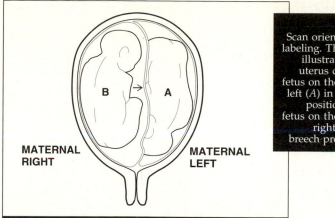

Fig. 22-8
Scan orientation and labeling. This coronal illustration of the uterus depicts the fetus on the maternal left (*A*) in the vertex position and the fetus on the maternal right (*B*) in the breech presentation.

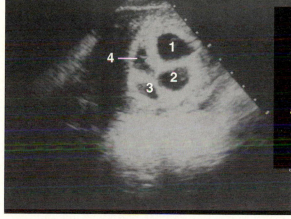

Fig. 22-9
Endovaginal image of a quintuplet pregnancy at approximately 5 weeks gestational age. The sonographer was able to demonstrate four of the sacs on this image (*1 to 4*). The fifth sac was located inferiorly.

or quintuplets. In the first trimester the sonographer can usually image and number all gestational sacs (Fig. 22-9). In the second trimester the examination requires constant landmark reorientation to ensure that all labeled images correspond to the same fetus.

The scanning protocol for the initial examination of the first-trimester multiple pregnancy is the same as that performed for a first-trimester singleton pregnancy (see Chapter 16). When feasible, the sonographer should obtain crown-rump length (CRL) measurements for each embryo and verify cardiac motion. If possible, the type of twinning should be documented. The adnexal areas should be examined to document the presence of a corpus luteum cyst or, more rarely, the presence of theca lutein cysts. **Theca lutein cysts** can develop in a normal multiple gestation as a result of excessive hormonal stimulation of the ovaries.

The scanning protocol during the second and third trimesters should include:
1. Determining and documenting the fetal number, presentation, and orientation in reference to maternal anatomy.

2. Documenting both fetal heads or trunks on the same image with appropriate labeling.
3. Documenting the amniochorionic membrane and the position of the placentae. If the placentae appear fused, the fetal sexes should be documented and the number of layers in the membrane should be determined.
4. Documenting the standard measurements for each fetus, including the biparietal diameter, head and abdominal circumferences, and femur length.
5. Performing the routine anomaly screen on each fetus, including the spine, brain, stomach, kidneys, urinary bladder, cord insertion, heart, and number of vessels in the umbilical cord.
6. Documenting the position and grade of each placenta.
7. Evaluating the amount of amniotic fluid.

The prime time for the initial sonographic examination is the same as recommended for a singleton pregnancy, between approximately 18 and 24 weeks. Accurate measurements for gestational age and accurate estimates of fetal weight are crucial, because discordant growth is a primary concern of the referring physician. For twins, a **concordant condition** means that a given trait affects both fetuses. A **discordant condition** means that the trait affects only one fetus. The breech presentation can produce less accurate measurements, even during the early second trimester, because the pressure of the uterine wall can produce fetal skull molding. This process can cause a dolichocephalic head shape, which produces a biparietal diameter (BPD) measurement that corresponds to a younger gestational age. The use of the head circumference or the cephalic index should reveal the presence of this head shape anomaly. The sonographer should make a notation for the interpreting physician when the fetal position has interfered with obtaining optimal measurements or anatomy survey scans. Multiple measurements on each fetus will increase the confidence that the measurements are accurate. Until approximately 26 to 28 weeks, twins grow at a similar rate in comparison with singleton pregnancies; consequently, the use of singleton growth charts should not cause significant errors in the gestational age and weight calculations. After this stage the twin growth rate declines in comparison with singletons, and the use of special growth rate tables for multiple pregnancies may assist in discriminating between a normal decrease in the growth rate and an abnormal decline related to intrauterine growth retardation (IUGR).[8]

COMPLICATIONS OF A MULTIPLE GESTATION

Intrauterine Growth Retardation

A **concordant growth rate disparity** means that the growth rate for both twins has declined by more than two standard deviations. This condition is not as common as discordant growth. The sonographer should determine the cause, such as placental infarction or abruption, or maternal factors, such as hypertension or diabetes. A maternal history of smoking or alcohol and other drug abuse may also provide a clue for the underlying cause of the concordant growth decline. During the third trimester the use of twin growth tables will allow a better discrimination between normal and abnormal growth rates.

Discordant growth rate disparity occurs when only one twin suffers from IUGR. Clinically this condition is defined when the birth weights of the twins vary by 25% or

more. On sonography a differ-
ence of 5 mm or more in the
BPD measurements is suggestive
of discordant growth.[1] Serial examinations are often necessary
for a definitive diagnosis.
Monozygotic twins who share a
common placenta are at a higher
risk for the development of discordant growth (Fig. 22-10). The
sonographer should verify the
presence and number of layers in
the membrane. The sonographer
should determine if the placentae are separate and located in
different areas of the uterine cavity or if they have merged with
one another. The determination
that both fetuses are the same
sex will serve as an additional
sign that they are monozygotic
twins. The sonographer should
search for additional signs of
IUGR, such as oligohydramnios
and a small, mature, placenta.
Doppler examination of umbilical cord flow may provide additional documentation.[11]

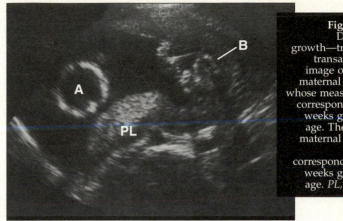

Fig. 22-10 A
Discordant
growth—transverse,
transabdominal
image of twin on
maternal right (A),
whose measurements
corresponded to 17
weeks gestational
age. The fetus on
maternal left (B) is
smaller,
corresponding to 14
weeks gestational
age. PL, Placenta.

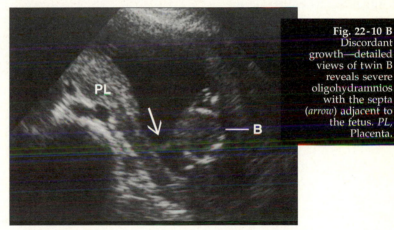

Fig. 22-10 B
Discordant
growth—detailed
views of twin B
reveals severe
oligohydramnios
with the septa
(arrow) adjacent to
the fetus. PL,
Placenta.

Twin-to-Twin Transfusion Syndrome

Monozygotic twins who share a
common or fused placenta may develop twin-to-twin transfusion syndrome. This
condition is a result of large subchorionic vascular connections that can cause an
imbalance in the vascular supply to both fetuses. The placenta supplies too much
blood to the fetus, which causes the development of nonimmune hydrops. The other
fetus does not receive an adequate vascular supply from the placenta and develops
IUGR. This syndrome begins to develop during the second trimester. In the early
stages, the sonographer may note growth retardation in one fetus before the development of hydrops in the other fetus. This is another reason that serial examinations are
necessary. The prognosis is poor for the fetus that develops full hydrops, characterized by ascites, pleural effusions, and skin edema (Fig. 22-11). The sonographer
may also note the presence of polyhydramnios. The prognosis for survival of the fetus
that has developed IUGR is better but depends on the severity of the vascular
compromise.[2]

Conjoined Twins

Conjoined twins can develop with monochorionic, monoamniotic, monozygotic twins. In this condition the embryonic disk does not completely separate into two embryos, resulting in several types of union. The most common site of union is at the sacrum and is termed **pygopagus twins.** Those joined at the chest are called **thoracopagus twins;** those joined at the head are termed **craniopagus twins;** and those with a union at the anterior abdominal wall are termed **omphalopagus twins.** For unknown reasons this condition affects girls more often than boys. The prognosis depends on the extent of the shared organs and the consequent risk of chronic medical problems.[3]

The first suggestive sonographic sign for this condition is often the lack of a membrane between twins that face one another. In the case of thoracopagus or omphalopagus conjoining the sonographer may see only one large abdomen or chest (Fig. 22-12). The sonographer should carefully perform the routine anatomy screen, noting if only one fetal heart, stomach, or bladder is demonstrated.[10] This type of information provides the first clue in the overall prognosis for the twins.

Congenital Anomalies

Monozygotic twins have a much higher risk factor for congenital anomalies than dizygotic twins. Compared with a singleton pregnancy, twins have a higher incidence of anomalies in the central

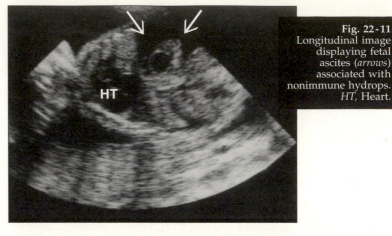

Fig. 22-11 Longitudinal image displaying fetal ascites (*arrows*) associated with nonimmune hydrops. *HT,* Heart.

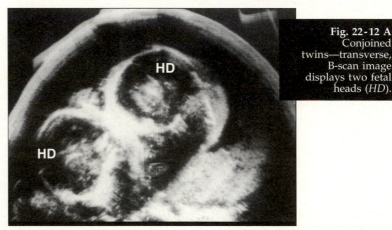

Fig. 22-12 A Conjoined twins—transverse, B-scan image displays two fetal heads (*HD*).

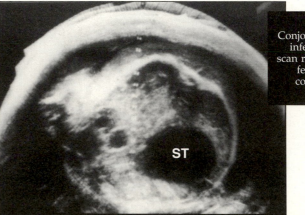

Fig. 22-12 B Conjoined twins—an inferior, transverse scan reveals only one fetal body with a common stomach (*ST*).

nervous, respiratory, cardiovascular, and gastrointestinal systems. Two-vessel cord and velamentous insertion also occur more frequently in monozygotic twins. Genitourinary tract anomalies occur less frequently than in singleton pregnancies.[10] An anomaly unique to monozygotic twins is the **fetus acardiacus,** or **"cardiac monster."** Experts theorize that this condition develops when one fetus does not receive an adequate blood supply during the early embryologic period. This severe vascular compromise produces deranged and disproportionate growth in the embryo. The most unique characteristics include a grossly deformed fetus that does not have a heart and an umbilical cord that may insert into any anatomic area.[12] The other twin usually appears normal and may measure LGA.[6]

The sonographer should always perform a thorough anomaly screen in every case of multiple gestation. The presence of monozygotic twins should always alert the sonographer that a more comprehensive anomaly screen is indicated.

Intrauterine Demise

Several conditions can cause the intrauterine death of one twin. An early disruption of the vascular supply can cause the death of one twin of either a dizygotic or monozygotic pregnancy. The death may lead to premature labor and delivery of both twins, or the pregnancy may continue with no obvious clinical symptoms. In the latter case the nonviable fetus may be partially reabsorbed and flattened by the enlarging twin, causing a disproportionately small second gestational sac and vestigial remnant of the fetus[7] (Fig. 22-13). At the time of the delivery of the normal fetus, close inspection of the placenta and membranes may reveal the small, mummified remains of the nonviable fetus. This condition is called **fetus papyraceous.**[3] This process can also occur with singleton pregnancies, usually related to a missed abortion that is never diagnosed. In one case a plain-film radiograph of an elderly woman revealed the presence of a fetus papyraceous in the uterine cavity.

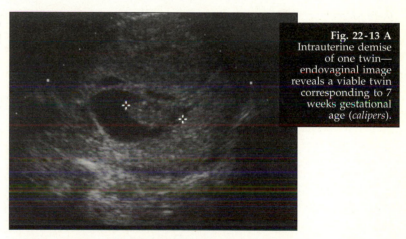

Fig. 22-13 A
Intrauterine demise of one twin—endovaginal image reveals a viable twin corresponding to 7 weeks gestational age (*calipers*).

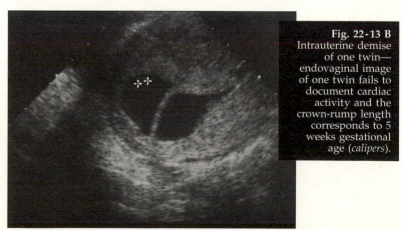

Fig. 22-13 B
Intrauterine demise of one twin—endovaginal image of one twin fails to document cardiac activity and the crown-rump length corresponds to 5 weeks gestational age (*calipers*).

TECHNICAL PITFALLS

Although rare, the sonographer may not initially identify all of the fetuses in a multiple gestation, particularly when performing the initial sonographic examination in the third trimester. With three or more fetuses, one fetus is often lying anterior to another, and the acoustic shadowing from the skull, ribs, spine, and extremities can mask the underlying fetus. The limited image size of current real-time systems can also promote "tunnel vision," if the sonographer does not meticulously scan the entire uterine cavity. Scanning from a lateral approach or having the mother lay on her side can also alleviate this pitfall.

The identification of polyhydramnios should lead the sonographer to perform a complete screening examination for congenital anomalies and to check the maternal history for signs of diabetes and other diseases that may produce this condition. However, polyhydramnios with multiple gestation often remains classified as "ideopathic," and the fetuses may have no signs of abnormalities.

After reading this chapter, the sonographer should fully appreciate the importance of imaging the amniochorionic membrane. This thin, hyperechoic band behaves as a specular reflector. In ultrasound physics a specular reflector is a large, smooth reflector that is **angle dependent.** This means that the sonographer must scan this type of reflector at approximately a 90-degree angle to visualize it. If the sonographer does not constantly change the scanning angle during the examination, a membrane may be present, yet the sonographer may not see it. Before determining that no membrane is present, the sonography should always scan from a lateral approach through the amniotic fluid and the fetal structures, with both a cephalic and caudal angulation. If no membrane materializes, the sonographer can be more confident that the nonvisualization is not related to the basic properties of a specular reflector.

A complete sonographic examination for multiple gestation requires an extended examination time. These mothers are more susceptible to compression of the inferior vena cava, because several babies can exert additional pressure. The sonographer should monitor the patient's condition frequently and permit her to lay on her side if she begins to feel light headed or nauseous. Even if the patient is experiencing no problems, allowing a 5- to 10-minute break every hour will give the sonographer an opportunity to maintain a high level of concentration and make the patient more comfortable.

SUMMARY

The sonographic examination of the multiple gestation requires a high level of concentration and meticulous technical skills. The sonographer must remember that this type of pregnancy is at risk for congenital anomalies and IUGR, as well as complications unique to a multiple gestation. As with singleton pregnancies, the patient should be referred to a high-risk perinatal laboratory, if the department does not have the capabilities to manage a multiple gestation with suspected or documented abnormalities.

REFERENCES

1. Barnes ER, Romero R, et al: The value of the biparietal diameter and abdominal perimeter in the diagnosis of growth retardation in twin gestation, *Am J Perinatol* 2:221, 1985.
2. Brennan JN, Diwan RV, et al: Fetal-to-fetal transfusion syndrome: prenatal ultrasonographic diagnosis, *Radiology* 143:535, 1982.

3. Dunnihoo DR: Fundamentals of gynecology and obstetrics, ed 4, Philadelphia, 1992, JB Lippincott Co, pp 564-578.
4. Finlay D, Dillon A, Heslip M: Ultrasound screening in a twin pregnancy with high serum alpha-fetoprotein, *J Clin Ultrasound* 9:514, 1981.
5. Fishbach F: A manual of laboratory diagnostic tests, ed 4, Philadelphia, 1988, JB Lippincott Co, pp 928-931.
6. Gibson JY, D'Cruz CA, et al: A cardiac anomaly: review of the subject with case report and emphasis on practical sonography, *J Clin Ultrasound* 14:541, 1986.
7. Gindoff PR, Yeh MN, Jewelewicz R: The vanishing sac syndrome. ultrasound evidence of pregnancy failure in multiple gestations, induced and spontaneous, *J Reproduct Med* 31:322, 1986.
8. Grumbach K, Coleman BG, et al: Twin and singleton growth patterns compared using US, *Radiology* 158:237, 1986.
9. Mahoney BS, Filly RA, Callen PW: Amnionicity and chorionicity in twin pregnancies: prediction using ultrasound, *Radiology* 155:205, 1985.
10. McLeod K, Tan PA, et al: Conjoined twins in a triplet pregnancy: sonographic findings, *J Diagn Med Songr* 4:9, 1988.
11. Nimrod C, Davis D, et al: Doppler ultrasound prediction of fetal outcome in twin pregnancies, *Am J Obstet Gynecol* 156:402, 1987.
12. Schinzel AAGL, Smith DW, Miller JR: Monozygotic twinning and structural defects, *J Pediatr* 95:921, 1979.

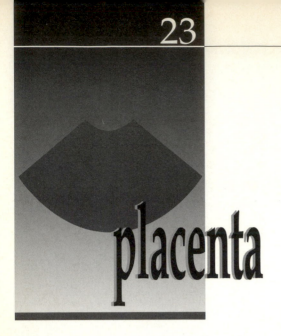

23

placenta

INSTRUCTIONAL OBJECTIVES

At the completion of this chapter, the reader will be able to:
1. Describe the clinical problems that are typical reasons for the sonographic evaluation of the placenta.
2. Discuss the anomalies of the placenta, including the succenturiate lobe and placenta accreta, increta, and percreta, and describe the clinical and sonographic significance of each.
3. Describe the sonographic placental grading system, and discuss the types of abnormalities associated with an abnormal grade for a given gestational age.
4. Describe the clinical symptoms and pathologic basis for the abnormalities of the placenta, including placenta previa, placental abruption, and neoplasms.
5. Identify on sectional sonograms the above-mentioned anomalies and pathologic conditions of the placenta, based on the sonographic appearance, the clinical history, and the results of other diagnostic procedures.
6. Describe several technical pitfalls associated with the sonographic evaluation of the placenta.

THE CLINICAL PROBLEM

A patient who has the clinical symptom of bleeding during pregnancy requires investigation. During the first trimester the differential diagnosis includes postimplantation bleeding, blighted ovum, spontaneous abortion, ectopic pregnancy, and hydatidiform mole. When bleeding occurs during the second and third trimesters, placental pathology becomes the prime suspect. The obstetrician should determine the cause and alleviate the bleeding, because significant blood loss can increase fetal morbidity and mortality. The most dangerous condition for both the fetus and mother is placental abruption, a true obstetric emergency, because it can result in massive hemorrhage. Sonography can provide the differential diagnosis in many patients who have the clinical symptom of bleeding.

Besides the abnormalities previously mentioned, the placenta is also involved in other fetal and maternal disorders. The placenta becomes abnormally thin with preeclampsia and abnormally thick in fetal hydrops; it attains an advanced grade early in the pregnancy with severe intrauterine growth retardation (IUGR) and may maintain an immature grade with diabetes. A thorough examination of the placenta during every sonographic examination is important; it often provides the first suggestion to the sonographer that something is abnormal. Correlating placental findings with other abnormal patterns will narrow the sonographic differential diagnosis.

ANATOMY AND PHYSIOLOGY

The placenta begins to develop early in the first trimester and has two components. The **fetal component** derives from the chorionic plate and the **maternal component** evolves from the decidua basalis. The **chorionic villi,** the functional unit of the placenta, develop from the chorionic plate. The chorionic villi invade the decidua basalis and produce wedge-shaped areas called **cotyledons,** each one containing several primary chorionic villi with smaller branches (Fig. 23-1). The **intervillous spaces** surround the chorionic villi. The maternal blood enters the inter-

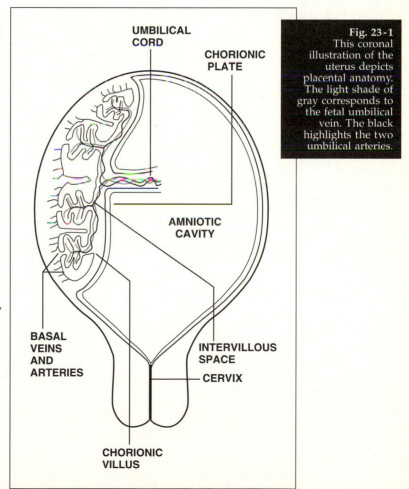

UMBILICAL
CORD

CHORIONIC
PLATE

AMNIOTIC
CAVITY

BASAL
VEINS
AND
ARTERIES

INTERVILLOUS
SPACE

CERVIX

CHORIONIC
VILLUS

Fig. 23-1
This coronal illustration of the uterus depicts placental anatomy. The light shade of gray corresponds to the fetal umbilical vein. The black highlights the two umbilical arteries.

villous spaces, coming in contact with the surface of the villi. Nutrients and metabolites are transported into the villus, but no significant mingling of the fetal and maternal blood occurs under normal conditions. This process works in both directions, as fetal waste products leave the villi and enter the intervillous spaces. This selective transfer is referred to as the **placental barrier.** In addition to nutrients and oxygen, other maternal substances that are permeable to the placental barrier include antibodies, vitamins, viruses, and many drugs and poisons. Bacteria are not normally transferred.[3]

The **spiral arteries** supply the maternal blood to the intervillous spaces, terminating in a series of capillaries at each villus. After oxygen and nutrients have entered the villus, the substances enter small veins, which ramify to form the **umbilical vein.** Deoxygenated blood leaves the fetus and travels to the placenta via the **umbilical arteries,** where they divide into numerous branches that lead to the chorionic villi. Once the exchange process has taken place, the maternal blood leaves the intervillous spaces through the placental venous system. The largest venous tributaries lie adjacent to the basal layer and the uterine wall.

CLINICAL LABORATORY TESTS

The results of several clinical laboratory tests can allow the differentiation between insignificant or normal placental sonographic findings and those that are abnormal. Although rare, an elevated maternal serum **alpha-fetoprotein (AFP)** may occur with placental pathology, such as intervillous thrombosis and chorioangioma.[6] In cases of immune hydrops the amniotic **bilirubin** level increases with fetal liver failure. Further correlation with the patient's clinical symptoms can allow a refined differential diagnosis of suspected pathologic conditions that cause abnormal placental signs.

RELATED IMAGING PROCEDURES

Other imaging techniques provide limited information on placental pathology. The radiographic plain film does not routinely visualize the placenta. Although seldom indicated, magnetic resonance imaging can provide additional information on placental location and appearance. However, sonography serves as the primary imaging technique for placental position and is the most widely used diagnostic procedure for the evaluation of abnormal conditions.

SCANNING PROTOCOLS AND TECHNIQUES

Documentation of the placental location in relation to the internal cervical os is included in the suggested routine sonographic examination of the second- and third-trimester pregnancies. In addition, the sonographer should note the placental grade. A summary of the routine protocol follows:

Fetal Age and Growth
1. BPD
2. Head circumference or cephalic index
3. Abdominal circumference
4. Femur length
5. Estimation of fetal weight

Fetal Anatomy

1. Cerebral ventricles to rule out hydrocephaly
2. Four-chamber heart and heart position within the thoracic cavity
3. Spine to rule out spina bifida
4. Stomach to access function and rule out anomalies
5. Kidneys to rule out anomalies and obstruction
6. Urinary bladder to access renal function and rule out obstruction
7. Umbilical cord insertion to rule out abnormalities of the anterior abdominal wall
8. Three-vessel cord
9. Fetal lie in relation to maternal longitudinal axis

Placenta and Maternal Anatomy

1. Anatomic location and grade
2. Position of placenta in relation to internal cervical os
3. Amount of amniotic fluid
4. Uterus for fibroids and other abnormalities
5. Adnexal areas to rule out masses

Additional measurements or anatomic areas may be required by the specific department protocol. Discovery of abnormal sonographic patterns typically requires a more extensive examination.

The sonographer should also document the placenta during a first-trimester sonographic examination. The placenta initially presents as a thicker portion of decidua, corresponding to the decidua basalis. By approximately the 10th week after the last normal menstrual period (LNMP), the sonographer can identify this homogeneously hyperechoic area (Fig. 23-2). By the second trimester the placenta presents as a prominent, homogeneous, hyperechoic area. The **chorionic plate,** or fetal surface, visualizes as a thin, smooth, hyperechoic line adjacent to the placental substance (Fig. 23-3).

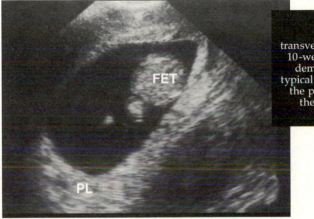

Fig. 23-2 Endovaginal, transverse image of a 10-week fetus (*FET*) demonstrating the typical appearance of the placenta (*PL*) in the middle of the first trimester.

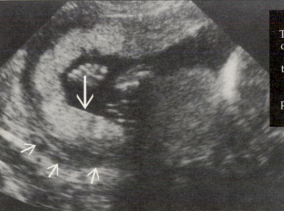

Fig. 23-3 Transverse sonogram of a second-trimester placenta depicting the hypoechoic basal area (*small arrows*) and the chorionic plate, or fetal surface (*large arrow*).

Cystic to hypoechoic circular and tubular structures may appear between the basal area and the uterine wall. Color or pulsed Doppler will reveal that these structures represent the branches of the maternal veins and spiral arteries.[8] The sonographer should always document the anatomic location of the placenta, such as anterior, posterior, or fundal. Usually a minimum of two images of the placenta, one transverse and one longitudinal, will record the placental position

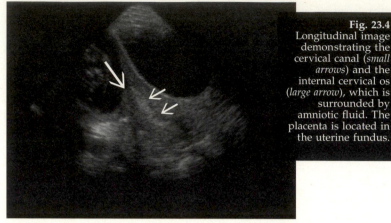

Fig. 23.4 Longitudinal image demonstrating the cervical canal (*small arrows*) and the internal cervical os (*large arrow*), which is surrounded by amniotic fluid. The placenta is located in the uterine fundus.

and the grade. The relationship of the placenta to the internal cervical os is always documented. These views require a full maternal urinary bladder. On a longitudinal scan the cervical canal appears as a moderately hyperechoic line in the less echogenic cervical myometrium (Fig. 23-4). The optimal cervical length usually ranges between 3 and 5 cm. The cervical canal terminates superiorly at the internal cervical os, which usually appears as an indentation between the anterior and posterior walls of the cervix. If the placenta is not close to the cervical os, one longitudinal view can document this abnormality. If the placenta is located adjacent to or over the cervical os, the sonographer should confirm this condition with both longitudinal and transverse images.

PLACENTAL ANOMALIES

Several placental anomalies are detectable with sonography and are clinically significant to the obstetrician. Some patients will develop a **succenturiate lobe,** which is an accessory lobe of placental tissue connected to the primary placenta by blood vessels. The diagnosis of a succenturiate lobe is important for several reasons. First, this lobe may remain in the uterus after delivery and cause postpartum hemorrhage and later infection. Second, the succenturiate lobe may cover the internal cervical os and produce bleeding during the pregnancy. Third, only the connecting vessels may cover the cervical os, which could rupture during delivery.[3] Usually the succenturiate lobe displays on sonography as a relatively small, hyperechoic mass of tissue located at a variable distance from the primary placenta (Fig. 23-5). The connecting vessels are usually indistinguishable with gray scale sonography, although color Doppler may allow the sonographer to document them. The sonographer may initially misidentify a **Braxton Hicks contraction** as a succenturiate lobe. However, the contraction usually disappears later during the examination.

A more rare group of conditions develop when the chorionic villi grow into the uterine layers. In **placenta accreta** the villi grow into the myometrium. With **placenta increta** the villi project through the entire myometrial layer. The most extensive condition, **placenta percreta,** occurs when the villi penetrate the uterine outer capsule. The most common factor that increases the risk for these conditions is a uterine scar from a previous cesarean section. Because the placental tissue is embedded in the uterine wall, the major complication with these conditions is retained placental tissue. Because placenta accreta, increta, and percreta are difficult to diagnose with sonography,[5] the sonographer must demonstrate the placenta adjacent to the uterine myometrium. In the second and third trimesters, the use of the maternal urinary bladder as an acoustic window for the myometrial and placental tissue can demonstrate the absence of a normally prominent myometrial

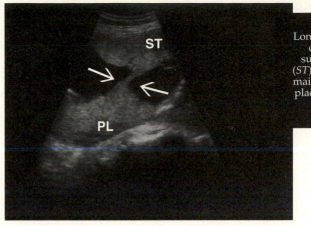

Fig. 23.5 Longitudinal image demonstrating a succenturiate lobe (*ST*) attached to the main portion of the placenta (*PL*) by its vascular supply (*arrows*).

layer. Obviously, if the placenta is not located in this position, visualization of the anterior or posterior myometrium is difficult.

PLACENTAL MATURATION AND GRADING

As the pregnancy advances, the development of calcified areas in the placenta occur as a result of normal physiologic processes. The development of **maternal lakes** and fibrin deposition appear to have no clinical significance. Maternal lakes visualize as anechoic or cystic areas, which may demonstrate vascular flow with color Doppler. Some researchers believe that these areas represent an early stage of fibrin development. **Perivillous fibrin deposition** appears to be the result of the maternal blood collecting in the intervillous spaces. These areas also present as cystic areas in the placental substance. Cystic areas adjacent to the chorionic plate usually represent **subchorionic fibrin deposition,** which also seem to be clinically insignificant.[12] These cystic areas typically appear during the third trimester, although some patients may develop these earlier. If a placenta contains a number of prominent cystic areas, the sonographer should evaluate the umbilical cord flow to the fetus with color or pulsed Doppler and search for signs of IUGR or fetal hypoxia. Large cystic areas extending from the placental substance to the basal area or chorionic plate may represent **intervillous thrombosis,** which has an increased incidence with Rh isoimmunization[10] (Fig. 23-6).

The **placental grading system** allows the sonographer to identify the normal stages in the maturation of the placenta during the pregnancy. Delayed or advanced maturation may indicate a pathologic process. During the first and second trimesters the placenta should adhere to the criteria for a **grade 0** classification. The criteria include a smooth, chorionic plate, no hyperechoic areas in the placental substance, and no linear hyperechoic regions adjacent to the basal layer (Fig. 23-7). By the early third trimester, approximately 30 weeks LNMP, the placenta may show evidence of a **grade 1** classification. These sonographic patterns include subtle indulations of the chorionic plate and a scattering of linear, hyperechoic areas in the placental substance, which course parallel to the chorionic plate (Fig. 23-8). There are no basal layer densities in a grade 1 placenta. At approximately 36 weeks LNMP, the patient may display the sonographic signs of a **grade 2** placenta. The criteria include marked indentations of the chorionic plate, intraplacental hyperechoic areas, and hyperechoic, linear areas in the basal layer, which course parallel with the length of the placenta (Fig. 23-9). At approximately the 38th week LNMP, the placenta may meet the criteria for a **grade 3** classification, which include hyperechoic linear densities that extend from the chorionic plate to the basal layer[9] (Fig. 23-10). By this stage the **cotyledons** may be distinguished sonographically as hypoechoic to anechoic areas located between the linear, hyperechoic borders.

A number of normal placentas will not progress through all these stages. The depiction of a grade 3 placenta does not allow the sonographer to determine if the vascular supply to the fetus is adequate or if it has been compromised. This becomes a potential problem with **prolonged pregnancy.** In this condition the pregnancy has extended beyond 40 weeks. For the patient with a reliable menstrual history, the clinical question that must be answered by the obstetrician is whether the placenta will continue to adequately support the fetus until labor begins. For this type of patient the sonographer often performs a biophysical profile to evaluate signs of fetal distress, to obtain an amniotic fluid index to determine the extent of oligohydramnios, and to grade the placenta. Even with a grade 3 placenta, if the fetus shows no signs of distress and the amniotic fluid is not severely decreased, the clinician can continue to delay inducing labor or

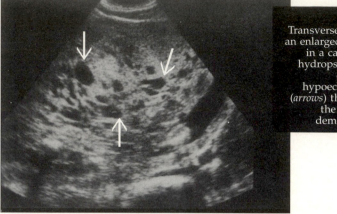

Fig. 23-6 Transverse image of an enlarged placenta in a case of fetal hydrops. Multiple cystic and hypoechoic areas (*arrows*) throughout the tissue are demonstrated.

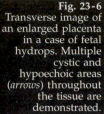

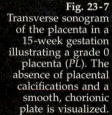

Fig. 23-7 Transverse sonogram of the placenta in a 15-week gestation illustrating a grade 0 placenta (*PL*). The absence of placental calcifications and a smooth, chorionic plate is visualized.

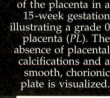

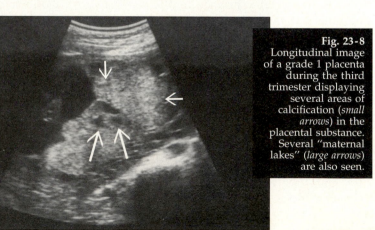

Fig. 23-8 Longitudinal image of a grade 1 placenta during the third trimester displaying several areas of calcification (*small arrows*) in the placental substance. Several "maternal lakes" (*large arrows*) are also seen.

performing a cesarean section. If the fetus shows signs of distress or hypoxia, the placenta may not have the ability to adequately support the fetus, and the obstetrician will alter the clinical management of the patient.

The sonographer should also evaluate placental thickness. The scaning plane should be perpendicular to the uterine wall. This will prevent an oblique section through the placenta, which may make it appear thicker than normal. The average placental thickness ranges between 3 and 4 cm. However the sonographer should also note the length of the placenta, because many normal variations occur. An **abnormally thick placenta** is typically 5 cm or greater. This condition may occur with maternal diabetes, immune and nonimmune hydrops, and other congenital anomalies. With diabetes the placenta may also show signs of delayed maturation, which may cause the placenta to fulfill grade 0 criteria during the third trimester. An **abnormally thin placenta** is typically less than 2 cm.[2] This condition may indicate preeclampsia or IUGR. With preeclampsia the patient is also at increased risk for the development of placental infarctions and retroplacental hematoma.

PLACENTAL PATHOLOGY

Placenta Previa

Placenta previa occurs when the placenta implants in the lower portion of the uterus. Normally the blastocyst implants in the upper third of the uterus, and the placental position roughly

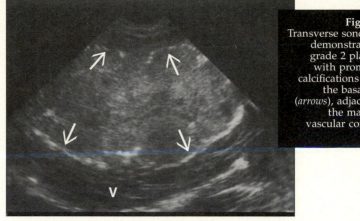

Fig. 23-9 Transverse sonogram demonstrating a grade 2 placenta with prominent calcifications along the basal area (*arrows*), adjacent to the maternal vascular complex (*V*).

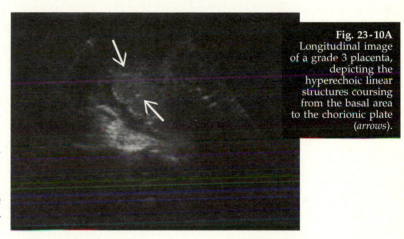

Fig. 23-10A Longitudinal image of a grade 3 placenta, depicting the hyperechoic linear structures coursing from the basal area to the chorionic plate (*arrows*).

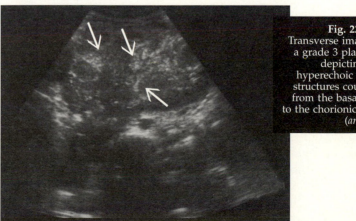

Fig. 23-10B Transverse image of a grade 3 placenta, depicting the hyperechoic linear structures coursing from the basal area to the chorionic plate (*arrows*).

corresponds to this superior implantation site. When implantation occurs in the lower portion of the uterus, the placenta can cover the internal cervical os and bleed either during the pregnancy or at the time of delivery. The diagnosis of a placenta previa is crucial to the obstetrician, because this condition requires a cesarean section to prevent hemorrhage during delivery, which could cause fetal distress or even death. The classic symptom is painless vaginal bleeding.

There are three clinical classifications of placenta previa. A **marginal previa** occurs when the placenta lies adjacent to the internal cervical os but does not cover any portion of it. With a **partial previa** the placenta covers a portion of the internal cervical os. In a **total previa** the placenta covers the cervical os (Fig. 23-11). In a **central previa** the entire placenta is located in the inferior portion of the uterus, with approximately equal halves of it lying on either side of the os[1] (Fig. 23-12).

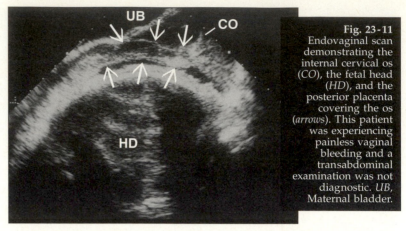

Fig. 23-11 Endovaginal scan demonstrating the internal cervical os (*CO*), the fetal head (*HD*), and the posterior placenta covering the os (*arrows*). This patient was experiencing painless vaginal bleeding and a transabdominal examination was not diagnostic. *UB*, Maternal bladder.

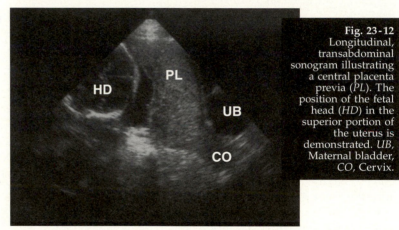

Fig. 23-12 Longitudinal, transabdominal sonogram illustrating a central placenta previa (*PL*). The position of the fetal head (*HD*) in the superior portion of the uterus is demonstrated. *UB*, Maternal bladder, *CO*, Cervix.

During the second trimester the sonographic demonstration of a placenta previa usually requires serial examinations. During the second and third trimesters the rapid growth of the fetus in a vertex or breech presentation causes a prominent expansion of the uterine myometrium. This expansion can change the position of the placenta in relation to the internal cervical os and has been referred to as **placental migration.** Because of this effect, the placenta may appear to cover the cervical os on an initial examination; a later examination may reveal that the placenta no longer covers the os. The only exception to this process is with a central previa, because the entire placenta is located in the lower portion of the uterus. This condition will typically persist throughout the pregnancy, and the usual clinical treatment is a restriction of physical activities and may include total bed rest.

The evaluation of a posterior placenta is a challenge for the sonographer. The fetal presenting part may obscure the relationship of the placenta to the cervical os. The use of the Trendelenburg position may displace the fetus superiorly and allow adequate visualization. If this technique fails, the sonographer may consider performing an endovaginal examination. When using proper endovaginal techniques, the risk of disturbing a previa and causing bleeding is minimal. However, the sonographer should adhere to the policies of the particular ultrasound department, which may include obtaining the clinician's approval for the endovaginal examination or may stipulate the presence of the physician or other medical personnel during the examination.

Placental Abruption or Retroplacental Hemorrhage

Placental abruption, or abruptio placenta, involves the premature separation of the placenta from the decidua. The size of the separation varies from quite small to the involvement of the total placenta. As mentioned previously, a severe placental abruption is an obstetric emergency, because massive hemorrhage can cause both fetal and maternal death. The symptoms range from vaginal bleeding with mild abdominal cramps to the development of a rigid, "boardlike" uterus and clinical signs of shock. The extent and location of the abruption is important to the clinician when planning the clinical management of the patient. The clinical prognosis depends on the size of the retroplacental hematoma, how much of the placenta has separated, and the amount of blood loss. A small abruption away from the central portion of the placenta may not interfere with the vascular supply of the fetus nor cause serious hemorrhage. A larger separation of 50% or more that is located adjacent to the central portion of the placenta represents a greater risk to the fetus and increases the potential for moderate to severe maternal hemorrhage.[1]

On examination the sonographer will note the presence of a cystic, complex or hypoechoic area between the placental substance and uterine wall (Fig. 23-13). An estimate of the percent of separation, as well as the size and location of the hematoma, is important information for the interpreting physician. The hematoma may be located some distance away from the placenta. The sonographer should evaluate the fetus for signs of distress or hypoxia. The most difficult sonographic pattern to identify is the hematoma that is isoechoic to the placental substance. If the patient has clinical symptoms suggestive of an abruption but the sonographic examination is within normal limits, the sonographer should not assume that a placental abruption has not occurred.[4] A repeat examination may allow the identification of the hematoma, since the pattern of blood can change as clotting occurs. However, the patient's clinical symptoms often allows the proper diagnosis.

Placental Neoplasms

Placental neoplasms are rather rare and include the hydatidiform mole, choriocarcinoma, chorioangioma, and teratoma. The hydatidiform mole and choriocarcinoma are discussed in Chapter 17. The **chorioangioma** is a benign neoplasm made up of capillary tissue from the pla-

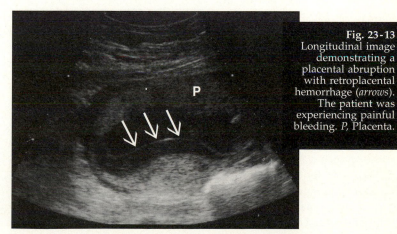

Fig. 23-13 Longitudinal image demonstrating a placental abruption with retroplacental hemorrhage (*arrows*). The patient was experiencing painful bleeding. *P,* Placenta.

centa. The size of the mass varies and may grow larger as the pregnancy advances. In rare instances there are multiple tumors. As in the case of many placental neoplasms, the sonographer may note polyhydramnios, which produces the correlating clinical category of a large-for-gestation age pregnancy. If the mass is located in the central portion of the placenta and interferes with the vascular supply to the fetus, IUGR may develop. If the neoplasm involves the chorionic villi, an arteriovenous shunt may develop. The fetal cardiovascular system may become overstressed, resulting in cardiomegaly and even hydrops. The sonographic pattern ranges from a solid to complex mass arising from the placenta[11] (Fig. 23-14). The sonographer should document the position of the neoplasm in relation to the central portion of the placenta and the umbilical cord anastomosis. The fetus should be evaluated for evidence of IUGR, cardiomegaly, and hydrops. Doppler evaluation of the umbilical cord vessels may provide further evidence of fetal vascular compromise or serve as the baseline examination for serial studies. Since these neoplasms can grow during the pregnancy, serial examinations are usually necessary.

The **teratoma** develops less frequently than the chorioangioma. Again the sonographic pattern ranges from solid to complex. The sonographer should always demonstrate the location of the mass in relation to the placenta. The use of Dop-

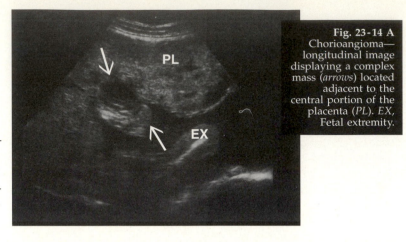

Fig. 23-14 A Chorioangioma—longitudinal image displaying a complex mass (*arrows*) located adjacent to the central portion of the placenta (*PL*). *EX*, Fetal extremity.

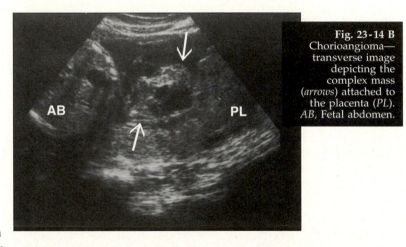

Fig. 23-14 B Chorioangioma—transverse image depicting the complex mass (*arrows*) attached to the placenta (*PL*). *AB*, Fetal abdomen.

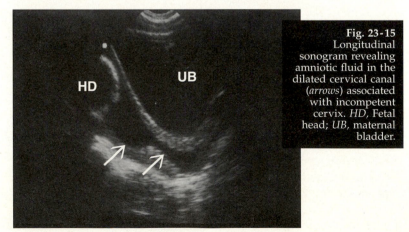

Fig. 23-15 Longitudinal sonogram revealing amniotic fluid in the dilated cervical canal (*arrows*) associated with incompetent cervix. *HD*, Fetal head; *UB*, maternal bladder.

pler can provide additional information, such as whether the neoplasm is interfering with the fetal vascular supply. The sonographer should again evaluate the fetus for signs of IUGR and hydrops.

Incompetent Cervix

In normal pregnancy the cervix does not start to dilate until late in the third trimester. Premature dilatation of the cervix is always an important clinical finding for the obstetrician. As discussed in previous chapters the cervix usually dilates when a spontaneous abortion occurs. Later in pregnancy the sonographer may find an enlarged cervical canal filled with amniotic fluid (Fig. 23-15). The patient may experience a vaginal discharge or be asymptomatic. An incompetent cervix is usually the result of cervical lacerations during a previous abortion or normal delivery, which weaken the cervical musculature.[7] The transabdominal sonographic examination may not always detect a dilated cervix, since the distended urinary bladder may exert enough pressure to obscure the anechoic lumen. If this condition is clinically suggested, an endovaginal examination may provide additional information.

TECHNICAL PITFALLS

When evaluating a patient for a possible placenta previa, the amount of urinary bladder distention plays a crucial role in a correct diagnosis.[13] Underdistention of the bladder will not allow adequate visualization of the internal cervical os. However, overdistention can compress the anterior and posterior layers of the lower uterine segment, and the unwary sonographer may misidentify the position of the internal cervical os. During the second trimester the walls of the lower uterine segment are prominent and often isoechoic to the cervical myometrium. Since this pseudocervix is located more superiorly than the actual cervix, a placenta located some distance away from the os initially appears to cover the pseudocervical os. Instructing the patient to partially void will usually reveal the true position of the cervical os. A Braxton Hicks contraction located in the inferior portion of the uterus may also be mistaken for placental tissue and may cause the erroneous identification of a placenta previa.

The demonstration of the chorionic plate is necessary to accurately grade the placenta and evaluate for evidence of infarctions, fibrin deposition, and neoplasms. Again, this linear, hyperechoic reflector is a specular reflector and, therefore, angle dependent. The sonographer must scan this interface close to a 90-degree angle for adequate visualization.

The maternal veins located in the basal layer of the placenta may appear prominent in some patients. Initially this pattern may appear similar to a retroplacental hemorrhage. Changing the scanning plane will usually prove that these patterns represent tubular structures. The use of color Doppler will also demonstrate normal venous flow, which is not seen with an abruption.

SUMMARY

The sonographer should always remember that the sonographic appearance of the placenta can provide the first clues to a number of fetal and maternal abnormalities. A thorough knowledge of maternal and fetal abnormal conditions will allow the sonographer to obtain the pertinent clinical history from the patient. The proper stage of maternal bladder filling continues to play a crucial role in the sonographic identification of placenta previa. When unsure that the sonographic criteria have been displayed for this condition, the sonographer should have the patient partially void and recheck the area. As in all areas of sonography, the sonographer should accept the responsibility to provide the highest quality diagnostic examination.

REFERENCES

1. Dunnihoo DR: *Fundamentals of gynecology and obstetrics,* Ed 2, Philadelphia, 1992, JB Lippincott, p535.
2. Hoddick WK, Mahoney BS, et al: Placental thickness, *J Ultrasound Med* 4:479, 1985.
3. Moore KL: *The developing human: clinically oriented embryology,* Ed 4, Philadelphia, 1988, WB Saunders, p104.
4. Nyberg DA, Cyr DR, et al: Sonographic spectrum of placental abruption, *AJR* 148:161, 1987.
5. Pasto ME, Kurtz AB, et al: Ultrasonographic findings in placenta increta, *J Ultrasound Med* 2:155, 1983.
6. Perkes EA, Baim RS, et al: Second-trimester placental changes associated with elevated maternal serum fetoprotein, *Am J Obstet Gynecol* 144:935, 1982.
7. Pernoll ML, Benson RC, editors: *Current obstetric and gynecologic diagnosis and treatment,* ed. 6th, Norwalk, Conn, 1987, Appleton and Lange, p643.
8. Smith DF, Foley DW: Real-time ultrasound and pulsed Doppler evaluation of the retroplacental clear area, *J Clin Ultrasound* 10:215, 1982.
9. Spirt BA, Cohen NN, Weinstein HM: The incidence of placental calcification in normal pregnancy, *Radiology* 142:702, 1982.
10. Spirt BA, Gordon LP, Kagan EH: Intervillous thrombosis: sonographic and pathologic correlation, *Radiology* 147:197, 1983.
11. Spirt BA, Gordon LP, et al: Antenatal diagnosis of chorioangioma of the placenta, *AJR* 135:1273, 1980.
12. Spirt BA, Kagan EH, Rozanski RM: Sonolucent areas in the placenta: sonographic and pathologic correlation, *AJR* 131:961, 1978.
13. Zemlyn S: The affect of the urinary bladder in obstetrical sonography, *Radiology* 128:169, 1978.

index